Teaching to the Test

A PANCE/PANRE REVIEW

Jackie Kazik, MA, PA-C

R & R Communications

Waukesha, WI

Teaching to the Test

Jacqueline Cox Kazik, LLC
P.O. Box 180292
Delafield, WI 53018
www.teachingtothetest.net

Teaching to the Test/ Jackie Kazik. —2nd ed.
ISBN- 13: 978-0-615-43329-5
ISBN- 13: 978-0-615-97363-0

Library of Congress Control Number: 2013908281

The medical content editor was Debra Cox Koetter, MPAS
The cover was designed by Marisa Krivitz
The copy editor was Jamie Lynn Schlax

Printing provided by R & R Communications, Inc.
Ordering Information:
Quantity sales. Special discounts are available on quantity purchases by corporations, associations, and others. For details, contact the author at the address above.

This book is dedicated to my two boys, Sam and Vinnie, who are the lights of my life.

They were my very first students.

Contents

Acknowledgments

First, I must thank my students, past and present, and all of the Physician Assistants that I have met over the years as attendees at the CME Resources review course and in the course of my own clinical practice. I have learned more from my fellow PAs than I have from any textbooks out there.

Next, I must thank my blog followers for many of the updates to this new edition. I thank them for suggesting topics, for "keeping me honest" when my information was not current enough, and for making me think about the best way to explain things so they make more sense and are easier to remember.

I will specifically thank the many PA's, both new graduates and old graduates, who I have worked with one-on-one and whom I feel have all become good friends, and superb colleagues of mine. They are instrumental in helping me hone my teaching skills. I am proud of each one who has jumped this hurdle, sometimes after multiple attempts. I am amazed at their tenacity, and the amount of work they have done, and am thrilled at each PASS!

Thanks to Jamie Lynn Schlax who took on the daunting task of fixing all the typos. I seem to have a propensity to forget the "end" parenthesis. She has no medical background, so this was a tough task, but she is a perfectionist, which is what this book needed in terms of dots, dashes, and formatting improvement. I will be grateful to her for eternity for all of her hard work on this edition.

In addition, a final thank you to my current students at Concordia University, Carroll University, UW-Madison, University of Arkansas (UAMS), and Massachusetts College of Pharmacy and Health Sciences. You are now my teachers!

It is always such a delight to work with PA students – they are the most dependable, responsible, enthusiastic students any professor could hope for!

“Seek opportunities to show you care.
The smallest gestures often make the biggest difference.”
— John Wooden

Introduction

I am not a scientist. I am not an expert. I am a PA. I am a teacher. I have been teaching for many years now, and my students are *my* teachers. In working with students, I have come to understand where they are stuck. In trying to explain things from various perspectives, I have come to know how best to get students to understand some basic principles that go a long way in allowing them to understand more complicated clinical problems.

Many of my explanations are not perfect in a pure, scientific sense. I utilize hyperbole and exaggeration to prove a point; I use anthropologic medicine to explain physiological concepts. In all cases, it is from these myriad explanations to class after class of PA students that I have been able to figure out the most effective way to teach these topics.

You will find that I have several sections in this book all formatted differently to maximize what I am trying to teach in this review. While I include every single topic in the NCCPA blueprint (and many more), they are not listed alphabetically as they are on the NCCPA website. Rather, I have them listed in the order that makes the most sense, either in terms of importance, in terms of understanding, or in terms of the best way to illustrate my point.

Likewise, the section that covers the content itself is not listed alphabetically, but in order of most import on the exam. Cardiovascular & pulmonary medicine comprises almost 30% of all the questions on the exam – as such, these are covered in detail and depth. Hematology, while important, is only 3% of all the questions, and is covered with emphasis on the most important hematology topics and with less focus given to the less significant.

This emphasis is intentional and important.

Pure and simple – I am teaching to the test.

SECTION ONE - UNDERSTANDING THE PANCE/PANRE

CHAPTER 1

Preparing To Take Your Test

Whether you are preparing to take the Physician Assistant National Certifying Exam (PANCE) or the Physician Assistant National Recertifying Exam (PANRE), you are already aware that this is a high stakes exam. The truth is, you are very likely to pass the exam. What I am hoping to do with this review book and my suggestions for preparing is help you pass this test on the first attempt.

I have taken the PANCE, and have now taken the PANRE for my fourth time. It is a difficult exam mainly because it encompasses all of medicine; questions at times do not reflect our clinical experiences; and frankly, we cannot hope to get the kind of exam scores that we expect from our experiences in PA school or in other standardized exams that we may have taken.

The typical mean score of 500, on either exam, represents an approximate 70-78% of questions correct overall, which is well above the pass score. I have been PA faculty for more than a decade now, and I can tell you that my experience has been that I want students to score far above these percentages on their exams in PA school. This is no longer PA school. The nature of this exam is altogether different. For this reason, there are specific things you can do mentally to prepare yourself to succeed in those moments during the exam when it feels as though you are doing poorly.

This book will educate you on the format of the exam to assist you in focusing your study and will illustrate for you the types of skills areas questions that may be asked. It will educate you about test item construction, refresh your basic medical knowledge, improve your clinical reasoning, and assist you in coming up with the most likely diagnosis given a particular patient scenario; even given minimal information.

Even with all that, the truth is you will simply have to choose to get some questions wrong. I know this goes against everything you have heard in the past, but the truth is that your goal is to PASS THE TEST; it is not to score an "A". The fact is that there is no grade given, no reward (except personal satisfaction), no promotion, not even a t-shirt for a super-high achieving score.

The PanceMaster code that allows you FREE access to PanceMaster, an online test question bank that will allow you access until you pass your test will be emailed to you if you select this option. This test-taking practice opportunity affords you as much time as you need to hone your skills at *online testing* – a skill set independent of the medical knowledge!

Our goal is to pass this test. So, let's get started...

Construction of the test

The PANCE (Physician Assistant National Certification Exam)

- 300 question multiple choice examination
- 5 blocks of 60 questions with 60 minutes allotted per session
- 45 minutes of break time

The PANRE (Physician Assistant National Recertification Exam)

- 240 question multiple choice examination
- 4 blocks of 60 questions with 60 minutes allotted per session
- 45 minutes of break time

The NCCPA's exam questions are developed by committees comprised of PAs and physicians who are selected based on their item writing skills, experience and references, and demographic characteristics (i.e., practice specialty, geographic region, practice setting, etc.). The test committee members independently write a certain number of test questions or items, referencing each to a recently published textbook –but not journal articles. Each item then goes through an intense review by content experts and medical editors from which only some items are selected for pre-testing.

Every NCCPA exam includes both scored and pre-test items, and examinees have no way of distinguishing between the two. This allows NCCPA to collect statistics about how the pre-test items perform on the exam, which informs the final decision about whether a particular question meets the standards for inclusion as a scored item on future PANCE or PANRE exams.
There are multiple but parallel, forms of the test. You will not know which form you have compared to your friend or neighbor taking an exam next to you.

All parallel forms must have the same content topics and tasks areas in the same proportions as in the exam blueprint. All forms of the exam must contain these psychometric properties (i.e. difficulty, reliability).

Each individual question is given a difficulty rating based on past performance; each form of the test then has a difficulty rating based on the cumulative difficulty rating of all the questions.

Scoring the test

Or as I am asked constantly, how do 65% of 300 questions end up being a score of 452?

When your exam is scored, you are initially awarded 1 point for every correct answer and 0 points for incorrect answers to produce a raw score. After the raw scores have been computed by two independent computer systems to ensure accuracy, the scored responses for your exam are entered into a maximum likelihood estimation procedure. This procedure is a sophisticated, mathematically-based procedure that uses the difficulties of all the scored items in the form taken by an individual examinee as well as the number of correct responses to calculate that examinee's proficiency measure. This calculation is based on the Rasch model and equates the scores, compensating for minor differences in difficulty across different versions of the exam. Thus, in the end, all proficiency measures are calculated as if everyone took the same exam.

Finally, the proficiency measure is converted to a scaled score so that results can be compared over time and among different groups of examinees. The scale is based on the performance of a reference group (some particular group of examinees who took the exam in the past) whose scores were scaled so that the average proficiency measure was assigned a scaled score of 500 and the standard deviation was established at 100. The vast majority of scores fall between 200 and 800. More details on the reference group for each exam and the calculation of scores will be provided in the form of Performance Interpretation Guidelines that you will receive with your exam results.

The NCCPA no longer publishes the percent correct level necessary to pass the examinations. Given that there are multiple test forms, this information would not be accurate since some test forms, while built to be exactly the same, are slightly different in their difficulty. Therefore, the percent correct is converted to a scaled score and report scores as well as the passing standard on that scale are reported to you.

Illustration:

There are two PAs taking a recertification exam. One has a slightly more difficult form (neither can tell that at the time, since both tests are very difficult). But when scored, all persons (overall mean) taking the easier form will get more Q's correct; and all persons (overall mean) taking the more difficult form will get more Q's wrong. Nevertheless, the mean is still the mean --- the mean is 500. Therefore, it becomes fair for all.

The amazing thing about statistics is that all things gravitate toward the mean. At the CME Resource review course, the same exam is given in all cities in the country to both new grads, and recerts. The mean is very consistent across all cities, participant demographics, and varies very little. That mean, on the CME resources exam, becomes a score of 500; and all participants are "graded" against that mean, much like the NCCPA does. This gives participants a very good idea of how they are doing compared to their peers, which gives you a very good idea of how you will do on the exam.

Now, I will say here that new grads perform better than the recerts. Why is that? They have been taking exams every week or two for the past two years, they are seasoned test takers. They also have just seen all the information over the grueling two or three years of PA school. The beauty of statistics is that that difference turns out to be small.

The Software

- Visit www.pearsonvue.com/nccpa
- Download the tutorial to your laptop (currently not available for Mac)
- Take the tutorial (also available at the testing center on exam day)
    - Make sure you know how to access the **Lab Values menu**
    - Know how to check your time (turn clock on or off)
    - Know how to answer questions
    - Know how to "mark" questions for later review
    - Know how to get back to those marked questions to review

The Content

- Visit https://nccpa.net for additional information on the content of the exam
- Click on either PANCE or PANRE under "Exams" (they are identical blueprints!)
- Review the content areas:
    - CV, pulm, GI, etc., to see individual topics covered (exam can include some not listed)
- Review the knowledge and skills/tasks areas:
    - Therapeutics, Clinical Intervention, Health maintenance (equally important and usually overlooked)

For Recerts Only

As of January 2011, you now must select an exam at the time of registration. The choices for exam include the "usual" Primary Medicine exam, which is the same we have always taken, with 100% of the questions coming from the entire NCCPA blueprint. New is the option to select an "Adult medicine" exam and a "Surgery" exam. Please check the NCCPA website and read the descriptions of all three options before selecting your option.

Primary care vs. Adult medicine vs. Surgery --- which one should you take?

Primary Care

- Same thing you have seen for the PANCE, or last PANRE
- All topics can potentially appear on the exam
- Pediatric percentages are still unknown
- Surgical percentages are still unknown
- There is no "geriatric" section per se

Adult Medicine

- Still 60% "primary medicine questions"
- No matter which exam you select, 60% of all questions (about 144) will come from all topic areas, as always
- If you select adult medicine, then 40% of all questions will be "adult-only", presumably without pediatric questions
- This is not a "specialty" exam
- There will be no record of which exam you took

Surgery

- Still 60% "primary medicine questions"
- No matter which exam you select, 60% of all questions (about 144) will come from all topic areas, as always
- If you select Surgery, then 40% of all questions will "have a surgical focus" and will include pediatric questions
- This is not a "specialty" exam
- There will be no record of which exam you took

So, once again, which one should you take?

The most important thing to realize is that no matter which you choose, 60% (144 questions) will be about all the content topic areas, i.e. women's health, dermatology, pediatrics, etc.

If you do not see pediatric patients, then you may want to select the Adult exam, as 40% of questions will not have pediatrics. Recall, however, that we have never been told how many pediatric questions will appear on the exam, so I have no way to guess at how much of a reduced pediatric presence the Adult medicine exam would have.

If you do surgery for a living, then you may want to consider the Surgery exam; however, and this is important: this is not an orthopedic surgery exam, nor is it a neurosurgery exam. The exam is still 60% (144 questions) on every single topic in the blueprint. The remaining 40% of questions will have a "surgical focus", but will contain pediatric surgical topics as well. Again, we have no idea how many pediatric questions are on the exam, so I have no way of predicting how many pediatric surgical questions you may be asked.

If this is worrisome to you, then my advice is to take the Primary medicine exam. It is what you have prepared for in PA school, and is what you took last time you took the PANRE. If you are truly frightened of pediatrics, then take the Adult medicine– but make certain to review pediatrics, because it will appear.

CHAPTER 2

Taking the PANCE or PANRE Exam

I have heard many myths about this exam. I have heard rumors that the exam is matching or fill in the blank. I even heard that if you "kill" the patient you get points deducted. I do not know where people come up with this stuff!

The NCCPA clearly spells out that this is a multiple choice format exam and there are five choices, one correct answer and four detractors, for each question. You get one point for each correct answer, and no points taken away no matter how badly you guess. You get a zero if you leave an answer blank, so **never leave an answer blank!** Put something in for an answer, and perhaps visit that question later after you have finished your block of questions.

Construction of Multiple Choice Questions:

The format of a multiple-choice question includes a stem, a question, and the five potential answers:

- *The "Stem"*
  - Presents the information needed to answer the question (and this is all you get!)
- *The Question*
  - Defines what is being asked of you (be careful, it may not be what you thought when you read the stem the first time!)
  - In a long wordy vignette, read the question being asked first, and then read the choices, and **then** read the vignette. You will avoid having to read this long vignette twice, and will save valuable time because you will already know the potential choices and be able to read with those in mind.
- *The Potential Answers*
  - The correct (keyed) answer & distractors (meant to distract you from the correct answer)
    - One choice obviously incorrect (it is very difficult to come up with four good distractors)
    - Two choices reasonable (but somewhat peripheral to the topic)
    - Two choices correct (one is the best answer, the other is "close")
    - The hard part is always figuring out which best answer the item writer thought was best! (Keep reading...)

What to Study

Or, how in the world does one study all topics of all medical specialties?

You don't! You study according to the NCCPA blueprint to maximize your study time and create a manageable study plan:

- Pay attention to the weight of the topic areas
    - CV 16%
    - Pulm 12%
    - GI 10%
    - Ortho/Rhem 10%
    - EENT 9%
    - OB/GYN 8%

- **TOTAL = 65% of all questions!**

Five topics are so much more manageable to study than all of medicine, don't you agree?

- Pay attention to the weight of the **knowledge & skills** areas:
    - Clinical Therapeutics 18%
    - Formulating the Most Likely Diagnosis 18%
- TOTAL = 36% of all questions!

These two tasks areas alone make up almost 40% of the questions you will see!

Since cardiovascular medicine is the most heavily weighted content area, and therapeutics is the most heavily weighted skills area, and CV has the most drugs of all the content areas, your best bet is to study **CV therapeutics**. Make sure you know the most important diagnoses in all the areas and the drugs used to treat those diseases.

That feels more manageable now, doesn't it? Nevertheless, there is more; human nature being what it is I have a few more caveats:

- *Do not* study what you know (or practice) – you already know more than the "average" PA in your particular area of practice
- *Do not* study what you love—the areas of medicine that you like tend to be the topics you review, or the journal articles that catch your eye; or the medicine that you talk about
- **Study** what you never liked or never really knew, especially if it is one of the above five topics!

Answering the Questions

You are not trying to score 100%, remember this as you go along:

- No question is worth any more than any other question
    - The more difficult questions do not count any more than the easy questions.

  - Also remember, there are actually easy questions on this exam too, do not fall into the trap of thinking all questions are a "trick". Some things all PA's are really expected to know, and if you know it, answer it!
- If you have no idea what the question is asking, answer something, *anything,* and then move on (you may get the next three correct)
- If you spend too much time on a question, you may run out of time, and 6 years later still not know the answer to that one silly question!
- If any question "scares" you (i.e. acid-base problem, ECG, x-ray), and you begin to get anxious, choose a letter, answer it, mark it and move on.
- When you have finished the 60-question block, if you have time, go back to your marked questions; you will be in a better mental place to come up with an answer to those questions now.
- There is usually more than one correct answer, but one that will be the best.
  - If you narrow your choices to two, you have a 50% chance of getting the answer correct. Those are good odds on this test on any individual question!
- Read the case carefully, most of the information there is vital to the correct answer.
  - Do not ignore ages, genders, pregnancy, ethnicities...they are usually pertinent.
  - Vital signs are frequently missed.
    - Sometimes just the elevated respiratory rate (RR) gives you the answer (but only if you notice it!)
- Sometimes the question is about priority or order (for example):
  - ABC (airway, breathing circulation); or recently changes to the CAB's
  - Physical exam of the abdomen is different from all other systems.
- Life threatening things should be ruled out first.
  - Look for the word *"initial"*
- History before Physical Exam before Diagnostics
- Answer the question being asked!
  - The detractor can be a true statement and still not answer the question that the exam is asking.
- Read the question *as is*...do not interject inferences....if it is not said, it is not happening.
- Do not panic if you see something you didn't anticipate (assume it's a question being tested)
  - If you see a word that you have never seen in all of your hard studying, it is probably not the correct answer.

Answer every question!

- If time is running out, and you have several questions left, pick a letter and use it throughout.
- Never leave a MCQ blank. You have a 20% chance of getting it right by simply guessing.
- There is no penalty for guessing; any blanks will be marked wrong.

Marking questions for later review – Which question should you mark after answering?

- Those that you have no clue
- Those where you have eliminated all but two (don't you hate these?)
- Those that are long and wordy, taking too long to read
- Any question at all that is making you anxious
- *But* -answer every question before marking it!

Long and wordy questions

- Long vignettes are more common than ever before, and that reading takes time.
- Don't you hate it when you read the question, and you say to yourself, "I know this is Grave's disease", and then you read the Q and it says: "The patient has Grave's disease, what is the most appropriate XXXX?"
- To make sure that you are not reading these long questions twice, make sure that you go to the end of the stem and read the **question being asked first.** Then read the stem.
- That way, you already know what it is the question is asking you about before you begin reading.
- This will save you valuable time!

ECG's and X-RAYS

- Look at the detractors first (this at least gives you a "clue")
- Then read the stem and the question (you may already have an answer)
- And then look at the image

When is it OK to change an answer?

- *Only when*
    - Something in a future question gave you a hint
    - Something was triggered in your memory
    - You recall one of those pearls above
- *But*
    - Don't do it in the middle of the test
    - Only when you go back to your marked questions
- *And remember*
    - "Answer changers" change answers to incorrect answers more often than to correct answers
    - If you are an answer changer, do this for me --- take an exam and record any questions that you change answers on, then go back and see how you did!

Educated Guessing

- Try to answer before you look at choice. If it is there, choose it and go on.
- If you don't know the answer, eliminate all the wrong choices, then make a guess from the remainder of choices
- If you know one is incorrect, you cannot choose "all of the above"
- If two or more are absolutely correct, it must be "all of the above"
- Once you decide on an answer....
    - Do not change an answer later unless you have a very compelling reason to do so! i.e., you misread the question, or you found an answer or clue in a later question.
- If you "knew" an answer, and it is not there, let it go, and choose the best of what you are given.
    - Remember, not all imaging modalities are available to everyone in every practice

  - Your favorite drug might be unique to your supervising doc, or your practice and may not be the "best" drug according to a textbook
  - The "way you do it" is not known to the item writer – have an open mind while taking this test

PEARL: You may note that I have just said the same thing four different ways because it is *so* important - ***never leave a question blank***!

Please at least guess and answer something, so that you have answered 60 questions at the end of 60 minutes!!!

What if guessing is your only alternative?

- *Clang association*
  - This works well with the therapeutics – instead of memorizing each individual drug, in the newer drugs, you just memorize the suffixes to identify easily the class of drugs. There are a few exceptions; however, particularly in the older antimicrobials (i.e. vancomycin and streptomycin (older antimicrobials) are *not* macrolides (i.e. azithromycin and clarithromycin) even though the suffixes are similar.
  - The good news is that most drug companies are now creating drugs whose suffixes are similar.
- *Longest detractor*
  - This worked well for my students – when trying to reduce ambiguity in an answer, and particularly in reworking that question so students would understand my meaning, the detractor becomes quite "wordy". Sometimes, if it all looks like gibberish and you are left with a complete guess, select the longest (wordiest) detractor.
- *When asked to identify two symptoms, or presenting findings;*
  - And you only know one for certain; at least give yourself a 50/50 chance and select the answer that has that one
    - Then mark it.
    - If possible, when you finish the exam section, go back and now look at all the options once more.
    - See if there is a second symptom, or finding, etc. that appears frequently among your choices – then select the answer that contains both.

In this example, use the "clang" association:

A 28 year old male with Type 1 DM has positive microalbumin during today's evaluation in the clinic. His BP is noted to be 148/88. What would be the most appropriate therapeutic agent to begin at this point?

A. propranolol
B. hydrochlorothiazide
C. lisinopril
D. atorvastatin
E. carvedilol

Answer: C. ACE inhibitor, i.e. lisinopril (or Enalapril, or captopril, or "anything"-pril

Discussion: In this question (and most questions about drugs), use the suffixes to help you identify the "class" of drug, and then select that agent. Propranolol is a beta-blocker, like sotalol, atenolol, carvedilol, and whatever-olol. Beta-blocker is a good drug for BP, but not the drug of choice for protecting the kidneys in a diabetic. Any whatever-statin would mean any HMG-CoA reductase. Atorvastatin might be necessary at some point to treat this patient's LDL, but we are talking in this question about protein loss from the nephrons.

In this example, select the longest (wordiest) answer:

S4 is described as:

A. A radiating aortic murmur
B. A radiating carotid bruit
C. A continuous murmur
D. The sound of blood striking a noncompliant, stiff or stunned left ventricular myocardium
E. A precordial thrill

Answer: D. Now, this is not always going to work for you – use it only if *guessing is your only alternative*

In this example, use the "most often appearing detractor" to select the two most appropriate answers:

What are the two most common presenting signs and symptoms in a patient presenting with congestive heart failure?

A. DOE[1] and orthopnea
B. paroxysmal nocturnal dyspnea and peripheral edema[1]
C. peripheral edema[2] and DOE[2]
D. DOE[3] and chest discomfort
E. peripheral edema[3] and fatigue

Answer: C is the correct answer; as you can see from my numbering, these two complaints are presented most often (to try to trick you, unfortunately), so are the most likely. Even if you have no idea what "DOE" is or means, it appears more frequently than the others appear and is most likely the correct answer.

Exam specifics

- There is a pull down menu for lab values (if you do not know what I am talking about, take the tutorial and find the pull down menu for normal lab values! see Chapter 1)
- Make sure to find both pages in the lab pull down menu!
- Most drugs are given as both generic and brand name (if not both, then generic). My advice to you would be to always memorize the generic names of the drug as this is most likely what you will see.

- If given a calculator, it will not be used. This only happened once to me, and the testing center person thought I was taking a physics exam.
- You will have a whiteboard on which to write and jot notes with dry erase markers.

Scheduled breaks

- Breaks are very important during the exam. Sitting for two or three hours is not conducive to performing well. You need both a mental and a physical break from the stress to improve your performance.
- Only while taking a "scheduled" break are you permitted to access personal items that have been stored in a locker during the exam.
    - I would suggest that you have water or juice and a couple of protein bars.
- I would also suggest that you get up and walk, either outside, or just walk in circles in the hallway; something to get your blood moving, and your tension down to improve your performance.
- You *should not* go to your car and look up answers on the test that you suspect you got wrong. You probably did, in fact, get them wrong, but proving it to yourself while in the exam mode is not conducive to confidence and a good performance
- You will have plenty of time to think about those questions for the next twenty years of your life.

Special Testing Accommodations (excerpt from www.nccpa.net)

The NCCPA complies with the Americans with Disabilities Act (ADA) and provides reasonable and appropriate accommodations that do not jeopardize exam integrity or security for examinees with documented disabilities and for other examinees with qualifying medical conditions that may be temporary or are not otherwise covered by the ADA, including those that require the use of any sort of medical device or medication during the exam.

If you require special testing accommodations for a documented disability covered under the ADA, you must indicate that special accommodations are needed when you apply for the exam.

Information on special accommodations and the required documentation is available online at https://nccpa.net

Irregular Behavior

NCCPA defines irregular behavior as any behavior that in the sole discretion of the NCCPA undermines or threatens the integrity of the application, assessment or certification processes of NCCPA, whether it occurs before, during or after an exam. NCCPA's Policies and Procedures for Disciplinary Review describe disciplinary actions taken based on irregular behavior. (https://nccpa.net)

Unauthorized retention, possession, copying, distribution, disclosure, discussion, or receipt of any examination question, in whole or in part, by written, electronic, oral or other form of communication, including but not limited to e-mailing, copying or printing of electronic files, and reconstruction through memorization and/or dictation, before, during, or after an examination, is strictly prohibited. In addition to constituting irregular behavior subject to disciplinary action such as revocation of certification, revocation of eligibility for future certification, and disciplinary fines, such activities violate the NCCPA proprietary rights, including copyrights, and may subject violators to legal action resulting in monetary damages.

If NCCPA determines that allegations of irregular behavior are true, it will impose sanctions against the offending individual, which may include temporary or permanent loss of eligibility for exams or certification, revocation of an existing certification, suspension of certification, invalidation of scores, fines or other sanctions as deemed appropriate. Such sanctions may include legal action against the offending individual.

PANCE/PANRE Procedures

You must complete the exam during your exam timeframe indicated on your exam acknowledgement that includes instructions on how to schedule your exam date with Pearson VUE. To obtain your preferred test center and date, it is in your best interest to schedule a test date as soon as possible.

If you are deemed eligible yet fail to take the exam during your exam timeframe as listed on your exam acknowledgement, you will forfeit your entire exam fee and have to reapply and pay for the exam.

Rescheduling or cancellation of your exam date during your exam timeframe as indicated on your NCCPA exam acknowledgement must be done through Pearson VUE at least 24 business hours prior to your scheduled exam date or you will lose your entire exam fee and will have to reapply and pay for the exam.

If you decide not to or cannot take the PANCE during your exam timeframe as indicated on your NCCPA exam acknowledgement you must submit a request in writing to NCCPA for the withdrawal of your exam eligibility/application from that exam timeframe. If an exam date has been scheduled, the written request must be received at least 24 hours prior to your scheduled exam date. If no exam date has been set, the request must be received on or before the last day of your exam timeframe as indicated on your NCCPA exam acknowledgement. Failure to request the withdrawal in writing to NCCPA within these timeframes will result in the forfeit of your entire exam fee and you will have to reapply and pay for the exam. Cancellation of your exam date with the testing vendor does not constitute withdrawal from the exam timeframe. This must be done by contacting NCCPA directly in writing (via mail, e-mail or fax).

You should arrive at the testing center 30 minutes before the scheduled testing time on the date of your exam. If you arrive later than the acceptable cut-off time, you will not be admitted to the test center. In that event, you will forfeit your entire exam fee and will have to reapply and pay for the exam

When you arrive at the test center, you must present two forms of valid and current identification (ID): One ID must contain a permanently affixed photo with your printed name and signature and the second ID must contain your printed name and signature. You will not be admitted to the test if the names on your ID do not match each other and your name as listed in NCCPA's record.

Once you begin the exam, you may not cancel or reschedule.

You are not permitted to keep written notes or record in any way the content of an exam. The only writing permitted by examinees while in the testing room is on the center Dry Erase boards.

SECTION TWO – KNOWLEDGE AND SKILLS

This is the least understood part of the blueprint. Most test-takers pay no attention to the weight in the "task" areas of the exam when preparing to take their exam. The exam is comprised of the content areas (i.e. cardiology, dermatology), but is also comprised of Q's related to tasks in medicine. These areas are tremendously important to focus on based on the weights assigned to each area. I am going to discuss these tasks areas in order of their magnitude on the exam:

CHAPTER 3

Formulating the Most Likely Diagnosis – 18%

Topics in this section as described in the NCCPA Blueprint:

- Significance of history as it relates to differential diagnosis
- Significance of physical findings as they relate to diagnosis
- Significance of diagnostic and laboratory studies as they relate to diagnosis
- Correlating normal and abnormal diagnostic data
- Formulating differential diagnosis
- Selecting the most likely diagnosis in light of presented data

These are the items that will end with the question, "Given xxxxx, what is the most likely diagnosis?"

Remember that when you see these words you are to use the information given to you in the stem to come up with the most likely diagnosis. The information is there, it is your job to recognize it and narrow your broad differential into the most likely single diagnosis. No small task!

For example: What is the differential diagnosis of chest pain? Huge!

- If we now make it a 6 year old with chest pain, the differential suddenly narrows to half a dozen things.
- If we make him a 64 year old smoking, hypertensive, diabetic, dyslipidemic with exertional chest pain, it's even easier!

So, find the words, the numbers (i.e. vital signs), the medications, the past medical history, the physical exam findings, i.e. the clues that point you toward the most likely diagnosis.

I have created a chapter with lists of diagnosis questions arranged by presenting symptoms combined with very brief clues from the history, physical and labs & diagnostics to help you begin to do this quickly (see Chapter 26)

Common Things Occur Commonly

PEARL: If you think about it, most of the time, the patient usually has the most common disease that causes "X" symptom, or has "X" PE findings, or has "X" lab finding. It is important, therefore, to know the commonality of disease states; particularly when the question stem seems quite vague and you don't feel like you have enough information. Throughout the content chapters, I will point out to you the commonality or the rarity of a disease (if it is significantly common or rare).

Here are the leading causes of death in the U.S. followed by leading causes of death worldwide. Be sure to read the question carefully to make sure you are answering what the item writer is asking, i.e. the most common cause of cancer is not the same as the most common cause of cancer death.

LEADING CAUSES OF DEATH IN U.S.

Centers for Disease Control and Prevention's National Center for Health Statistics (NCHS) as of November 8, 2011

1. Ischemic Heart disease
2. Malignant neoplasms
3. COPD/Asthma
4. Cerebrovascular diseases (stroke)
5. Accidents (unintentional injuries)
6. Alzheimer's disease
7. Diabetes mellitus
8. Nephritic and nephrotic syndrome
9. Influenza and pneumonia
10. Intentional self-harm (suicide)
11. Septicemia
12. Chronic liver disease and cirrhosis
13. Essential hypertension and hypertensive renal disease
14. Parkinson's disease
15. Aspiration pneumonia

LEADING CAUSES OF CANCER IN U.S. (MEN))

1. Prostate
2. Lung
3. Colorectal

LEADING CAUSES OF CANCER IN U.S. (WOMEN)

1. Breast
2. Lung
3. Colorectal

LEADING CAUSES OF *CANCER DEATH* IN U.S.

1. Lung
2. Colorectal
3. Breast/Prostate

LEADING CAUSES OF *CANCER DEATH* WORLDWIDE (note the difference!)

(According to the World Health Organization 2010 (WHO)

1. Lung
2. Gastric
3. Liver
4. Colorectal
5. Breast
6. Cervical

About 70% of all cancer deaths occurred in low- and middle-income countries. Deaths from cancer worldwide are projected to continue to rise to over 13.1 million in 2030.

Most Common vs. Most Life-Threatening

PEARL: Another way to decide on the *most likely* diagnosis from a list of five options is to ask your self these two questions:

- Given these five options (or the three that you have narrowed it to), is one of these much more common than the others?
- Given these five options (or the two that you have narrowed it to), is one of these going to kill your patient quickly if you do not recognize it?

A 34 year old patient presents with dyspepsia for the past three weeks. Abdominal exam is normal; DRE shows brown stool, however, the stool guaiac is positive for occult blood.

What is the most likely diagnosis?

A. Duodenal Ulcer
B. GERD (Gastroesophageal Reflux Disease)
C. H. Pylori Infection
D. Gastric Ulcer
E. Pancreatic Cancer

Answer: A. Duodenal ulcer

Discussion: I quickly eliminate pancreatic cancer and GERD, because those two diagnoses, as they stand, would not cause GI bleeding in and of themselves in a patient. Next, I eliminate H. pylori infection, because the infection with H. Pylori does not cause bleeding, the ulcers that result from the infection cause the bleeding. I am left with duodenal ulcer and gastric ulcer.

Here is where thinking can go wrong. I am much more concerned that any patient may have a gastric ulcer because it can be cancerous or it can cause massive GI bleeding. This patient does not have massive GI bleeding since you are told that the bleeding is "occult", i.e. not black tarry stool, but instead is brown stool that is positive for blood. She is not really the typical age for a gastric carcinoma, and duodenal ulcer is much more common than gastric ulcer (6:1). So, given this particular information, A is the best answer.

A 78 year old man with coronary artery disease requiring bypass grafting and bilateral endarterectomy presents with severe abdominal pain. He is tachycardic and hypotensive. The pain is severe and constant; radiates into his back and into his groin. He is diaphoretic and feels like he is going to die.

What is the most important diagnosis to rule out first?

A. Ureteral Stone
B. Abdominal Aortic Dissection
C. Acute Pancreatitis
D. Mesenteric Ischemia
E. Bowel Perforation

Answer: B. Abdominal Aortic Dissection

Discussion: In this question, I can eliminate ureteral stone (typically, it is unilateral, colicky, and not going to kill our patient quickly). The rest are problematic, and all are in my differential, and all are concerning. The diagnosis that could kill our patient in 5 or 50 minutes is acute dissection. Keep all these four (dissection, acute pancreatitis, mesenteric ischemic, bowel perforation) in your differential, as they all will kill your patient if not managed. The question is clearly asking for the first to rule out.

Acute vs. Chronic

PEARL: An important distinction to keep in mind is whether a problem presented in a question is an acute problem for the patient or a chronic problem for the patient. Depending on acute vs. chronic, the differential diagnosis changes. Just recognizing acute vs. chronic might enable you to get the answer correct, even if you do not know the nuances of the disease being presented.

A 28 year old female presents with c/o fatigue, shortness of breath and pelvic pain.

On physical exam her BP is 88/52, her HR is 128. Exam of her nails and skin are wnl. She exhibits no significant pallor.She has a Grade II/VI systolic ejection murmur. She has LLQ pelvic discomfort with soft mass, which is tender.

What is the most likely diagnosis?

A. Menorrhagia
B. Thalassemia
C. Ruptured ovarian cyst/ectopic pregnancy
D. Spherocytosis
E. Autoimmune hemolytic anemia

Answer: C

Discussion: In evaluating this question, there is not enough information given (in my mind), but that's the way it goes! This is all you have. (I would like a pregnancy test result)

Given the limited information, the fact is that she exhibits none of the signs of a chronic anemia, i.e. koilonychia, cheilitis, glossitis. She exhibits signs of a fairly acute volume depletion (she is hypotensive and tachycardic.) Given just this information, she must have an **acute** loss of blood or volume. All of the detractors are chronic problems except C.

I have created similar examples in Chapter 26, Diagnosis by Symptoms for acute vs. chronic GI blood loss, for acute vs. chronic pancreatitis, for acute vs. chronic cough, for acute vs. chronic dyspnea, for acute vs. chronic fever, etc. (You get the point!)

Here are some very basic examples of acute vs. chronic medical presentations:

GI disease

- **Liver disease**
  - *Acute hepatitis*
    - Normal albumin
    - Normal coag (INR/PT)
    - Markedly high ALT/AST
  - *Chronic hepatitis*
    - Low albumin
    - High INR/PT
    - Modest elevation of ALT/AST
- **Diarrhea**
  - *Acute diarrhea*
    - With blood = dysentery (shigella, salmonella, campylobacter)
    - Without blood = viral, giardia
  - *Chronic diarrhea*
    - With blood = ulcerative colitis
    - With weight loss = Crohn's, chronic pancreatitis; celiac disease
    - Without weight loss/no blood = IBS, lactose intolerance, celiac disease

Nephrologic disease

- *Acute renal failure*
    - High BUN levels relative to elevated creatinine (BUN : creatinine >20:1)
    - Normal albumin
    - Normal hemoglobin/hematocrit
- *Chronic renal failure*
    - Higher creatinine level relative to BUN (BUN: creatinine < 20:1)
    - Low albumin (with all its comorbidities – see Chapter 10 for info on albumin)
    - Low hemoglobin/hematocrit

Neurologic disease

- *Acute neurologic abnormality*
    - No atrophy
    - No skin changes
    - Sudden and severe abnormalities
- *Chronic neurologic syndromes*
    - Atrophy of muscles
    - Chronic changes in skin
    - Progressive worsening of conditions

Hematologic disease

- *Acute anemia*
    - Tachycardia
    - Shortness of breath/leg cramping/dyspnea on exertion
    - No skin changes
- *Chronic anemias*
    - Only mild tachycardia or normal heart rate
    - Asymptomatic (or minimally symptomatic)
    - Cheilitis; pallor; koilonychia

Dermatologic disease

- *Acute dermatologic abnormalities*
    - No secondary skin changes (except maybe excoriations)
    - Normal skin thickness
- *Chronic dermatologic conditions*
    - "Secondary" skin changes, i.e. lichenification, atrophy, straiae

Orthopedic disease

- *Acute orthopedic injuries*
    - Traumatic; vascular or neurologic issues
- *Chronic orthopedic syndromes*
    - Overuse; pain is main feature with performing the activity that caused it

Cardiovascular disease

- **Peripheral vascular disease**
    - *Acute occlusion* = white, cold, painful foot
        - Etiology = atrial fibrillation (embolism)

- *Chronic arterial insufficiency* = skin changes, claudicating pain with walking
    - Etiology = atherosclerosis causing plaque development
- **Pericardial effusion**
    - *Acute* = only 100 cc can cause death (tamponade)!
        - Jugular venous distention; high diastolic BP; low systolic BP
        - Low voltage on ECG
        - Etiologies = rupture of aorta, bleed after surgery,
    - *Chronic* = 500-2000 cc.
        - Patient may be relatively asymptomatic
            - Enlarged cardiac silhouette on CXR (water bottle heart)
            - Etiology = chronic liver failure; chronic renal failure
- **Congestive heart failure**
    - *Acute onset* = new presenting event, i.e. AMI, new drug
    - *Chronic* = fatigue, vague symptomatology; well compensated

<u>Pulmonary disease</u>

- **Cough**
    - *Acute x 2-3 days* = bronchitis, pneumonia, allergic/asthma
    - *Chronic x months* = cancer, TB, sarcoid, ACEI, pulmonary edema/htn
- **Shortness of breath**
    - *Acute x 20 minutes* = Pulmonary embolism; hyperventilation (panic)
    - *Acute x 2-3 days* = pulmonary embolism, myocardial infarction, CHF, hemorrhage, metabolic acidosis (see acid-base),
    - *Chronic* = COPD, pulmonary fibrosis/hypertension/edema, sarcoid
- **Hemoptysis**
    - *Acute* = acute pulmonary edema (MI, ARDS, severe valve disease)
    - *Chronic purulent* = bronchiectasis, TB

<u>Urologic disease</u>

- **Hematuria**
    - *Acute* = cystitis, stone, supratherapeutic INR
    - *Chronic* = bladder cancer, renal cancer,nephritic syndrome, idiopathic
- **Prostatitis**
    - *Acute* = bacterial infection
    - *Chronic* = "fibromyalgia of the prostate"
- **Cystitis**
    - *Acute* = bacterial infection
    - *Chronic* = "fibromyalgia of the bladder" (interstitial cystitis)

<u>Infectious disease</u>

- **Acute bacterial infections**
    - Fever, *acute onset*, constitutional symptoms
    - Typical pathogens for the condition (see each ID section)
- **Chronic bacterial infections**
    - *Persistent symptoms* of acute infection, or more insidious in onset
    - Atypical pathogens (but those typical for *chronic* infection)
        - Staph aureus
        - Fungal infections

PEARL: How many antibiotics does it take to cure a fungal infection?
Correct! If the patient has a chronic infection, your clinical intervention may include obtaining a culture to make sure you are treating the appropriate pathogen! No "empiric" therapy should be the answer for chronic infections!

Pay Attention to the Vital Signs

The most frequently skimmed over information, and sometimes the most important information given to you is the temperature, HR, BP, RR, and pulse ox. Sometimes, just that information is all you need to get the question correct.

- If you are answering a question about acid-base the respiratory rate and pulse ox are crucial to getting the question correct.
- Tachycardia usually means something significant is going on (recall that Cardiac Output (CO)= Stroke Volume x HR; so if the CO is decreased because of an acute MI, CHF, hemorrhage, dehydration, sepsis, anaphylaxis, etc., the HR will be increased. Do not ignore tachycardia!
- Similarly, if you are given orthostatic vital signs, pay careful attention to whether these are normal (normal CO) or abnormal (decreased CO). This alone will help you make an educated guess from the five choices given you, even if you are moving quickly and do not have time to read the entire stem.

Order is important

Sometimes the question is about order:

- History is performed before physical exam, which is done before ordering labs and before imaging.
- The order of the abdominal exam is different from that of all other body systems, i.e. auscultation comes after inspection.
- Life-threatening illness may need immediate intervention prior to complete evaluation.
- The order in providing medications is sometimes very important.
    - Adding a beta-blocker only after you have given a diuretic and ACE inhibitor and the patient is euvolemic is important in a patient with CHF.
- Basic Life Support
    - ABC = airway, breathing, circulation (in that order)
    - Now CAB = circulation (compressions), airway, breathing

I assume that C-A-B will be the new order of things from now on –so be prepared!

CHAPTER 4

Clinical Therapeutics - 18%

Topics in this section as described in the NCCPA Blueprint:

- Mechanism of action
- Indications for use
- Contraindications
- Side effects
- Adverse reactions
- Follow-up and monitoring of pharmacologic regimens
- Risks for drug interactions
- Clinical presentation of drug interactions
- Treatment of drug interactions
- Drug toxicity
- Methods to reduce medication errors
- Cross reactivity of similar medications
- Recognition and treatment of allergic reactions
- Selecting appropriate pharmacologic therapy for selected medical conditions
- Monitoring pharmacologic regimens and adjusting as appropriate
- Evaluating and reporting adverse drug reactions

Introduction to the Clinical Therapeutics Chapter

In terms of how to study for this task area, there are three main areas of therapeutics:

- Cardiovascular drugs
- Antimicrobial drugs
- Psychotherapeutic/neurologic drugs

Of course, each area of medicine has its own list of medications as well, i.e. dermatology has steroid and antifungal creams; endocrine has cabergoline and bromocriptine; but taken as a whole, these three areas, studied well, will provide you with the best opportunity to get the most questions correct. In trying to decide what to leave in and what to leave out, I have to make some assumptions. Those assumptions are that the drugs we use the most are going to be asked about the most.

It is important to memorize the generic (or chemical) names of the medicines, as there is no guarantee that brand names will be given to you.

Focus primarily on the indications for the drug and the contraindications. Keep in mind, however, that rarely will the question frankly state, "Which of the following is a contraindication for the use of "X" drug?" More likely, something in the stem (i.e., the HR of 54, or the SBP of 92) will be your clue that a contraindication exists. So, **pay attention to what is given to you!**

Drugs not mentioned here are covered in each individual content topic chapter (Chapters 11-24) specific to the disease entity or symptom being discussed.

PEARL: Basic terminology for pharmacology review:

Tachyphylaxis

- This describes a patient's tolerance for a drug that develops rapidly after starting the medication, i.e. Opiate, benzodiazepines, nitrates
    - This causes the patient to have to continue to increase the dosage to get the same effect
- The way to prevent tachyphylaxis is to limit the regular use of the drug (in the case of opiates and benzodiazepines); in the case of nitrates, remove the paste at night, and reapply in the morning to maintain good efficacy

Allergy vs. Sensitivity

- Patients often get this confused:
    - Nausea from morphine is *not* an allergy, it is a common side effect
    - Rash from tetracycline after sun exposure is *not* an allergic reaction, it is a sun sensitivity problem that the drug causes
    - Rash from amoxicillin given to a patient with infectious mono is *not* an allergy; it is a sensitivity that the patient gets from taking the med with mono
- Remember --- if a sensitivity reaction, you can give it to the patient if necessary.

Narrow Therapeutic Window

- This has to do with drugs that are very toxic at just over the normal therapeutic range
- Drug levels should be checked regularly; and if the patient has any symptoms whatsoever that may be due to the drug's toxicity.
    - *The most common examples:*
        - Digoxin
        - Theophylline
        - Epileptic drugs (valproic acid)

Dose-Efficacy Curve

- This concept has to do with the fact that increasing the dose of a drug does not necessarily increase its effectiveness, and may, instead, increase the side effects
- This is the reason that there is a maximum dose beyond which we should not increase dosage levels, i.e. side effect risk will exceed any benefit

PEARL: The CYP System

The cytochrome P450 (CYP) enzyme family plays a dominant role in the biotransformation of a vast number of structurally diverse drugs. Many drug interactions are a result of either the inhibition or induction of CYP enzymes.

- CYP enzymes are concentrated in the liver, but are also present in lesser amounts in kidneys and lungs.
- Drugs may competitively inhibit the enzymes that metabolize a second drug if they engage the same CYP enzyme subtypes, thereby increasing the plasma levels of the second drug.
- Conversely, a drug may induce the action of an enzyme, thereby making it more efficient at metabolizing the second drug and reducing that drug's bioavailability.
- In order to avoid dose-related side effects, some of these interactions may need dosing adjusted (increased or decreased) to take into account CYP interactions.
- Determining the appropriate dose of a drug has to take into account comorbid medical conditions that can such as liver failure and renal failure which can decrease the rate of the drug's metabolism.
- For the most part, we assume that the elderly are slower metabolizers of drugs, in general, compared to younger patients. That is why you should always start low and titrate up.
- Not all CYP drug-drug interactions are actually clinically significant. Know the most important (given to you below).
- Of the CYP enzymes, the CYP3A4 drugs have the most important effect on drug metabolism, as most drugs are metabolized in the liver utilizing the CYP3A4 enzymes.

50% of all drugs are metabolized by the CYP3A4 system:

- The following are *strong inhibitors* (will increase plasma concentrations of other CYP3A4 metabolized drugs):
  - Macrolides (azithromycin, clarithromycin, erythromycin)
  - Ketoconazole
  - Verapamil
- The following are *strong inducers* (will decrease plasma concentrations of other CYP3A4 metabolized drugs):
  - Rifampin
  - St. John's Wort
  - Carbamazepine
  - Phenytoin

25% are metabolized by CYP2D6:

- SSRI's (fluoxetine, paroxetine, sertraline)
- SNRI's (Effexor)
- Tricyclics (amitriptyline, nortriptyline)

15% are metabolized by CYP2C9:

- Warfarin
- NSAID's

- ARB's (valsartan, losartan)

<u>10%</u> are metabolized by CYPsC19:

- PPI's (proton pump inhibitors, i.e. omeprazole, lansoprazole, pantoprazole)
- Benzodiazepines

Cardiovascular Therapeutics

BETA BLOCKERS (BBs)

- **Drugs in class**
    - Propranolol
    - Nadolol
    - Atenolol
    - Metoprolol
    - Labetalol (both alpha & beta blockade)
    - Carvedilol (both alpha & beta blockade)
    - Timolol (main use as an eye drop in chronic glaucoma)
    - Pindolol (Cat. B in pregnancy)- sympathomimetic effect too (better in Raynaud's)
- **Drugs in terms of cardiac "selectivity" (i.e. does it block B2 receptors in bronchioles?)**
    - *Nonselective (both B1 and B2 – avoid in asthma)*
        - Carvedilol
        - Labetalol
        - Nadolol
        - Propranolol (shorter half-life, crosses blood-brain barrier, less cardioselective)
        - Pindolol
    - *Selective B1 blockers*
        - Atenolol (more cardioselective than propranolol)
        - Metoprolol ***(most cardioselective of all)***
        - Bisoprolol
        - Esmolol
        - (I would still be hesitant to use these on the exam in patient with reactive airway disease!)
- **Main Effects**
    - Slows conduction at the AV node
    - Negative inotrope (decreases contraction, but increases LV compliance)
    - Decreases renin release
- **Mechanism of action**
    - Blocks beta-adrenergic receptors (review Chapter 10, *The Autonomic Nervous System*) Lowers HR
        - Lowers BP
        - Reduces contractility of the heart
        - Decreases myocardial oxygen demand

        - Constricts bronchioles
- **Indications for use**
    - Hypertension
    - Post-MI
    - Angina
    - Systolic congestive heart failure (carvedilol or metoprolol succinate)
    - Diastolic heart failure (HCM, LVH)
    - Aortic aneurysm prophylaxis
    - Tachyarrhythmias
    - Migraine prophylaxis
    - Grave's disease (propranolol) blocks peripheral tissue conversion T3 to T4
- **Contraindications**
    - Bradycardia (HR < 60)
    - Hypotension (SBP <100)
    - AV blocks
    - Reactive airway disease
- **Side effects**
    - Hypoglycemia "unawareness" in Diabetes Mellitus
        - Beta-blockers should be used with caution in diabetics because of their ability to block sympathetic response to hypoglycemia and thus make proper awareness more difficult
        - Benefit in patients post MI still outweigh risk
        - If BB only being considered for hypertension, I would not recommend it --- use ACEI instead!
    - Fatigue, exercise intolerance
    - Depression
    - Erectile dysfunction
- **Follow-up and monitoring of pharmacologic regimens**
    - Symptoms of dyspnea may worsen initially when begun for congestive heart failure.
- **Risks for drug interactions**
    - Other cardiac drugs that have negative inotropic and chronotropic activity
        - Verapamil/diltiazem
- **Good to know**
    - Propranolol –in hyperthyroidism slows conversion of T3 to T4 in peripheral tissue
    - Carvedilol – drug of choice in stage 3 & 4 CHF
    - Labetalol – blocks both alpha and beta sympathetic system
        - Prevents "unopposed" alpha stimulation

ALPHA ADRENERGIC BLOCKERS

- **Drugs in Class**
    - Prazosin
    - Doxazosin
    - Tamsulosin (Flomax)
- **Mechanism of action**
    - Blocks α receptors which then causes smooth muscle relaxation, therefore, arteriolar dilatation

- **Main Effects**
  - Reduces afterload (systemic vascular resistance)
  - Lowers BP
- **Indications for use**
  - Hypertension
  - BPH (benign prostatic hyperplasia)
  - Usually used with a diuretic (HCTZ)
- **Contraindications**
  - Hypersensitivity/allergy
  - Hypotension
- **Side Effects:**
  - "First dose" syncope
  - Titrate from lowest dose; give first dose at night (at h.s.)
- **Risks for drug interactions**
  - Avoid with Beta Blockers (can cause significant hypotension)
- **Good to Know**
  - Use in patients with BPH (prostate enlargement)
    - Does not shrink size of prostate and will not decrease PSA levels
    - Relaxes smooth muscle of urethra and provides better flow

CALCIUM CHANNEL BLOCKERS– Dihydropyridines and Non-dihydropyridines

- **Drugs in class**
- **Dihydropyridines**
  - Nifedipine
  - Amlodipine
- **Non- dihydropyridines (has more depressive effects on myocardium)**
  - Diltiazem
  - Verapamil

- **Main MOA of all CCB's– interferes with Ca^{++} influx into the cell membrane – causes smooth muscle relaxation** *(muscles need Ca^{++} for "tone" – that's why hypocalcemia causes "tetany" kinds of reactions, i.e. Chvostek's and Trousseau's sign. *See endocrine chapter for more about calcium*)*
  - Dilatation of the main coronary and systemic arteries
  - Decreases myocardial contractility (nifedipine more than amlodipine)
  - Increases blood flow and oxygen delivery to the myocardial tissue
  - Decreases total peripheral resistance

Dihydropyridines – Nifedipine and Amlodipine

- ***Indications* for use – for both**
  - Hypertension
  - Angina
- ***Contraindications* for both**
  - Avoid in renal dysfunction, may increase proteinuria
- **Short acting nifedipine only**

- **<u>***Do not use in immediate post-MI period – increased mortality!!!***</u>**

- **Side effects**
  - Reflex tachycardia (see notes on beta blockers vs. calcium channel blockers below)
  - Constipation (especially in the elderly)
  - Increased peripheral edema
- **Adverse reactions**
  - *Nifedipine*
    - Reflex tachycardia
    - Peripheral edema
  - *Amlodipine*
    - Peripheral edema (see PEARL below)
  - Give with ACEI.
- **Good to know**
  - Amlodipine does not worsen LV function (use in congestive heart failure patients if needed).
  - Nifedipine should not be used immediately post-MI.

PEARL: Peripheral edema occurs most often with amlodipine and is infrequent with the other CCBs. It is felt to be due to redistribution of fluid from the vascular space into the interstitium. Amlodipine causes arteriolar vasodilation without venodilatation that allows more of the systemic pressure to be transmitted to the capillary circulation. Treatment of this form of edema with a diuretic will not relieve the edema.

This edema is much less common when amlodipine is given with an ACE inhibitor. This effect is likely related to venodilation by the ACE inhibitor that helps remove the fluid sequestered in the capillary bed from the arteriolar dilation caused by the amlodipine.

<u>Non-dihydropyridines – Diltiazem & Verapamil</u>

- **Mechanism of action**
  - Slows AV Node Conduction
  - Potent negative chronotropic effect (slows HR- both)
  - Both have some negative inotropic effects (decreased contractility)
    - *Diltiazem* – less effect, less hemodynamic compromise
    - *Verapamil* – more potent negative inotrope – so *do not use* in CHF
  - Coronary vasodilation (or, reverses coronary vasospasm!)
- ***Indications* for use - for both**
  - Atrial fibrillation with rapid ventricular response
  - SVT/PSVT
  - Hypertension
- ***Contraindications* - for both**
  - Wolff-Parkinson-White Syndrome with Atrial Fibrillation *(*see **PEARL** below)
    - Risk of progression into ventricular fibrillation
  - Ventricular Tachycardia
    - Risk of severe hypotension
    - May progress into ventricular fibrillation
  - Sinus Node or AV Node dysfunction without Pacemaker

        - AV Block
        - Sick Sinus Syndrome
    - Severe congestive heart failure
    - Concurrent intravenous beta blocker use
- **Side effects**
    - May decrease contractility and increase congestive heart failure symptoms of dyspnea
- **Adverse reactions**
    - Worsening congestive heart failure sxs (dyspnea on exertion, peripheral edema)
    - Hypotension
    - Constipation
    - V Fib may occur when verapamil/diltiazem is given to WPW patient in A fib
- **Risks for drug interactions**
    - Verapamil increases Digoxin levels.

PEARL: Verapamil/diltiazem in WPW with atrial fibrillation:

- *Atrial fibrillation (AF)* is a medical emergency when rapid antegrade conduction over an accessory pathway occurs (Wolff-Parkinson-White (WPW) syndrome).
- In WPW syndrome, antegrade conduction occurs over the accessory pathway (the Bundle of Kent). If AF develops, the normal rate-limiting effects of the AV node are bypassed, and the flow through the accessory bundle may be exceedingly fast (sometimes as high as 200 to 240 beats/min) and may lead to ventricular fibrillation.
    - *The treatment of choice is direct current (DC) cardioversion.*
- The usual rate-slowing drugs used in AF are not effective, and digoxin and the nondihydropyridine calcium channel blockers (e.g., verapamil and diltiazem) are **contraindicated** because they may increase the ventricular rate and cause ventricular fibrillation.
- If cardioversion is impossible, IV amiodarone is preferred because it will prolong the refractory period of the accessory bundle. (Amiodarone always seems to be the answer, yes?)

PEARL: BB's vs. CCB's

The beta sympathetic system's main action is to increase HR, BP and contractility of the heart in a *"fight or flight"* response to a stimulus.

Beta-blockers, therefore:

- Block the sympathetic "flight or fight" response system, reversing effects on HR & BP resulting in:
    - Decreased HR
    - Decreased BP
    - Decreased cardiac contractility

Calcium channel blockers, on the other hand, block the voltage gated calcium channels (which exist in cardiac smooth muscle and blood vessel smooth muscle) and decreases intracellular calcium needed for contraction:

CCB's, therefore:

- Decrease cardiac contractility
- Decrease smooth muscle contraction of arteriolar vessel walls, i.e.
  - Decrease total peripheral vascular resistance
  - Decrease BP

In other words, both beta-blockers and calcium channel blockers have similar results but from completely different mechanism of action.

Because the CCB will not be blocking the sympathetic nervous system as it reduces the BP, there may be beta adrenergic system stimulation(due to decreased cardiac output), which will cause a "reflex" tachycardia (since the beta system has not being blocked). You could negate this by giving the patient both a CCB and a BB but this may have deleterious effects on cardiac contractility since both drugs have negative inotropic activity on the myocardium!

ANGIOTENSIN CONVERTING ENZYME INHIBITORS (ACEIs)

- **Drugs in Class**
  - Captopril
  - Lisinopril
  - Enalapril
  - "Anything" pril
- **Mechanism of action**
  - Blocks the R-A-A-S system. (see Chapter 10 section on cardio-renal physiology)
- **Indications for use**
  - *Hypertension*
    - Not very useful in low renin patients (esp. African-American ethnicity who will respond better to thiazides and CCB's)
  - *Myocardial Infarction*
    - Early ACE Inhibitor in AMI – within 24 hours
    - Significant reduction in congestive heart failure and death
    - Significantly lower mortality at 1 year
  - *Congestive Heart Failure*
  - *Diabetic Nephropathy*
  - *Renal insufficiency* (but **not overt** renal failure)
- **Contraindications**
  - *Absolute* Contraindications
    - Angioedema: even if not due to ACE Inhibitor
    - Pregnancy
    - Renal artery stenosis
  - *Relative* Contraindications
    - Aortic stenosis
    - Hypertrophic cardiomyopathy
    - End stage renal failure (GFR < 5)
- **Side effects**

  - *Cough* (dry and irritating)
    - Occurs in 5 to 20% of patients
    - More common in women
    - More common in African-American patients
    - Not dose related
    - Stops within 4 days of medication cessation
  - *Hyperkalemia* (5% of patients)
    - Associated with renal insufficiency, Diabetes Mellitus
  - *Teratogenicity in second or third trimester*
    - Fetal injury or death
    - Pregnancy Category C if discontinued in first trimester
  - *Renal Insufficiency*
    - Renal artery stenosis (see monitoring below)
    - No specific creatinine level is an absolute contraindication
    - Baseline Serum Creatinine <3.0 mg/dl is safe
  - Hypotension
    - Restart ACE Inhibitor at half the prior dose.
    - Decrease or hold dose of any concurrent diuretic.
- **Adverse Reactions**
  - Angioedema –in up to 3% of African-American patients (see PEARL)
  - becoming more common in patients overall

ANGIOTENSIN RECEPTOR BLOCKERS (ARBs)

- **Drugs in Class**
  - Losartan
  - Irbesartan
  - Valsartan
- **Mechanism of action**
  - Blocks the R-A-A-S system at angiotensin receptor site (let the words in the class name help you on the exam!)
- ***Indications* for use**
  - Proteinuria control is equivalent to ACE Inhibitors.
  - Not as effective as ACE Inhibitors in MI prevention but still:
    - reduces cardiovascular risk & stroke risk
- ***Contraindications***
  - Same as ACEI's

PEARL: ACEI-induced & ARB-induced angioedema

Angiotensin converting enzyme (ACE) inhibitors are the leading cause of drug-induced angioedema in the United States because they are so widely prescribed. Patients most commonly present with swelling of the lips, tongue, or face. Urticaria and itching are notably absent.

This is not an allergic reaction due to histamine release. Instead, it is related to bradykinin production. This is why the angioedema can happen months to years after taking the medication.

In the 1980s, life-threatening airway obstruction requiring intubation was reported in up to 22% of angioedema cases caused by ACE inhibitors, with an overall mortality of 11%. These mortality numbers have declined dramatically during the past decade at least, in part, due to earlier intervention in the course of an angioedema episode. If severe, FFP (fresh frozen plasma) and intubation are indicated.

DIURETICS

The diuretics are generally divided into four major classes, which are distinguished by the site at which they impair sodium reabsorption :

- Thiazide-type diuretics in the distal tubule and connecting segment (and perhaps the early cortical collecting tubule)
- Loop diuretics act in the thick ascending limb of the loop of Henle
- Potassium-sparing diuretics in the aldosterone-sensitive principal cells in the cortical collecting tubule
- Acetazolamide and mannitol act at least in part in the proximal tubule

Thiazides

- **Hydrochlorothiazide**
  - *Main Effect*
    - Decreases preload
  - *Mechanism of action*
    - Blocks sodium reabsorption at renal tubule
    - Causes depletion of both sodium and potassium.
  - *Indications for use*
    - Hypertension
    - Mild to moderate water retention
    - Congestive heart failure –systolic
  - *Contraindications*
    - (Relative): hyperuricemia, hyperglycemia, hypercalcemia, hyperlipidemia
    - (Absolute): hypokalemia, pregnancy
  - *Side effects*
    - Hypokalemia, volume depletion, impotence, precipitates gout
  - *Good to know*
    - Not effective when GFR is < 30 ml/min --- i.e. in severe congestive heart failure or ESRF
    - There is one diuretic that works with poor GFR = **metolazone**
    - Causes tubules to reabsorb calcium – good for patients with osteoporosis
    - Flat dose response curve
      - Do not exceed 25 mg per day
      - Increased side effects without improved efficacy

Loops

- **Furosemide**

- **Bumetanide**
  - *Main Effect*
    - Decreases preload
  - *Mechanism of action*
    - Blocks sodium channels in the Loop of Henle
  - *Indications for use*
    - Systolic congestive heart failure
    - Severe fluid retention (better at reducing volume than thiazide, but not any better at BP reduction)
  - *Contraindications*
    - Hypovolemia/dehydration
    - Pregnancy
  - *Side effects*
    - Hypokalemia
    - Erectile dysfunction
    - Dehydration (elevated creatinine)
  - *Good to Know*
    - Better activity in patients with renal failure than thiazides

<u>**Spironolactone/Eplerenone**</u>

- *Main Effect*
  - Loss of sodium
  - Decreasing preload ("where sodium goes, so goes water")
- *Mechanism of action*
  - Aldosterone receptor blocker
    - Aldosterone is released by adrenal due to angiotensin 2 effects
    - Causes sodium to be reabsorbed (to increase ECF volume)
    - These drugs **block** the excretion of sodium by the tubule
    - In exchange, potassium is reabsorbed
    - Hence, a "potassium sparing diuretic"
  - Blocks conversion of androstonedione to testosterone in peripheral tissue
- *Indications for use*
  - CHF
  - Spironolactone : acne/hirsutism in women (dermatology and GYN for PCO syndrome)
- *Contraindications*
  - Hyponatremia
  - Hyperkalemia (renal dialysis patients should NOT be given spironolactone!)
- *Side Effects*
  - Hyponatremia & hyperkalemia
  - Not a potent antihypertensive
- *Good to know*
  - Because men like to have testosterone in their body, and this blocks conversion, eplerenone may be used in men (much more expensive)

Mannitol/Acetazolamide

- *Main Effect*
    - Removal of "fluid" from the body
- *Mechanism of action*
    - Osmotic diuresis
- *Indications for use*
    - Increased CSF pressures
    - Acute angle closure glaucoma
- *Contraindications*
    - Hypovolemia
    - hypotension

NITRATES

Nitroglycerin

- *SL, IV, transdermal*
    - SL is immediate release
    - IV is quick action
    - Transdermal is slow release
- *Main Effect*
    - Decreases preload through venodilation
    - Reduces left ventricular end diastolic pressure (LVEDP)
    - Dilates coronary arteries
    - Decreases cardiac muscle O2 demand
- *Mechanism of action*
    - Smooth muscle relaxation
    - Causes "pooling" of volume in venous system in legs
- *Indications for use*
    - Angina
    - AMI
    - Systolic heart failure
- *Contraindications*
    - Hypotension (SBP<100mm Hg)
    - Right ventricular wall MI
- *Side effects*
    - Headache
    - Hypotension
- *Risks for drug interactions*
    - ED drugs (sildenafil)
        - Profound hypotension
        - Treatment of hypotension if occurs
            - IV fluids

Nitroprusside

- *Mechanism of Action*

- Causes release of nitric oxide, therefore vasodilatation
- Reduces both preload and afterload
- Rapid onset

- *Main Uses*
  - IV therapy
  - ICU use only
- *Side Effects*
  - May cause severe rebound hypertension
  - May cause cyanide poisoning

POSITIVE INOTROPIC AGENTS

Digoxin (digitalis)

- *Main effects*
  - Positive inotrope – improves contractility
  - Slows AV nodal conduction
- *Mechanism of action* - unknown
- *Indications for use*
  - Class 4 CHF (see Chapter 11; CHF section re: classes of heart failure)
    - To improve quality of life
  - Class 3 or 4 CHF with atrial fib with rapid response
- *Contraindications*
  - AV blocks
  - Bradyarrhythmias
- *Adverse reactions / Drug Toxicity*
  - Nausea, gi upset
  - Tachyarrhythmias
- *Follow-up and monitoring of pharmacologic regimens:*
  - Get Digoxin levels whenever you think of it for any symptoms the patient may have.
- *Risks for drug interactions*
  - Many – just assume it may be a problem if patient is on Digoxin.
- *Drug toxicity*
  - Important, very narrow therapeutic window
    - Especially with hypokalemia
- *Good to Know*
  - Hypokalemia can induce Dig toxicity symptoms
  - Does not prolong life – only improves QOL
- *Treatment of Dig toxicity*
  - Cardiac monitoring
  - Hold dose (long half-life, so this takes days)
  - Digibind

Dobutamine (given IV)

- Positive inotropic effects
- Peripheral vasodilatation (some vasoconstriction as dopamine, but net vasodilatory effect)
- Used – as a pressor and to increase myocardial O2 demand in pharmacologic stress testing

Dopamine (given emergently as IV drug)

- Affects all adrenoreceptor sites
- Positive inotropic activity, but vasoconstriction at higher doses
- Used – as a pressor

ALDOSTERONE RECEPTOR BLOCKERS

- **Drugs in class**
    - Spironolactone
    - Eplerenone
- **Mechanism of action**
    - Block aldosterone receptor site
        - Kidneys excrete Na^+ in exchange for K^+
    - Not potent diuretics in terms of water, (that would be furosemide) but reduces salt retention (and therefore, some water goes with the Na)
- **Indications for use**
    - Systolic CHF
- **Contraindications**
    - Hyperkalemia
    - Hyponatremia
- **Side effects**
    - Spironolactone reduces conversion of androstenedione to testosterone in peripheral tissues (potential risk of feminization of male fetus in pregnancy; may cause gynecomastia)
    - Eplerenone does not have this effect, but is much more expensive
- **Follow-up and monitoring of pharmacologic regimens**
    - Monitor potassium
    - Make sure that sodium is normal before beginning this drug!

DIRECT ARTERIOLAR DILATORS

- **Drugs in class**
    - ***Minoxidil***
        - Should only be used to grow hair (potent vasodilator with many side effects)
    - **Adverse effects**
        - Pericardial effusions
        - Myocardial ischemia
    - ***Hydralazine***
        - *Main Effects*
            - Lower BP
        - *Mechanism of Action*
            - Direct peripheral arteriolar vasodilator
            - Slow onset of action

        - *Side effects*
            - Used to be used first-line in pregnancy
                - Risk of maternal hypotension – fallen out of favor
            - Labetalol and nifedipine are better
            - Can induce lupus-like illness with positive ANA (stop drug and sxs resolve)
    - ***Hydralazine + HCTZ = Bidil***
        - Best effects in African-American patients

CENTRALLY ACTING ADRENERGIC INHIBITORS

- **Drugs in class**
    - Clonidine
    - Methyldopa
- **Main effects**
    - Lower BP
    - Reduce CO
- **Mechanism of action (for all in this class)**
    - Interferes with sympathetic control of the vasomotor center in the medulla
    - Reduces level of sympathetic activity therefore vasodilatation
- **Indications for use**
    - Hypertension
    - Methyldopa is safe to use in pregnancy
    - Clonidine has an off label use for opiate withdrawal
    - Clonidine has off label use for "hot flashes" in menopause
- **Adverse reactions**
    - Dry mouth, constipation, drowsiness

PEARL:

Sudden cessation of clonidine is important cause of hypertensive crisis – should be weaned over two weeks to avoid --- think clonidine (cessation) in a patient on exam in hypertensive crisis.

Cardiovascular Drugs in Medical Context

IN ACUTE MYOCARDIAL INFARCTION

- **Remember M-O-N-A (B)**
    - **M**orphine
    - **O**xygen
    - **N**itroglycerin
    - **A**spirin
    - +/- **B**eta blocker

<u>However, do it in this order:</u>

- Aspirin
- Then oxygen
- Then NTG (if SBP > 100 mm Hg)
- Morphine for pain (if SBP > 100 mm Hg)
- If reasonable cardiac function, beta-blocker given within 24 hours of infarct improves mortality. (DO NOT give if concern for cardiogenic shock now or in the near future)
- Do not use short-acting nifedipine in immediate post-op period; increases mortality!

IN CONGESTIVE HEART FAILURE

- **If fluid overloaded** *(JVD, peripheral edema, and rales)*:
  - Loop diuretic
- **For RAAS inhibition:**
  - ACEI, ARB, Aldosterone blocker
- **When euvolemic:**
  - Add carvedilol or long acting metoprolol succinate
- **Consider ICD** *(implantable cardiac defibrillator)* **if EF < 35%**
- **Digoxin at end of life**

IN ARRHYTHMIAS

- **Atrial fibrillation -most common sustained arrhythmia *(See Chapter 11 for details on mgmt.)***
  - Rate control = diltiazem (if no h/o WPW)
  - Can use beta-blockers, digoxin (best if severe CHF)
  - Cardioversion if unstable (risk of stroke, embolization)
    - DC cardioversion
    - Amiodarone for pharmacologic (or Flecainide)
- **Atrial flutter - second most common arrhythmia**
  - To control rate
    - Atenolol, metoprolol, propranolol
    - Diltiazem (usually preferred) or verapamil (careful in CHF)
  - Cardioversion if unstable of < 48 hour onset
  - <u>***Treatment of choice*** *(better than the others)*</u>
    - *Radiofrequency ablation by Electrophysiologist*
- **Supraventricular tachycardia**
  - Valsalva and carotid massage (not if bruits or concern for carotid disease!)
  - <u>Adenosine 6 mg IV push</u> (rapid infusion)
  - Cardioversion if unstable
- **Ventricular tachycardia**
  - Amiodarone
  - Lidocaine/procainamide
  - Prevention of VT

        - Atenolol
- **Ventricular fibrillation** – ***defibrillate!***
    - Superior to any drug treatment
- **Bradyarrhythmias**
    - Atropine
    - Pacemaker

IN HYPERTENSION

- **Behavior Modification** – do not forget that this is an important part of health maintenance *(10% of the exam questions!)*
    - Weight reduction
    - DASH eating plan
        - High K, Ca
        - Low Na
        - Decrease ETOH
        - Exercise
    - ***1600 calorie DASH plan has effects similar to single drug therapy***
- **Drug Therapy**
    - According to JNC VII (the latest available Joint National Commission Statement):
        - Thiazide diuretics should be considered in treatment hypertension in any patient
        - If BP >160/100 – start with two agents (one being a thiazide)
- **However, there are many compelling reasons to use a different drug, or add another drug:**
    - In patients with *ischemic heart disease and CHF*, the following medications, if used, would lower BP as well:
        - Beta blockers
        - ACE inhibitors
        - Angiotensin receptor blockers (ARB's)
        - Spironolactone
    - *In diabetic nephropathy:*
        - ACEI, or ARB, or both
        - Thiazide may be used in diabetic patients at low doses (6.25 mg, 12.5 mg)
    - *In preventing recurrent stroke:*
        - Thiazide PLUS
        - Beta Blocker or
        - ACE inhibitor or
        - ARB or
        - CCB (amlodipine or nifedipine)

ADVANTAGES TO USING A PARTICULAR ANTI-HYPERTENSIVE DRUG:

- **Thiazides**
    - Slows demineralization in osteoporosis
- **Beta-Blockers**
    - Control atrial tachyarrhythmias, i.e. SVT

- Migraine prophylaxis
- Thyrotoxicosis
- Benign Familial Essential Tremor

- **CCB's (Nifedipine, Amlodipine)**
  - Useful in Raynaud's
- **Alpha blockers (tamsulosin, doxazosin, prazosin)**
  - BPH

DISADVANTAGES TO USING A PARTICULAR ANTI-HYPERTENSIVE DRUG:

- **Thiazides**
  - Not in gout
- **Beta-Blockers**
  - Not in HR < 60 bpm
  - Not in SBP < 100 mm Hg
  - Not in asthma, reactive airways disease
  - Not in second or third degree AV block
- **ACEI's and ARB's**
  - Not In Pregnancy

Pulmonary Drugs

ACUTE ASTHMA TREATMENT

Acute asthma treatment (as occurs in clinic, urgent care and ER) is very different from the chronic management of the actual disease process. Most importantly, corticosteroids *do not* provide immediate relief and are used for acute exacerbations but in the *post*-treatment care.

The most important historical clue to elicit from the patient is the severity of previous attacks:

- Prior intubation
- Prior hospitalization
- Prior need for steroids

The order of the list above is important -with intubation suggesting more severe disease than the patient who has never been hospitalized, but has been on steroids.

The most important management of an acute asthma exacerbation is to document lung exam, perform peak flows, give inhaled or nebulized albuterol, and then repeat the peak flows and lung exams to document effect.

If improved, but not completely, another nebulized treatment followed by peak flows

- This is repeated x 3; if no improvement, then hospitalization, IV steroids, possibly ABG's and intubation would be warranted)
- Let the vital signs and description of the patient lead you to the appropriate clinical intervention.

Drugs in acute asthma exacerbation:

- **Short acting beta agonist** (SABA)
  - *Drugs in class:*
    - Albuterol
    - Levobuterol (Xopenex)
    - "Duoneb" – albuterol + ipratropium (below)
    - *Can be given as three nebulized treatements (15 min each) or a single one hour continuous nebulized treatment*
  - *Mechanism of Action*
    - Beta 2 agonist effects
    - Peak in 30-60 minutes; last 3-5 hours
- **Anticholinergic agents**
  - *Drug in class*
    - Ipratropium
  - *Mechanism of Action*
    - Dries mucous secretions
- **Oral corticosteroids (short course, high dose, i.e. 50 mg. x 5 days)**
- **Others**
  - *Magnesium sulfate*
    - Dose: 40-75 mg/kg IV (up to 2 grams) for 1 dose
    - Smooth muscle relaxant and histamine release inhibitor
    - Variable efficacy
    - Monitor for sedation, hypotension, loss of reflexes (DTR's)

PEARL: Remember – if the respiratory rate is high (which it usually is during an asthma attack or any other reason for difficulty breathing) and the stem of the question tells you that ABG's show a normal pH; this is not a good thing (the patient should be alkalotic, from blowing off all that CO_2!) Do not be fooled by a normal pH in a patient who is hyperventilating!

CHRONIC ASTHMA MANAGEMENT

Chronic asthma management is aimed at preventing acute exacerbations and improving lung function. *(See Chapter 12, Pulmonary Medicine, for appropriate step-wise addition of asthma medications).*

Drugs used in chronic management of asthma ***(but not to be used in acute asthma attack!)***

- **Long acting beta agonist** (LABA)
  - *Drugs in class*
    - Salmeterol
  - *Mechanism of action*
    - Beta 2 agonist
    - Relaxes bronchiole smooth muscle
    - Slow onset; lasts 12 hours
- **Inhaled corticosteroids**
  - *Drugs in class*

        - Beclometha**sone** (QVAR)
        - Triamclinol**one**
        - Flunisolide (Nasalide)
        - Fluticа**sone** (Flovent Diskus, Flovent HFA)
        - Bude**son**ide (Pulmicort Flexhaler or Respules)
        - Momenta**sone** Furoate Inhalation Powder (Asmanex Twisthaler).
    - *Mechanism of Action*
        - Steroids are the most potent anti-inflammatory agents.
        - Inhaled forms are topically active, poorly absorbed, and least likely to cause adverse effects.
        -
- **Leukotriene inhibitor**
    - *Drug in class*
        - Zafir**lukast**
        - Monte**lukast**
    - *Mechanism of action*
        - Inhibits leukotriene at receptor site
        - Leukotriene causes bronchoconstriction, mucus production, edema of bronchioles
- **5-lipoxygenase inhibitor**
    - *Drug in class*
        - Zileuton
    - *Mechanism of action*
        - Inhibits leukotriene formation
- **Mast cell stabilizer**
    - *Drugs in class*
        - Cromolyn sodium
    - *Mechanism of action*
        - Stabilizes mast cell membranes
        - Prevents histamine release from the mast cell
- **Monoclonal antibodies**
    - Omalizumab
- **Methylxanthines**
    - Theophylline
    - Bronchodilator
    - Very narrow therapeutic index
        - Problem with toxicity
        - Rarely used

COPD MANAGEMENT

Chronic management of COPD

- **Much like asthma there are several components to the pathophysiology of the disease**
    - Abstruction to air flow (bronchiolar constriction)
    - Inflammation
    - Mucous production
- **Smoking cessation is the key**
- **Oxygen is often needed chronically**

- **Beta agonist "rescue" inhalers (see asthma above)**
    - Albuterol
    - Bronchodilators/smooth muscle relaxation
- **Long acting beta agonist inhalers**
    - Salmeterol
    - Bronchodilators/smooth muscle relaxation
- **Other Bronchodilators**
    - Anticholinergics
        - Ipratropium (Atrovent)
        - Reduces mucous production
    - Theopylline
- **Anti-inflammatory agents**
    - Corticosteroids
        - Short course, not used anymore for long courses
        - Reduces inflammation
    - PDE-4 inhibitor - Roflumilast
        - New
        - Only used if FEV1 < 50% predicted or frequent exacerbations of chronic bronchitis
        - Must be used with bronchodilator (no bronchodilating effect)

Acute exacerbation of COPD/acute bronchitis

- If fever, worsening dyspnea and increased sputum production with discoloration
    - Treatment with both steroids and antibiotics is indicated
        - Reduces repeat occurrences
        - Reduces hospitalization and length of stay
    - (see more in Chapter 12- Pulmonary Diseases)

PEARL: The most important PEARL in the therapeutic chronic management of COPD is that nothing except **oxygen** has been found to impact the scope and severity of the disease, and the length of time the patient is alive with the disease.

That said, chronic COPD symptoms are improved with pulmonary therapeutics.

Bugs & Drugs

ORAL ANTIBIOTICS

Beta-Lactams

- **Penicillins**
    - Pen VK
    - Amoxicillin
    - Dicloxacillin
- **Augmented Penicillins**
    - Amoxicillin/Clavulanic Acid

- **Cephalosporins**
    - Cephalexin (Keflex)
    - Cefuroxime (Ceftin)
    - Cefaclor (Ceclor)
    - Cefprozil (Cefzil)
    - Cefpodoxime
    - Cefixime (suprax)
    - Cefdinir (Omnicef

Macrolides *(careful with this "clang" association, clindamycin and vancomycin are NOT macrolides!)*

- Erythromycin
- Clarithromycin
- Azithromycin

Tetracyclines

- Tetracycline
- Minocycline
- Doxycycline

Quinolones

- Ciprofloxacin
- Levofloxacin
- Ofloxacin
- Moxifloxacin

Sulfonamides (with trimethoprim)

- TMP-SMZ (Bactrim)

Lincosamides

- Clindamycin

Glycopeptides

- Vancomycin (PO good in c.dificile)

Nitroimidazoles

- Metronidazole

Nitrofurans

- Nitrofurantoin (Macrobid)

IM / IV ANTIBIOTICS

Beta-Lactams Penicillins

- Pen G
- Penicillin G benzathine (im)
- Penicillin G procaine (iv)
- Nafcillin (iv)
- Ampicillin (IV)

Augmented Penicillins

- Ampicillin/sulbactam (Unasyn)
- Piperacillin/tazobactam (Zosyn)

Cephalosporins

- Cefazolin (IM/IV) <Ancef>
- Ceftriaxone (IM/IV) <Rocephin>

Macrolides

- Azithromycin

Tetracyclines

- Doxycycline
- Tetracycline

Sulfanomides

- TMP/SMZ (Bactrim)

Quinolones

- Ciprofloxacin
- Levofloxacin
- Moxifloxacin

Aminoglycosides

- Gentamycin
- Tobramycin
- Streptomycin
- Amikacin

Lincosamides

- Clindamycin

Glycopeptides

- Vancomycin

Nitroimidazoles

- Metronidazole

Carbapenems

- Imipenem *(pseudomonas coverage)*
- Meropenem *(pseudomonas coverage)*
- Ertapenem ***(no pseudomonas coverage)***

Monobactam *(pseudomonas coverage)*

- Aztreonam

MOA OF MOST ANTIBIOTICS (Scientific Concept/Therapeutics)

- **Inhibit cell wall growth**
  - *Beta-lactams*
    - Penicillins/cephalosporins
  - *Glycopeptides*
    - Vancomycin
- **Inhibit protein synthesis**
  - *Macrolides*
    - Azithromycin, clarithromycin,
  - *Aminoglycosides*
    - Tobramycin/gentamycin
  - *Tetracyclines*
    - Doxycycline/minocycline

- **Inhibit DNA/RNA synthesis**
  - Fluoroquinolones
  - Metronidazole
- **Inhibit Folic Acid synthesis *(therefore, DNA synthesis)***
  - Trimethoprim/sulfamethoxazole

ANTIBIOTIC RESISTANCE

- **Bacteria produces enzyme that inactivates drug**
  - Beta-lactamase (inactivates beta-lactams!)

Bacteriocidal *(use in immunocompromised or infections where host defenses are not ideal)*

- Beta-lactams
- Monobactams
- Glycopeptides
- Aminoglycosides
- Luoroquinolones
- Metronidazole

Bacteriostatic

- Tetracyclines
- Macrolides
- Ketolides
- Sulfonamides
- Lincomides

Against Intracellular Organisms

- Tetracyclines
- Macrolides
- TMP-SMZ
- Fluoroquinolones

LIVER VS. RENAL EXECRETION OF DRUGS

Liver

- Ceftriaxone
- Macrolides
- Sulfamethoxazole
- Metronidazole
- Clindamycin
- Nafcillin

Renal
- Beta lactams (except for ceftriaxone and nafcillin)
- Trimethoprim
- Vancomycin
- Aztreonam

Mixed
- Fluoroquinolones
- Tetracyclines

ANTIBIOTICS FOR OTHER INFECTIONS

Mycobacterial infections
- **Isoniazid**
  - Drug of choice in latent TB (9 month course)
- **Rifampin**
  - Also in prophylaxis for meningitis
- **Pyrazinamide**
  - Also useful in hyperuricemia
- **Ethambutol**
  - Side effect of optic neuritis (ethambutol and eye start with an "e")

Viral Infections
- **.....cyclovir**
- **Amantadine**
- **Oseltamivir (Tamiflu)**

Fungal Infections
- **Amphotericin B**
- **Nystatin**
- **....azoles**

Treatment Recommendations Based on Source for Severe Sepsis

GENERAL GUIDELINES
- Start IV antibiotics within one hour of recognition of severe sepsis
- Obtain blood cultures (x 2 in adults, x 1 in children) PRIOR to starting antibiotics
- Use MAXIMUM FIRST DOSE; (consult pharmacist to adjust based on renal or liver function)
- Drain all abscesses, debride all necrotic tissue; remove all infected drains or lines
- If infected invasive line site: obtain culture from line or culture the tip

RISK FACTORS FOR MULTIDRUG RESISTANT BACTERIA
- Any patient who has had IV antimicrobial therapy in the past 90 days

- Hospitalization in the preceding 90 days for 2 days or more
- Current hospitalization for more than 5 days
- Residence in nursing home or extended care facility
- Current dialysis
- Home wound or infusion therapy
- Outpatient with family member with a multidrug resistant organism

SELECTING ANTIMICROBIAL ACCORDING TO SOURCE

- **Unknown; Neutropenic patient**
  - Vancomycin Plus
  - Tobramycin plus
  - Cefepime or Meropenem or Aztreonam
- **Pneumonia**
  - *To medical floor*
    - Azithromycin, PLUS
    - Ceftriaxone
  - *Aspiration suspected (alcoholic; loss of consciousness)*
    - Above (azithromycin and ceftriaxone) PLUS
    - Clindamycin
  - *To ICU*
    - Pseudomonas coverage needed plus above
    - Always cover cystic fibrosis patient for pseudomonas
- **Abdominal infections**
  - Cipro PLUS Metronidazole (preferred)
  - Ceftriaxone (if pen allergic, aztreonam) PLUS metronidazole
- **Pyelonephritis**
  - Ceftriaxone (if pen allergic, Aztreonam)
- **Skin and Soft tissue *(MRSA suspected)***
  - Vancomycin PLUS
  - Clindamycin PLUS
  - Cefepime or aztreonam
- **Meningitis**
  - Ceftriaxone (if pen allergic, meropenem) PLUS
  - Vancomycin
- ***Remember*** – Penicillin allergy that would not allow you to use cephalosporin must be an anaphylactic reaction (not just a rash – if rash, select cephalosporin if appropriate for the infection)

Drugs affecting the Sympathetic Nervous System

If necessary, review the physiology chapter 10 about the sympathetic and parasympathetic nervous systems in order to understand how these agents work.

ADRENERGIC NEUROTRANSMITTERS Catecholamines)

- **Norepinephrine (NE)**
  - Stored in granules inside nerve endings

  - When adrenergic receptor is stimulate, NE is released
  - Travels to cardiac muscle and smooth muscle receptors and causes fight or flight response
  - Passes back into the nerve ending after stimulating receptor (this is called *"reuptake")*
  - It then is reused, or will be destroyed by monoamine oxidase (MAO)
- **Epinephrine (EPI)**
  - Stored in adrenal medulla
  - Stimulates adrenergic receptors much like NE
  - Very similar to NE in action
  - Specifically, it relaxes smooth muscle in bronchioles (more oxygen available then for fight or flight)
- **Effects of both NE and EPI (all designed to get you ready to fight or flee your "enemy")**
  - *Alpha-adrenergic receptors*
    - Arteries and veins of body (vasoconstricts to move blood from the periphery to the heart, brain and kidneys (increases BP by increasing systemic vascular resistance)
    - Pupil of eye (dilates it so you can see your enemy better)
  - *Beta-adrenergic receptors*
    - Heart (Beta-1 specifically)
    - Increase in contractility (inotropy)
    - Increase in heart rate (chronotropy)
    - Improves AV conduction
    - Bronchial smooth muscle (Beta-2 specifically)
    - Bronchodilatation (so you have more oxygen)
    - Vasodilatation in skeletal muscle (so you can run)

So now, take this information and carefully read the words in the stem or in the question, and make sure that you know if the question is asking about an alpha-adrenergic drug (neosynephrine) or an alpha *blocker* (terazosin); likewise, beta-adrenergic drug (albuterol) or beta *blocker* (propranolol)?

These adrenergic agents would have opposite effects to the blocking agents, yes?
Be careful here on the test!

EXAMPLES OF ALPHA-ADRENERGIC AGENTS

- **Levophed (norepinephrine)** – IV drug to drive BP up in a hypotensive patient
- **Ephedrine** – nasal decongestant
- **Phenylephrine** – nasal decongestant
- **Pseudoephedrine** – nasal decongestant
- **Tetrahydrozoline (visine)** – ophthalmic drop to shrink blood vessels (so eyes are not red)

(?) **What do you think would be the #1 side effect of using these ocular and nasal vasoconstrictive agents?**

Answer: Elevated BP -- so very cautious use in hypertensive patients. The next most common side effect is tachyarrhythmias – as would be expected.

In fact, phenylpropanolamine has been removed from the market; and all of the medicines that are OTC (over the counter) are restricted in pediatric use.

EXAMPLES OF ALPHA BLOCKING AGENTS

- **Doxazosin (Cardura)** – treatment of HTN; and for BPH (relaxes smooth muscle in urethra too)
- **Prazosin (Minipress)** – treatment of HTN (relaxes smooth muscle in arterioles, decreases BP)
- **Tamsulosin (Flomax)** – main use now in BPH
- **Terazosin (Hytrin)** – used in lowering BP

What should your biggest concern be if you decide to start tamsulosin on an elderly gentleman with BPH whose BP in the clinic is 130/72?

Answer: Major concern is for *syncope*, especially when getting up quickly in the middle of the night because of his enlarged prostate!

EXAMPLES OF BETA ADRENERGIC AGENTS

- **Epinephrine** – see above, most frequent use in anaphylaxis (see shock chapter XXX)
- **Isoproterenol** – both a cardiac stimulator and a bronchodilator (but not used much)
- **Terbutaline** – bronchodilator (also used in OB to reduce contractions, relaxes smooth muscle in the uterus)
- **Albuterol** – the "rescue" drug for asthmatics – relaxes smooth muscles in the bronchioles
- **Salmeterol *(Serevent)***– a long acting form of albuterol

What would be the expected side effect on all patients using any of these drugs? or to whom you have just given this drug in the ER or clinic?

Answer: Elevation of the BP and HR!

EXAMPLES OF BETA BLOCKING AGENTS

Nonselective (blocks both B1 and B2 receptors)

- Propranolol (Inderal)
- Labetalol

- Nadolol (Corgard)
- Carvedilol (Coreg)
- Timolol

What is the main contraindication unique to nonselective beta blocking agent in patients?

Answer:

SBP < 100 mm Hg
HR < 60 bpm
AV nodal blockade
COPD/Asthma – reactive airway disease

You cannot use any beta blocking agent in patients with SBP <100; P < 60 or AV nodal block. Theoretically, you could cautiously use a selective agent in a COPD/asthmatic patient, but do not use a nonselective agent in these patients.

B1 selective Beta-blockers

- Atenolol (Tenormin)
- Metoprolol (Toprol/Lopressor)
- Bisoprolol

(Theoretically, B1 selective BB's avoid the problem of the asthmatic or COPD patient who would have constriction of their bronchioles from the blocking action of this drug on the beta-receptors in the lungs; however, if another class of drug would work as well, I would still select that over any BB).

OTHER DRUGS:

- **Methyldopa (Aldomet)** -my go-to drug in treating pregnant women with hypertension!
    - interferes with the synthesis of NE (so acts like a blocker of the sympathetic system)
- **Reserpine**
    - Prevents storage of NE inside the storage granules of the nerve endings
- **Guanethedine**
    - POTENT – use only for severe hypertension – long half life
    - Prevents release of NE
    - Depletes NE from storage granules

Drugs affecting the Parasympathetic Nervous System

General Principles – parasympathetic response is used to "shut off" the sympathetic response; therefore, lowering HR, lowering BP, constricting pupils, and constricting bronchioles (you survived your fight or flight, so you can calm down now)

- The neurotransmitter of the parasympathetic system is **acetylcholine (ACH).**
- ACH is produced and stored within the cholinergic nerve endings
- Receptors are in the smooth and cardiac muscle membranes and are the **cholinergic receptors.**

- **"Cholinergic drugs"** are those that produce similar effects to ACH – parasympathetic effects
- Acetylcholinesterase inactivates ACH when it is outside the nerve ending, but does *not* block it at the receptor site itself.
- Inactivation of ACH is very quick, so the actual effects of ACH last only seconds (as long as the patient has acetylcholinesterase!)

There are three "types" of cholinergic receptors:

- Muscarinic receptors – on smooth muscle and cardiac muscle
- Nicotinic-neural (Nn) receptors – on smooth and cardiac muscle
- Nicotinic-muscle (Nm) receptors – on skeletal muscle

CHOLINERGIC DRUGS AND THEIR MAIN USES:

- **Main use:** *Miosis of the pupil*
  - In treating glaucoma
- **Drug:**
  - Acetylcholine
  - Pilocarpine
- **Main use:** *Myasthenia gravis*
- **Drug:**
  - Edrophonium
  - Neostigmine
- **Main use:** *Alzheimer's dementia*
- ***Drug:***
  - Donepezil (Aricept)
  - rivastigmine (Exelon)
- **Other Uses of an cholinergic drug in general:**
  - As an antidote to anticholinergic drug overdose
  - Treatment of urinary retention (nonobstructing)

These drugs are usually called *"anticholinesterase drugs"*; so think of them as allowing more ACH at the receptor site by blocking ACH's breakdown.

What are the most common side effects associated with using such a scary and powerful drug as an anticholinesterase drug??

Answer: Low BP (hypotension and shock), paralysis of skeletal muscles (used in the OR intentionally) but more scary, paralysis of respiratory muscles – called *"cholinergic crisis"*

What would be the antidote then for a cholinergic crisis?

Answer: An anti-cholinergic drug like atropine!

ANTICHOLINERGIC DRUGS AND THEIR MAIN USES:

- **Main use:**
  - Used to increase HR in bradycardia
  - To treat enuresis (bedwetting)
  - Biliary colic
  - By optho as a mydriatic and cycloplegic (dilates and paralyzes the pupil)
- **Drug:**
  - Atropine
- **Main use:** *reduces bowel motility (helps with cramping)*
- **Drug:**
  - Hyoscyamine (levsin)
- **Main use:** *the "cruise" patch; helps with motion sickness*
- **Drug:**
  - Scopolamine
- **Main use:** Overactive bladder; urge incontinence
- **Drug:**
  - Oxybutynin and tolterodine

Psychiatric/Neurological Drugs

DRUGS FOR ANXIETY RELATED DISORDERS

Benzodiazepines – Pregnancy Category D – Do Not Use!

- *Drugs in Class*
  - Diazepam (Valium)
  - Triazolam (Halcion)
  - Temazepam (Restoril)- intermediate – 8-10 hours
  - Flurazepam (Dalmane) – long acting – used for sleep but sedation during day
- *Mechanism of Action*
  - Inhibits GABA; decreases neuronal excitability
  - Lipid soluble; readily enters CNS
  - Well absorbed orally
  - Eliminated by kidneys
- *Main Use*
  - Anxiety – generalized anxiety disorder; panic attack
- *Other Uses*
  - Sedation (insomnia – not the best drug to use, though!)
  - Hypnotic effects
  - Muscle relaxant (muscle spasm)

- *Main Side Effects*
  - Tachyphylaxis – rapid tolerance to drug effects, requiring higher and higher doses for same effect
  - Addiction
- *Contraindications*
  - Pregnancy/nursing
  - Acute open angle glaucoma
  - Respiratory impairment
- *Overdose*
  - Flumazenil is a benzodiazepine receptor antagonist
    - It has multiple complications and is almost never used to marked problems
  - Supportive therapy is much less risky
- *Good to Know*
  - Drug interaction with antifungals (ketoconazole) due to impaired metabolism (high benzodiazepine drug levels) due to CYP3A activation.
  - Sudden cessation of benzodiazepines can cause seizure, status epilepticus, and can cause death; patients must be weaned from their drug if addicted/dependent

PEARL: Antipsychotic Drugs - How/Why Do They Work?

The main effects of the antipsychotics are to reduce bizarre behaviors; hallucinations; and irrational thought without significantly depressing intellectual function. Most take 1-2 weeks to have full development of effects.

General principle: antipsychotic drugs act on subcortical areas of the brain; i.e. thalamus and limbic system (which control behaviors), to block neurotransmitters from exhibiting their effects.

Dopamine appears to be the most important neurotransmitter:

- It is necessary for the synthesis of catecholamine neurotransmitters (epinephrine and norepinephrine).
- Most drugs for schizophrenia and other psychoses involve blocking dopamine receptors; these are called the "neuroleptic" agents as they have side effects that mimic seizure activity.
- Dopamine is a monoamine neurotransmitter (hence, this is why MAO inhibitors work!)
- Dopamine is responsible for "reward driven" learning.

Too much dopamine:

- Highly addictive drugs, like cocaine and methamphetamine, act directly on the dopamine system by inhibiting the re-uptake of dopamine, therefore, more is available.
- Schizophrenia is known to cause increased levels of dopamine in the limbic pathways and prefrontal cortex.

Not enough dopamine:

- Parkinson's disease causes flat affect; depressed mood, tremor and motor impairment due to loss of dopamine-secreting neurons in the substantia nigra.

- ADD and restless leg syndrome is thought to be due to decreased dopamine activity.

PEARL: So, if you were to want to treat Parkinson's, ADD or restless leg syndrome, you would select a drug that increases dopamine secretion. But, if you want to treat behavioral or schizophrenia disorders, you would select a drug that decreases dopamine secretion.

Effects of drugs that reduce dopamine activity (neuroleptics/antipsychotics):

- Impaired concentration
- Reduced motivation
- Anhedonia (inability to experience pleasure)
- Tardive dyskinesia (which can be irreversible)
- Sexual dysfunction
- Weight gain

Typical Antipsychotics

Phenothiazines

- *Mechanism of action*
  - Blocks dopamine, histamine, is anticholinergic and alpha blocking too!
- *Drugs in Class and their "other" uses*
  - Chlorpromazine (Thorazine) – antipsychotic & antiemetic
  - Prochlorperazine (Compazine) - antiemetic
  - Promethazine (Phenergan) –antihistamine & antiemetic, motion sickness
  - Thioridazine (Mellaril) - antipsychotic
- *Main Side Effects*
  - Sedation
  - Dry mouth
  - Rash, photosensitivity
  - Blood disorders
  - Liver toxicity
- *Good to Know*
  - NMS (neuroleptic malignant syndrome) is associated with the antipsychotic drugs
  - hyperthermia, rigidity, catatonia, nervous system instability
  - Stop antipsychotic immediately; most require ICU admission, mortality is high!!!

Butyrophenones

Haloperidol (Haldol)

- *Indications for use*
  - Highly agitated; manic patients
- *Main Side Effects*
  - More movement disturbance
  - Causes less anticholinergic, antihistaminic SE than phenothiazines
- *Contraindications*
  - Extrapyramidal effects in the past (these are sometimes not reversible)
- *Good to Know*
  - More potent; much lower doses used

Thioxanthines

Thiothixene (Navane)

- *Main Side Effects*
  - Somnolence
  - Postural hypotension
  - Parkinsonian syndrome (neuroleptic movements)
- *Contraindications*
  - Allergy = dermatitis, obstructive jaundice; anemia and leukopenia

Atypical Antipsychotics

Drugs in class with main side effect:

- **Clozapine (Clozaril)**
  - Sedation, hypotension
- **Risperidone (Risperdal)**
  - Sedation
- **Olanzapine (Zyprexa)**
  - Well tolerated
  - Sleepiness, constipation, weight gain, dry mouth
- **Quetiapine (Seroquel)**
  - Sedation (less than most of the others)
  - Also used in depression (as add-on drug)

PEARL: The atypical antipsychotics block serotonin in addition to dopamine; therefore there is less trouble with dyskinesis.

It should be noted that all the above drugs are indicated in the treatment of psychotic disorders, but are frequently used alone or with other drugs in the management of bipolar disorder and major depression.

BIPOLAR DISORDER TREATMENT

Lithium – Category D in Pregnancy – Do Not Use!

- *Main Use*
    - Most commonly used drug for the treatment of mania in bipolar disorder
    - Used in combination with antidepressants or antipsychotics
- *Mechanism of action*
    - SImilar in chemical makeup to sodium
    - Sodium is required for nerve conduction; but lithium inhibits it
    - Decrease therefore in excitability of nerve tissue
    - Increases reuptake (therefore decreased release) of NE and dopamine
- *Main Side Effects*
    - Nephrogenic DI (diabetes insipidus)
- *Contraindications*
    - Not in patients with thyroid disorders
- *Good to Know*
    - Very narrow therapeutic window (*toxic* if above normal range)
    - Blood levels should be measured regularly
    - Patient needs adequate sodium intake for proper urinary excretion of the drug
    - ****Hyponatremia is dangerous for patient on lithium – check level!!****
    - SIgns of toxicity: vomiting, diarrhea, ataxia, tinnitus, polyuria; death
    - Treatment – force fluids and make them urinate it out; increase intake of sodium

Aripiprazole (Abilify)

- *Mechanism of action:*
    - Partial dopamine agonist (3rd generation, newer drug)
- *Main use:*
    - Schizophrenia in adults
    - Also used in bipolar disorder and major depression
- *Neuroleptic drug*

THERAPEUTICS FOR MAJOR DEPRESSION

Selective Serotonin Reuptake Inhibitors

Newest in the antidepressant classes of drugs

- *Mechanism of Action*
    - SSRIs inhibit reuptake of serotonin into the presynaptic cell,
    - Thereby, increasing the level of serotonin in the synaptic cleft available to bind to the postsynaptic receptor
- *Indications*
    - Main clinical use is in depression
    - Has been used in OCD; performance anxiety; generalized anxiety & panic, PTSD
- *Drugs in class*
    - Citalopram
    - Fluoxetine
    - Paroxetine

- Sertraline
- *Major Side Effects*
  - Serotonergic syndrome
    - Hyper-reflexia, seizures
    - Mania/hypomania in undiagnosed bipolar disorder
  - Sexual dysfunction (usually orgasmic, and not ED)
  - Increased suicide risk – especially in children and adolescents
- *Contraindications*
  - MAOI's – cause serotonergic syndromes
- *Good to know*
  - Withdrawal can occur
  - Wean patient from medication over several days to weeks

Tricyclic Antidepressants - *developed some time after MAOI's – late 1950's*

- *Mechanism of Action*
  - Cyclic antidepressants block the absorption (reuptake) of the neurotransmitters serotonin and norepinephrine making more in the brain.
  - This seems to help brain cells send and receive messages, which in turn boosts mood.
  - Developed from antihistamines (remember these side effects which are similar)
- *Drugs in class*
  - Amitriptyline
  - Amoxapine
  - Desipramine
  - Doxepin
  - Imipramine
  - Nortriptyline
- *Indications*
  - Major depression
  - Because of side effects, and newer SSRI's, these are not used as often, but are an option in patients who do not respond to SSRI.
- *Other*
  - Migraine prophylaxis
  - Sleep disorders (side effect of drowsiness helps with that)
  - Chronic pain disorders
- *Side Effects*
  - Similar to anticholinergics (antihistamines, antimuscarinic)
    - Dry mouth
    - Somnolence
    - Urinary retention
    - Constipation
    - Hyperthermia
    - "dry as a bone, mad as a hatter, hot as a hare, red as a beet"
  - Block sodium and calcium channels
    - Therefore, lethal cardiac arrhythmias with overdose
- *Good to know*
  - "withdrawal" syndromes – wean the patient to prevent symptoms

Monoamine oxidase inhibitors (MAOIs) - *introduced in the 1950s as the first antidepressant*

- *Drugs in class*
    - Isocarboxazid
    - Phenelzine
    - Tranylcypromine
    - Selegiline
- *Indications*
    - Not used often because of hypertension reaction with tyramine-containing foods.
    - Used only now in recalcitrant depression or panic disorder
    - Occasionally used in Parkinson's disease in conjunction with the dopamine precursor levodopa.
- *Mechanism of action*
    - Blocks enzyme monoamine oxidase, which metabolizes neurotransmitters such as dopamine, norepinephrine and serotonin.
    - By blocking this action, the neurotransmitters remain at high levels in the brain, which is thought to boost a person's mood.
- *Major Side Effect*
    - Tyramine-containing compounds can cause malignant hypertension
    - Strict diet is needed; and close monitoring
    - Aged cheeses, red wine
- *Good to know*
    - Most MAOIs are available in tablet form.
    - A skin patch is now available as well (applied daily)

PSYCHOMOTOR STIMULANT DRUGS

- *Drugs in Class*
    - Adderal (dextroamphetamine/amphetamine)
    - Ritalin (methylphenidate)
    - Concerta (methylphenidate)
- *Main uses*
    - ADD/ADHD
    - Narcolepsy
- *Contraindications*
    - Tourette's syndrome
    - Pregnancy
    - Stimulant drug use
    - Hypertension
    - Cardiac disease
    - Substance Abuse Aides

Immunosuppressive Agents

See physiology chapter (XX) on immune response to review normal immune function and understand how these agents work on the immune system

Corticosteroids

- ***Corticosteroid Indications***
    - *Endocrine Disorders (Adrenal Insufficiency)*
        - In adrenal insufficiency, daily replacement dose needed
    - *Rheumatic Disorders (Psoriatic arthritis, RA, OA...)*
        - Now most often used for flares; high dose, short course
    - *Collagen Disease (SLE, Dermatomyositis...)*
        - Usually longterm
        - Treat for sequelae (DM, dyslipidemia, hypertension, etc)
    - *Dermatologic Disease*
        - Topical
        - If large surface area, consider oral, short course
    - *Allergic Disorders*
        - Topically for small areas of skin
        - Oral high dose, short course (e.g., poison ivy)
        - IV (angioedema)
    - *Ophthalmic Disorders*
        - Steroid drops best ordered by ophtho
        - Can worsen conditions if wrong etiology
    - *Respiratory Disorders*
        - Inhaled
        - Short course, high dose
    - *Hematologic Disorders (ITP...)*
        - Suppresses immune response in immune-mediated problems
    - *Neoplastic Disorders*
        - Especially brain cancer; dexamethasone reduces cerebral edema
    - *GI Disease*
        - Enterocort (oral or rectal)
- ***Mechanism of action of corticosteroids:***
    - *Anti-Inflammatory Effects*
        - Suppresses the activation of T-lymphocytes
        - Suppresses the production of cytokines by activated T-helper cells (cytokines are pro-inflammatory and activate eosinophils)
        - Decreases the release of various chemical mediators of inflammation (histamines, prostaglandins, leukotrienes) released by mast cells & eosinophils
        - Stabilizes lysosomal membranes of neutrophils, preventing the release of catabolic enzymes
        - Reduces vasodilitation and plasma extravasation
    - *Inflammatory Pathway*
        - They suppress inflammation & immune dysfunction associated with diseases that affect every organ in the body.
        - They suppress inflammation caused by allergic and autoimmune reactions.

        - Due to their lymphotoxic effects, they are used in the treatment of lymphocytic leukemia and lymphomas.
        - They are used as immunosuppressants to prevent organ graft rejection.
- ***Prescribing Tips:***
    - For all steroids, use lowest possible dose for treating conditions.
    - High potency corticosteroids evoke a longer-lasting stimulation of gene transcription than do lower potency corticosteroids.
    - Topical and inhalatory administration is preferred when possible due to decreased systemic absorption.
- ***Glucocorticoids raise plasma glucose levels during stress to provide energy for fight/flight.***
    - Corticosteroids may cause- euphoria, insomnia, mood swings, personality changes, severe depression, or psychosis.
- ***Adverse reactions:***
    - Raise the blood pressure through vasoconstriction
    - Exacerbate peptic ulcers due to the stimulation of gastric acid and pepsin
    - Reduce the secretion of TSH and FSH from pituitary
    - Cause subcapsular cataracts and glaucoma
    - Mask bacterial or mycotic infections
    - Cause growth retardation in children.
    - Osteoporosis due to increased bone catabolism and antagonizing the effect of Vit D on Ca^{+2} absorption
    - Supraphysiological doses for more than two weeks:
        - "Cushingoid" sign & symptoms due to tissue and metabolic changes:
            - "Buffalo hump", supraclavicular fat pads, weight gain, muscle wasting of legs, weakness, hirsutism, bruising, acne, striae
        - Hyperglycemia, glucose intolerance
        - Hypertension
- ***Hydrocortisone (short-acting, low potency)***
    - Duration of action 8-12 hours, with equal glucocorticoid and mineralocorticoid effects
    - *Preferred glucocorticoid for replacement therapy in adrenal insufficiency*
    - Used for anti-inflammatory effects, but more potent glucocorticoids often preferred for treating inflammatory, allergic and autoimmune disorders
    - Oral, topical and parenteral formulations
- ***Prednisone (Intermediate acting/medium potency)***
    - Often used for systemic treatment.
        - In the body, prednisone is rapidly converted to prednisolone.
        - Duration of action 12-36 hours, with the glucocorticoid potency approximately 5x higher than the mineralocorticoid potency.
        - Used to treat cancer, inflammation, allergy & autoimmune diseases
        - Only in oral formulation
        - Usual PO steroid dose- 5 days of 20-60mg/daily
- ***Methylprednisolone (intermediate acting/medium potency)***
    - Often used for systemic treatment
    - Duration of action 12-36 hours, with the glucocorticoid potency approximately 10x higher than the mineralocorticoid potency
    - Used to treat cancer, inflammation, allergy & autoimmune diseases
    - Oral, topical and parenteral formulations

- ***Dexamethasone (long acting/high potency)***
  - Used in diagnostic dexamethasone suppression tests and a variety of neoplastic, infectious and inflammatory conditions.
  - Duration of action 24-72 hours, with high glucocorticoid and zero mineralocorticoid effects
  - Oral, topical and parenteral formulations

OTHER IMMUNOSUPPRESSIVE AGENTS

Azathioprine

- **MOA**
  - *Cytotoxic* --- inhibits synthesis of adenine and guanine needed for synthesis of DNA/ cell replication
  - Decreases circulating lymphocytes (and most rapidly dividing cells)
- **SE's**
  - Potent immunosuppression with opportunistic infections

Cyclophosphamide

- **MOA**
  - Alkylating agent
  - Kills and suppresses function of lymphocytes

Cyclosporine

- **MOA**
  - Suppresses T cell function, especially helper cells
  - Inhibits production of interleukin-2
  - Results in inhibition of normal T cell function
  - When drug is stopped, T cells start doing their thing again

Monoclonal antibodies

- I don't think it's as important to know the names of these drugs as to know the concept of producing antibodies, injecting them into the human and let them "compete" with the problem agent at the receptor site – only most common are mentioned here

TNF alpha inhibitors

- **MOA**
  - Poorly understood as well, but thought to bind to specific antigens on cancer cells and kill them directly

Monoclonal antibody binds to and inhibits activity to TNF-α

- Blockers of interleukin

T cell blockers

Immunostimulant agents (used in treatment of cancers)

Dermatologic Drugs

In trying to decide what to study for Dermatology, consider antifungals (fungal infection), antimicrobials (bacterial infection) and steroids (immune response).

This is *much* easier on the exam than in clinical practice:

- ***Fungal* infections: treat with anti*fungal***
  - Will be relatively chronic (toenails) or over a couple days (tinea)
  - Will have positive KOH scraping!
  - Lesions will be pruritic
- ***Bacterial* infections: treat with anti*microbial***
  - Will be acute in onset
  - Will have positive gram stain
  - Will have purulent d/c
  - Patient will be febrile
  - Lesions will be tender
- **Immune: treat with steroid**
  - Will be chronic
  - KOH and gram stain negative
  - Will be pruritic
  - May have other symptoms (allergic rhinitis, conjunctivitis)
  - History of contact (nickel allergy)

ANTIFUNGALS

- **Nystatin**
  - Least expensive
  - Powder form, can be reconstituted as swish & swallow
- **Miconazole/Terconazole**
  - Miconazole – Candida albicans
  - Terconazole – Candida albicans, glabrata and tropicalis
  - Typically a topical or vaginal cream
- **Fluconazole**
  - Diflucan
  - Oral form
    - Once time dose for vaginal yeast infection
    - Daily for week or more for esophageal. etc
- **Griseofulvin (oral only)**
  - treatment of choice for scalp fungus
- **Terbinafine**
  - Lamisil
  - Use in fingernail and toenail fungus
  - Oral or "polish"

STEROIDS

- **Potency is important!**
    - Typically the question will be about potency and not actual name of drug
    - Adding an emollient increases potency
    - Occluding the area increases potency
    - Larger surface area increases systemic absorption
    - Steroids long-term cause atrophy (wrinkling and thinning of skin)
- **Treating Derm Conditions**
    - Used in: *dermatitis, pruritis, psoriasis*
        - Low potency steroids preferred for thin skin and folds. & pediatric pts.
            - Face, genitalia, neck (i.e. thin skin)
        - Low/Medium potency for ears, trunk, arms legs, scalp.
        - Medium/High potency for thick skin (palms, soles, knees, elbows)
    - Ointments best for dry, cracked, scaly, hardened skin.
    - Lotions & Creams for moist, weepy lesions and intense inflammation.
    - Lotions & Gels for hairy areas.

ANTIMICROBIALS - Remember, abscess cannot be treated with medicine, **needs I & D**!

- **For MRSA**
    - *Sulfamethoxazole/trimethoprim (SMX-TMP/Bactrim)*
- **For other Staph**
    - *Cephalosporin (Keflex)*
- **For impetigo**
    - *Mupirocin (Bactroban ointment)* – is as good as oral unless disseminated

---

Select Drug Concerns

Alendronate = Jaw osteonecrosis

Quinolones = Spontaneous tendonitis and tendon rupture

Azithromycin, clarithromycin = QT prolongation on ECG
(also erythromycin, quinidine, amiodarone, ketoconazole)

Nifedipine = Increases death and incidence of re-infarct in immediate post-MI period

Rosiglitazone = Increase CV disease and incidence of MI

Pioglitazone/cytoxan = Increased risk of bladder cancer

CHAPTER 5

History & Physical Exam- 16%

Topics in this section as described in the NCCPA Blueprint:

- Pertinent historical information associated with selected medical conditions
- Risk factors for development of selected medical conditions
- Signs and symptoms of selected medical conditions
- Physical examination techniques when pertinent, you will be alerted to any particular techniques in the content sections
- Physical examination findings associated with selected medical conditions
- Appropriate physical examination directed to selected medical conditions
- Differential diagnosis associated with presenting symptoms or physical findings
- Conducting comprehensive and focused interviews
- Identifying pertinent historical information
- Performing comprehensive and focused physical examinations
- Associating current complaint with presented history
- Identifying pertinent physical examination information

Introduction to the History & Physical Exam Chapter

In the old days, PAs had to perform an **OSCE** *(observed skilled clinical exam)* on a "patient" as part of our Certification process. We were given a chief complaint, brief history, and then had to:

- Select the appropriate focused physical exam components to perform, and then
- Perform those components using appropriate instructions to the patient, appropriate draping and proper technique and use of the instruments.

You will not have to do this; however, you are not off the hook. Sixteen percent of all the questions on the exam will be about performing these skills in clinical practice.

This is where the new graduates excel, and those of us out practicing for some time get a little rusty.

In the next section, I will brush off the cobwebs and remind you how a "Bates" physical exam should be done. I will focus on those areas that are "technical" and not always performed in actual clinical practice. In addition, besides just performing the exam, we need to review what those findings on that exam mean for the patient, and how you use findings to narrow that differential to the "most likely" diagnosis.

Eliciting the History

Recall that an appropriate history includes:

- ***Chief complaint (CC):*** Usually in the patient's own words, may be colloquial, but usually just one or two words
- ***The history of present illness (HPI):*** Use the acronym "oldcarts"
  - Onset, location, duration, character, aggravating & alleviating factors, radiation, timing or therapies tried
- ***Past medical history (PMH):*** Recall that the medication list is one way to establish the patient's PMH.
- ***Medications:*** Pay special attention if the question tells you that a new med was started; and remember that the medications are a good clue to the PMH (if PMH was not provided specifically in the stem)
- ***Allergies:*** Recall that allergy is not the same as intolerance to a drug – hallmark of taking a good allergy history is to ask what the reaction was to establish a true allergic reaction (rash vs. Angioedema vs. Anaphylaxis)
- ***Social history:*** Smoking, alcohol use, sleep patterns, occupation
- ***Family history:*** Usually only first-degree relatives except in some clear genetic disorders
- ***Chief concern:*** Many times different from the chief complaint, the patient may be worried about something that makes no clinical sense to you, but unless addressed, the concern is not ever cleared up for the patient.

The above list, in the appropriate order, is worth memorizing again. Many questions will allude to one of these historical components being missing, or may give you a component as a "clue" in establishing the "most likely" diagnosis

REVIEW OF SYSTEMS (ROS)

When the patient has an entirely positive review of systems, this indicates a disease state that affects all systems, i.e. endocrine etiology, autoimmune etiology, or psychogenic (somatoform disorder), look for this in your choice of answers.

Basic Review of PE for the main content areas:

General Principles:

The physical exam questions on the exam could either be about the "normal" PE findings expected, i.e. where is the normal PMI? , or could be questions about having you recognize a finding that is not normal, i.e. "the patient's PMI is at the 8th intercostal space at the mid-axillary line" (suggests a huge heart)

Physical examination is done in *this* order:

- Inspection
- Palpation
- Percussion
- Auscultation

Except in the abdomen where auscultation occurs prior to palpating and percussing the patient.

THE CARDIAC PHYSICAL EXAM

The cardiac exam begins in the EYES:

- Inspect the retina on fundoscopic exam for:
    - AV nicking which occurs when the BP is high, the arteriole sits on top of the vein and can "pinch it off", causing occlusion, or leaking of fluid/protein/blood from the vein which in turn causes:
    - Copper wire – light reflected off a "tense" arterial --- also suggests hypertension
    - Cotton wool spots, hard and soft exudates and flame shaped hemorrhages of either/both hypertension or diabetes.

Then the **NECK**:

- Inspection, palpation and auscultation of the **carotids**:
    - Delayed and decreased pulses = *aortic stenosis*
    - Big pulses = *aortic regurgitation/insufficiency*
    - Auscultate for bruits = *carotid plaques*
        - Recall that the murmur of AS often radiates into the R carotid and can sound an awful lot like a bruit

Inspection and measurement of the **internal jugular pulsation** (to estimate central venous pressure):

The exam is performed with the patient on the table at 30-45 degrees, a ruler on the "angle of Louis", and a straight edge is placed from the top of the jugular venous column to your ruler.

(Your ruler lies 5 cm above the right atrium by convention).

The normal CVP is 8-10 cm H20, so if the ruler sitting on the chest is already 5 cm above the right atrium, then the ruler should read somewhere between 3 and 5 cm. which would be a normal JVP (i.e. the 5 cm which is invisible to you is added to the ruler's 3cm (3+5=8) or the 5 cm invisible is added to the 4 cm on the ruler = 9, etc.

If the ruler reads 8 cm. then the CVP is 13, which is too high - the patient has too much "volume", and will need diuresis.

A 68 year old patient presents with DOE. On physical exam, you evaluate his jugular venous pulsation with the above physical examination technique. What is the normal range that would be noted on the "ruler" that you place on the patient's chest at the angle of Louis?

A. 1-3 cm.
B. 3-5 cm
C. 5-7 cm
D. 7-9 cm
E. 9 cm

Answer: B. The R atrium (by convention) lies 5 cm. below your ruler; 5 + 3 = 8 cm.; 5 + 5 = 10 cm; normal JVP or CVP

A 68 year old man presents with DOE. On PE, you note a JVP which measures 8 cm. on a ruler placed at the 2nd intercostal space on the manubrium at the top of the venous pulsation measured with a straight edge. This represents:

A. A normal measured JVP
B. An increased JVP
C. Is only accurate when performed in conjunction with the hepatojugular reflex
D. Is not pertinent to the patient exam if he has no peripheral edema
E. I have no idea what you are talking about

Answer: B. 5 + 8 = 13 cm; an elevated JVP

Next the PRECORDIUM:

Inspect for hyperdynamic pulsations, vibrations, and lifts/heaves (all suggesting abnormal action of the heart)

Palpate the precordium in the main four areas: base, pulmonic, LSB, and apex:

- Lifts/heaves (you can feel the heart "hitting" your hand as you hold it on the patient's chest which suggests a "hyperdynamic contraction)
- Thrills (you can feels a vibration from a "murmur" or the flow of blood through an abnormal valve
    - Put your hand on your chest and hum, *that* is a thrill (but without the humming part☺)

Palpate the PMI (point of maximum impulse) --- normal is at the 5th (or 6th) intercostal space at the mid-clavicular line

Percuss the heart border (no one ever actually does this), but presumably you are percussing for enlargement of the heart

Auscultate:

The bell: Used for low pitched and soft sounds – the bell sits lightly on the chest wall, many times used with the patient in left lateral decubitus to bring the heart closer to the stethoscope (these are usually mitral (or tricuspid) murmurs which are under much lower (diastolic) pressures and therefore softer sounds (S3 & S4)

The diaphragm: Used for high pitched and loud sounds – the diaphragm is pressed tightly against the skin of the chest wall. For almost all other sounds in the chest, i.e. rubs, bruits, lung sounds, harsh murmurs of aortic stenosis, and aortic regurgitation/insufficiency. The diaphragm will miss the low-pitched, soft murmurs of some mitral valve problems, and will miss S3 and S4.

A 32 year old pregnant female presents for dyspnea on exertion. On physical exam you note 1) a hyperdynamic pulsation at the PMI with no displacement; 2) a "thrill" at the apex, and 3) a loud murmur at the apex radiating into the axilla. Which of the following is the most likely true statement?

A. This is a normal physiologic variant in pregnancy
B. This represents a significant physical exam finding and warrants echocardiogram
C. This represents a minor physical exam findings and should be observed
D. This represents a common change in pregnancy due to increased blood volumes.
E. I have no idea what this represents

Answer: B. The constellation of signs with her symptom of DOE is concerning. A loud murmur with a thrill is never "physiologic" and warrants evaluation.

Finally, the PERIPHERAL VASCULAR SYSTEM

Inspect for abdominal aortic pulsations (suggests aortic aneurysm)

Palpate the abdominal aortic pulsation (if >3 cm, suggests aneurysm – needs US for evaluation in an asymptomatic patient)

Palpate the femoral, popliteal, dorsalis pedis, posterior tibialis (there is no percussion of the peripheral arteries and check capillary refill in the nail beds.

Auscultate the abdomen for intra-abdominal bruits (besides the renal arteries, aorta and iliacs, remember auscultation also occurs in the femoral arteries)

THE PULMONARY PHYSICAL EXAM

Inspection for:

- *Contour of thoracic cage*
  - Increased AP diameter (barrel-chest) = COPD/emphysema
- *Respiratory rate*
- *Depth of breathing*
- *Pattern of breathing*
  - Increased expiratory phase compared to inspiration = obstructive airway disease
- *Work of breathing*
  - Increased work of breathing
  - Intercostal retractions
  - Accessory muscle use
  - Speaking in shortened word strings

Palpation for:

- *Subcutaneous emphysema* = rice krispies sound
  - Emphysema, pneumothorax
- *Tactile fremitus (ninety-nine)* ** sound travels best in water, i.e. "fish finder" in fisherman's boat
  - Increased volume with consolidation (pneumonia)
  - Decreased if air in chest (pneumothorax, COPD)

Percussion for:

  - *Diaphragmatic excursion*
    - Elevated hemidiaphragm/paralyzed diaphragm
  - *Decreased or dull sound*
    - Fluid (consolidated pneumonia; pleural effusion)
    - **Could also represent an elevated hemidiaphragm – no way to tell without CXR**
  - *Resonance*
    - Dull
      - Fluid or consolidation

        - <u>Normal</u>
            - Normal lung filled with normal air: parenchyma
        - <u>Hyperresonant = too much air</u>
            - Pneumothorax
            - Emphysema

<u>**Auscultation** for:</u>

- *Tracheal breath sounds*= upper airway sound
- *Bronchial breath sounds* = large airway sound
    - Lower pitched, rhoncherous
- *Vesicular sounds*
    - This is the normal sound you should hear throughout most of lung fields
- *Stridor* = Upper airway sound
    - Foreign body aspiration
    - Tracheal narrowing (croup)

PEARL: Breath sounds are decreased when there is too much air (sound travels best in fluid and worst in air)

- Breath sounds become more "bronchial" (and louder) when there is fluid in the parenchyma (i.e., pneumonia)
- It is not normal to hear bronchial breath sounds in the lung parenchyma (should be vesicular); likewise, it is not normal to hear tracheal sounds anywhere but over the trachea. Bronchial sounds in the lung parenchyma usually suggest bronchitis at the least, pneumonia otherwise.

SPECIAL SOUNDS

- **Whispered pectoriloquy**
    - increased volume of whisper
        - Suggests consolidation (pneumonia)
- **Vocal fremitus**
    - Again, increases if water present (or consolidation)
- **Egophany**
    - "EE" vocalized by patient is heard as "AY" in a consolidation
- **Wheezing** – (sounds like a creaky door, squeaking)
    - Airway obstruction in small airways (*not stridor*)
- **Rales** (crackles – crunch cellophane near your ear to hear what this sounds like)
    - Fluid in alveolar air spaces (pulmonary edema)
- **Rhonchi** (gurgling, low pitched)
    - Pneumonia
    - COPD exacerbation
    - Bronchitis occasionally
- **Rubs** (sounds like Velcro ripping)
    - *Pleural vs. pericardial* === have the patient hold breath – if stops, it is pleural (when the patient stops moving the pleura the "velcro" sound of pleura rubbing on pleura stops, but if it is pericardial, not breathing will have no effect on the rub)

•

PEARL: Pathologic conditions will alter fremitus. In particular:

- Lung consolidation (pneumonia) is the normally air filled lung parenchyma engorged with fluid or pus, most commonly in the setting of pneumonia. Sound travels better in fluid than in air; so in consolidation, vocal and tactile fremitus becomes more pronounced. Egophany will be present. Fluid will make percussion dull, as normally you are tapping over air-filled lung.
- Pleural fluid collects in the potential space that exists between the lung and the chest wall, displacing the lung upwards. Even though sound would travel better through this fluid, there are no bronchials at all in that "space" and so the sound, while louder, essentially goes "nowhere" – not to your stethoscope anyway. There will be decreased tactile and vocal fremitus over the area of the effusion. Egophony would not be present either, except perhaps in the compressed lung tissue *above* the fluid. Fluid will make the percussion dull, just like in consolidation.

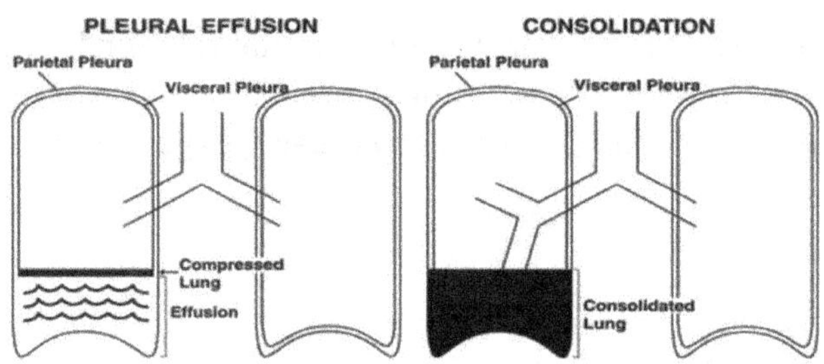

In general, fremitus is a pretty subtle finding and should not be thought of as the primary means of identifying either consolidation or pleural fluid. It can, however, get you that "one more question right" that you need to pass this test.

While examining a patient's chest you discover an area with absent breath sounds, increased tactile and vocal fremitus and egophony. Which of the following conditions do these findings most likely represent?

A. Pleural effusion
B. Pneumothorax
C. Pneumonia
D. Pulmonary hypertension
E.Pulmonary edema

Answer: C. These physical exam findings most often correlate with an increased density of the pulmonary tissues. This would most commonly be caused by a consolidation secondary to pneumonia.

Which of the following physical exam findings would be most likely in a patient with a pleural effusion?

A. Dullness to percussion with decreased tactile fremitus
B. Hyperresonant to percussion with decreased tactile fremitus
C. Dullness to percussion with increased tactile fremitus
D. Hyperresonant to percussion with increased tactile fremitus
E. Dullness to percussion with egophany

Answer: A. Due to the increased density presented by the effusion the percussion note will be dulled and transmission of speech vibration will be reduced. In contrast, emphysema with its increased lung volume will cause hyperresonance and increased fremitus.

PHYSICAL EXAMINATION FINDINGS OF COMMON PULMONARY CONDITIONS

	Pleural Effusion	Pneumonia	Tumor	Pneumothorax
Trachea	Midline/shifted if large	midline	Midline/shifted in large tumor	Midline/shifted in tension
Excursion	Reduced	Normal	Normal (or reduced if lg)	reduced
Fremitus (Tactile/Vocal)	Decreased	increased	Normal or decreased	none
Percussion	Dull	Dull	Normal (dull if large)	hyperresonant
Breath Sounds	Decreased	Increased	Normal or decreased if lg	None
Rubs	Sometimes	None	None	None
Egophany	Band above effusion	Present	None	None

THE ABDOMINAL EXAM

Inspection
- For scars, pulsations, obvious masses.

Auscultation (this is a different order than in any other organ system!)
- For bruits, bowel tones & pitch

Percussion
- For tympanic sound (most of bowel filled with gas) or dullness (liver border), or shifting dullness (ascites)

Palpation
- Lightly
- Deeply
- In all four quadrants and the periumbilical area and epigastrium

REMEMBER: Disorders in the chest often manifest with abdominal symptoms; pneumonia often causes back and abdominal pain; acute myocardial infarction often manifests as epigastric discomfort and generalized nausea – *so pulmonary exam and cardiac exams should be done on all patients who present with GI complaints!*

Let the anatomy of the abdomen help you answer the questions:

Differential Diagnosis by Location

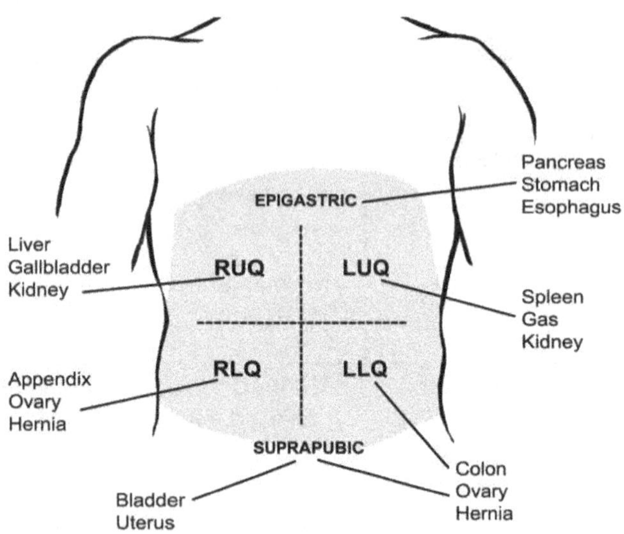

RUQ = liver, GB, biliary tree, pancreas

- Normal liver "span" should be 6-12 cm; tip just palpable, percuss for dullness from top to bottom and bottom to top (this dullness is the liver span)
- GB should *not* be palpable

- Pancreas head should *not* be palpable

LUQ = splenic flexure; spleen

- spleen tip should not be palpable and percussion here should be tympanic

LLQ = sigmoid and descending colon, L ovary in female, inguinal ring in male

RLQ = appendix, ascending colon, R ovary in female, inguinal ring in male

RUQ = GB, liver, lower lung base, sometimes pancreas

Epigastrium = Stomach, pancreas, lower esophagus, heart

THE MOST COMMON ABDOMINAL "SIGNS"

RUQ

Murphy's sign– a sign of acute cholecystitis

- The patient is asked to take a breath while you gently palpate the RUQ; then have him exhale; as the diaphragm comes down, the GB is brought closer to your waiting hand and the patient "splints" or catches his breath to prevent the tender GB from hitting your hand – this is done both on PE and during an US exam.

Courvoisier's (palpable gall bladder) sign – a sign of pancreatic cancer

- The patient's RUQ is palpated and a mass is felt. This could represent a calcified gall bladder from chronic inflammation; but more worrisome is that it represents a tumor on the head of the pancreas. If associated with jaundice, think *pancreatic tumor.*

RLQ

McBurney's point – pain here is a sign of acute appendicitis

- This point is on the right side of the abdomen, one-third of the distance from the anterior superior iliac spine to the navel. This point roughly corresponds to the most common location of the base of the appendix where it is attached to the cecum.

Psoas Sign

- Place your hand above the patient's right knee.
- Ask the patient to flex the right hip against resistance.
- Increased abdominal pain indicates a positive psoas sign.

Obturator Sign

- Raise the patient's right leg with the knee flexed.
- Rotate the leg internally at the hip.
- Increased abdominal pain indicates a positive obturator sign.

LLQ

Rovsing's – a sign of acute appendicitis

- The patient's abdomen is palpated; obviously, a patient with an acute appendicitis will have pain in the RLQ; but if the patient has pain referred to the RLQ when you palpate the LLQ, that is a rovsing's sign; also called "referred pain" suggesting peritoneal irritation.

Nonfocal, but equally important other abdominal findings:

Signs of peritoneal inflammation

- Rebound tenderness
- Cervical motion tenderness (CMT) on pelvic exam

Signs for peritoneal fluid (ascites)

- *Shifting dullness*
    - Percuss for areas of dullness and tympany
    - Have the patient roll to one side
    - Percuss again, see if the dullness has shifted to areas that used to be tympanic
- *Fluid wave*
    - Put hand in middle of abdomen and percuss at lateral edge; fluid wave will hit your hand, suggesting ascites

A 58-year-old woman presents with complaint of jaundice, dark-colored urine, and light-colored stools for the past several days. She has no history of jaundice or gallstone disease.

With the exception of a palpable gallbladder, the physical examination of the abdomen is unremarkable. Computed tomography of the abdomen reveals a mass in the head of the pancreas, a dilated proximal biliary duct, and a severely distended and elongated gallbladder.

What is the most likely diagnosis?

A. Porcelain gall bladder (chronic cholelithiasis)
B. Hepatitis
C. Chronic pancreatitis
D. Pancreatic carcinoma
E. Acute cholecystitis

Answer: D. Pancreatic carcinoma

Discussion: All of these options could be entertained. Even if you have no prior history of gall bladder disease, at any point in time you could develop it. The most concerning and important point in this question is the palpable "gall bladder", i.e. Courvoisier's sign, and finding of tumor on head of pancreas on CT. The pancreatic tumor is compressing the common bile duct extrinsically (by pushing on it, and causing it to become obstructed). This causes similar symptoms to cholecystitis but without any actual abnormality of the gall bladder, except from the pressure the tumor is putting on the duct.

THE GYN EXAM

The pelvic exam begins with inspection, but then is completely different from the other systems.

Speculum examination:

Inspect the vaginal walls, the "cuff" if S/P hysterectomy, and for discharge (normal white odorless discharge is "normal leukorrhea"). If Ph is done, should be acidic (if alkaline, there is a pathogen)

Inspect the cervix (should be smooth and pink), the os – nulliparous (never dilated) or multiparous (after a baby or dilatation procedure). "Friable" cervix suggests infection; leukoplakia suggests cancer or pre-cancer

Bimanual examination:

Palpate a 4-week (maybe 6 in someone who has had some kids) sized, freely mobile uterus that can be anteverted, midposition or retroverted (makes no difference medically). There should be no cervical motion tenderness, *no* adnexal tenderness, and *no* adnexal masses. Enlargement of the uterus beyond "6-week sized" is not normal. Irregular contour suggests fibroids.

A normal ovary measures < 5 cm. *Anything > 5 cm. should have an ultrasound. Any irregular mass should have an ultrasound.*

Rectovaginal palpation should be done in order to examine the "pouch of Douglas or cul de sac" for masses (dermoids, ovarian cancer), or nodularity (endometriosis), or bulging (ruptured ectopic pregnancy or free fluid)

THE ORTHOPEDIC EXAM

Inspection:
- Skin for abrasions, lacerations, injury, bruising, redness
- Joints for swelling
  - Red, warm, boggy = infection/inflammation
  - Swelling without redness and warmth = osteoarthritis
- Deformity in trauma

Palpation:
- Warmth and "bogginess"
- Deformity
- Point tenderness over tendon insertions (overuse syndromes), over boney deformities (fractures), over bursa

Active range of motion:
- always performed first – patient moves joint without assistance (if possible)
- measure the ROM and compare to normal

Passive range of motion:
- Done after AROM – if no trauma

- if trauma, and patient unable to move, obtain radiograph before moving joint
- PROM is compared to AROM; in some overuse syndromes (rotator cuff tear), patient has limited AROM but you are able to move the shoulder through normal ranges of motion passively.
- *Septic joint will hurt with both active and passive ROM*

Special tests (All special tests are covered in the ortho section (Chapter 14).

THE NEUROLOGIC EXAM

Mental status:
- Level of Consciousness
- Attention
- Speech
- Perceptual difficulties
- Orientation to person, place, date & time, situation
- Memory
- Language (expressive and receptive)
- Visual
- GCS (Glascow coma scale)

- The Glascow Coma scale comprises three tests: eye, verbal and motor responses.
- The three values separately as well as their sum are considered.
- The lowest possible GCS (the sum) is 3 (deep coma or death), while the highest is 15 (fully awake person)
- 3= does not open eyes, does not move, does not make a sound (patient gets one single point for not doing each of these things)

	1	2	3	4	5	6
Eyes	Does not open eyes	Opens eyes in response to painful stimuli	Opens eyes in response to voice	Opens eyes spontaneously	N/A	N/A
Verbal	Makes no sounds	Incomprehensible sounds	Utters inappropriate words	Confused, disoriented	Oriented, converses normally	N/A
Motor	Makes no movements	Extension to painful stimuli (decerebrate response)	Abnormal flexion to painful stimuli (decorticate response)	Flexion / Withdrawal to painful stimuli	Localizes painful stimuli	Obeys commands

Table X: The Glascow Coma Scale

The Cranial nerves – On Old Olympus' Towering Tops a Finn and German Viewed Some Hops

I – Olfactory

- *Sensory*- (sinusitis; nasal congestion; basilar skull fracture)

II – Optic

- *Sensory*
- Visual acuity, visual fields by confrontation (wiggling fingers); fundoscopic exam of optic cup and nerve

III, IV, VI – Oculomotor, Trochlear, Abducens

- *Motor* – Extraocular movements (EOM's); direct, consensual light response and accommodation
- CN III has the most activity in terms of allowing sight, so it is probably the nerve to select if you are purely guessing
    - Opens eyelid
    - Pupil direct and consensual response
    - Corneal eyeblink reflex (closes eye when cornea touched with cotton wisp)
- CN IV moves the eyeball up and down (very basically) and obliquely; palsy will cause a vertical diplopia
- CN VI moves it laterally (hence the name abducens, like ab-duction)

V – Trigeminal

- *Both sensory & motor*:
- *Sensory*
    - There are three divisions for pain and sensation --- ophthalmic; maxillary, mandibular
        - Ophthalmic branch often involved in trigeminal neuralgia
        - Ophthalmic branch, when involved with zoster poses a risk to dendritic lesion on the cornea)
- *Motor*
    - Temporal and masseter strength (clenching teeth); lateral movement of the jaw

VII – Facial – motor & sensory

- *Sensory* –taste on anterior 2/3 of tongue
- *Motor* – facial symmetry – smile, frown, puff cheeks, squeeze eyelids shut

VIII – Acoustic – sensory

- Cochlear branch - hearing – impairment causes sensorineural hearing loss
- Vestibular branch – sense of balance (in concert with the cerebellum) – damage to either the cranial nerve or the cerebellum may cause ataxias

IX & X – Glossopharyngeal / Vagal nerve – tested together

- Gag reflex; symmetric rise of the soft palate

XI – Spinal Accessory

- *Motor*
- Elevate shoulders against resistence; turn head against resistance (traps and sternocleidomastoid m. strength)

XII – Hypoglossal

- *Motor*
- Tongue movement; strength

PEARL: This is not the time to spend a week re-memorizing the cranial nerves. Your time is best spent on a topic with a greater percentage of questions. That said, there are a few cranial nerves that are affected more often than others are, i.e. CN VII in Bell's palsy.

The extra ocular movements involve CN III, IV, and VI. This is worth noting in general, so you can make an "educated guess" if you cannot recall exactly which one moves the eye inward or downward, etc.

Here is an image to help you remember (for the rest of your life) which CN opens and closes the lid.

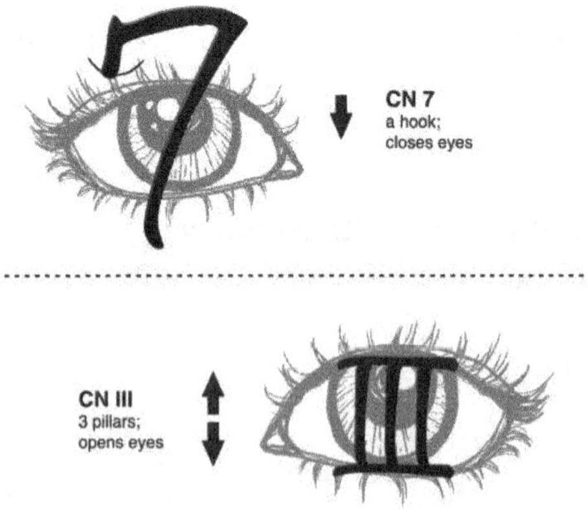

CN III – opens the lid – therefore, if a CN III palsy (diabetes is most common, but brain tumor must be considered), the eyelid will not open (patient will have a ptosis)

CN VII – closes the lid – therefore, if CN VII palsy, the lid cannot close

Bell's palsy vs. Stroke = In a facial nerve (CN VII) paralysis, the forehead will not move, the lid will not close -- the facial nerve is responsible for TOTAL facial muscle movement; in a stroke (upper motor neuron deficit), the forehead is "spared", and forehead wrinkles are symmetrical and lid closes appropriately

PEARL: Accommodation is part of "PERRLA" – pupils are equal, round, reactive to light (implied direct & consensual) and *accommodation*

The truth is, we rarely actually make the patient do "accommodation" – that entails having them look at your finger (with each eye individually) observe for pupillary constriction; then have them look at a distant point (each individually) and look for pupillary dilatation

What is the reason we have a patient focus on a distant object during fundoscopic exam?

Answer: To dilate the pupil a bit so we can see the retina better.

MUSCLE STRENGTH AND TONE

- Upper motor neuron abnormalities- increase in tone; spasms; hyper-reflexia with clonus; abnormal Babinski
- Lower motor neuron abnormalities – decrease in tone; flaccidity; loss of reflexes

DTR's

- C5 & C6 = biceps
- C6 & C7 = triceps
- L2,3,4 = patellar
- S1 = ankle

SENSATION

- Check for dermatome distribution loss of sensation to pain; temperature; vibration; position (proprioception)
    - **C6** = thumb
    - **T4** = level of nipple
    - **T10** = level of umbilicus
    - **L5** = great toe
    - **S2,3,4** = anal sphincter

CEREBELLAR TESTING

Recall that the reason we learned many ways to do this, is so that we can test the cerebellum on a bedridden patient!

- *If able to stand/walk* -- Romberg; gait and tandem gait (tightrope walking)
- *If in bed* – Rapid alternating movements; finger to nose; heel down shin

A 29-year-old male presents after motorcycle accident with closed head trauma. No helmet was found at the scene. He does not open his eyes to painful stimulation, is making no noise, but pushes his arms away stiffly as IV is inserted.

What is his GCS?

A. 1
B. 3
C. 4
D. 5
E. 15

Answer: C. 4

Discussion: 1 point for no eye movement; 1 point for no noise; 2 points for decerebrate posturing with pain = 4

Which disease is associated with no pupillary response to either direct or consensual light testing; but normal response to accommodation?

Answer: Tertiary syphilis

Discussion: This was told to me by an ophthalmologist – "The Prostitute Analogy"

A prostitute will not respond but will accommodate ☺

THE DERMATOLOGIC EXAM

History

- *What to pay attention to in the stem of the question*
  - Itchy?
  - Painful?
  - Recent in onset? Or several weeks/months? (acute vs. chronic)
  - Fever, weight loss, or other constitutional symptoms?
- *Personal history*
  - Comorbidities
    - Dlabetes, autoimmune disease, etc.
- *Family history*
  - Allergic, genetic, ethnic
- *Occupational history*
  - Contact exposure; inhalant exposures
- *Other systemic symptoms?*
  - CV, pulm, GI, neuro, etc
    - Kawasaki's = rash + CV complications
    - Zoster = rash + neurologic/optho concerns
    - Dermatitis herpetiformis = GI complaints, i.e., celiac disease

Inspection & Palpation (No percussion or Auscultation!)

- *Overall general appearance and vital signs*
    - Fever? suggests infectious origin
    - Hygiene
    - Chronic nature of skin changes/abnormalities
    - General sense of health of patient
- *Skin examination (including all skin surfaces, mucous membranes, hair and nails):*
    - Description of primary lesion
    - Description of secondary changes
    - Color
    - Margins/borders
    - Shape
- *Palpation*
    - Consistency
    - Temperature
    - Mobility
    - Tenderness
    - Depth
- *Number*
    - Single; multiple; too numerous to count
- *Arrangement*
    - "Christmas tree distribution"; dermatome distribution
- *Confluence*
- *Distribution*
    - Scalp (seborrhea, tinea capitus, lice, alopecia)
    - Face (perioral dermatitis, rosacea, erysipelas (most common face, neck, ears)
    - Hands only (contact, dishydrotic eczema, maceration from hand washing)
    - Includes palms and soles (Kawasaki's, syphilis)
    - Web spaces of hands (scabies)
    - Neck (contact from nickel, lotions, perfumes)
    - Sun exposed areas (drugs, porphyria, lotions)
    - Entire body (drug eruption, viral exanthema, secondary problem, i.e. Autoimmune)
    - Trunk only (tinea, pityriasis rosea)
    - Inguinal folds (tinea cruris, hidradenitis suppurativa)

Multiple, 1mm skin-colored, discrete papules with central umbilication located on the upper chest and left axilla of a 5-year-old child. They are not itchy; but they seem to be increasing in number over the past several weeks. He has no other symptoms, and no other lesions.

What is the most likely diagnosis?

A. Molluscum contagiosum
B. Condlyomata accuminata
C. Verrucous lesions (plain warts)
D. Folliculitis
E. Early psoriasis

Answer: A. Molluscum contagiosum

Discussion: This is the typical presentation, typical appearance of the lesions, and the typical distribution pattern of molluscum. In children, it is typically on the upper body; in sexually active adults, it presents more as a sexually transmitted virus in the skin of the mons, lower abdomen and thighs. Condylomata and plain warts are both part of the "human papilloma virus" category which can cause the venereal warts called condyloma and the simple warts of plantar warts and other skin warts. These do not have umbilicated centers. They are papules, so are in the differential diagnosis of a papular rash. Folliculitis is pustular, so not in this differential diagnosis. Early psoriasis could, present like this – the papular lesions of psoriasis are associated with Koebner's phenomenon, but again, these do not have umbilicated centers that are the *hallmark* of molluscum.

Pay careful attention to every word describing the symptoms, presentation, appearance, and distribution of the rash or lesion. Also, remember acute vs. chronic!

PRIMARY LESIONS

- **Macules** = Circumscribed area of change in skin color which is not palpable
- **Papules** = Superficial, raised, solid lesion, generally considered <0.5cm in diameter
- **Plaques** = Plateau-like elevation above the skin surface, usually formed by confluence of papules; often well-defined
- **Nodules** = Large papule; palpable, solid round or ellipsoidal lesion
- **Vesicles** = Circumscribed, elevated, containing fluid, <0.5cm
- **Bulla** = Large vesicle, >0.5 cm
- **Pustules** = Circumscribed, elevated, contains a purulent exudate
- **Wheals** = Irregular elevated edematous skin area, often changes in size and shape

SECONDARY SKIN CHANGES

- **Crusts** = Serum, blood or purulent exudate dried on the skin surface
- **Scales** = Flakes of stratum corneum
- **Lichenification** = Thickened skin with accentuated skin markings
- **Excoriation** = Shallow, hemorrhagic excavations resulting from scratching
- **Erosions** = Defect of the epidermis as a result of physical abrasions/vesicles/bullae
- **Ulcer** = Skin defect that extends into the dermis or deeper

- **Fissure** = Deep skin split extending into the dermis
- **Macerated** = From moisture/water exposure
- **Atrophy** = Decreased skin thickness due to loss of underlying dermis

CHAPTER 6

Labs & Diagnostics – 14%

Topics in this section as described in the NCCPA Blueprint:

- Indications for initial and subsequent diagnostic or laboratory studies
- Cost effectiveness of diagnostic studies or procedures
- Relevance of common screening tests for selected medical conditions
- Normal and abnormal diagnostic ranges
- Risks associated with diagnostic studies or procedures
- Appropriate patient education related to laboratory or diagnostic studies
- Using diagnostic equipment safely and appropriately
- Selecting appropriate diagnostic or laboratory studies
- Collecting diagnostic or laboratory specimens
- Interpreting diagnostic or laboratory studies results

Introduction to the Labs & Diagnostics Chapter

General Principle: First, it is important to remember that labs and diagnostics should be selected only after the history and physical exam have been done.

It is the findings in the H & P that dictate which labs and diagnostics are indicated. So when the question asks you "what initial test....?", or "what appropriate diagnostic imaging study...?" your selection of that test is based on the information given to you in the stem. These lab and diagnostic results lead you to the likely diagnosis.

If a single test will narrow the differential from 20 things to 2 things and has little harmful effects to the patient, this is likely the best initial test to order.

- For example, if a patient presents with joint arthralgias, a sed rate (while very nonspecific) if negative, will essentially rule out an inflammatory or infectious process. If positive, of course, all you know is that there is an inflammatory or infectious process going on, and you have to take it from there.

- Mr. Jones, our 60-year-old diabetic, hypertensive, dyslipidemic male has chest pain again. ECG and cardiac enzymes, if negative, give you a lot of information, and a lot more time to try to figure out what is causing his chest pain. Missing the "tombstones" on his ECG and his 10 fold elevated Troponin because it was not what you thought to do as an "initial" diagnostic, would be bad for poor Mr. Jones.

The most common labs (in terms of diagnosing common and lethal illnesses) are included in this section. It will not encompass all possible labs (any specifics will be in the content areas themselves).

Remember - normal values here are for illustrative purposes only - there is a pull-down menu for you on the test to find normal lab values in the lower left corner of the screen during the exam (discover it during the tutorial!)

Dermatologic evaluation is quite different from all the rest and is at the end of this chapter.

The most common imaging modalities and very general information about less common imaging will be in the final section.

Laboratory Evaluation

All diseases discussed in this section about interpreting a CBC are discussed in greater detail in Hematology, Chapter 23.

CBC WITH DIFFERENTIAL AND PLATELET COUNT

The White Blood Cells

Normal WBC count = 5,000-10,000 (this is the total of all the various types of WBC's)

- ***Elevated*** *= Leukocytosis*
    - Bacterial infection
    - Leukemia
    - Steroids (recent steroid use can elevate WBC)
    - Stress reaction (just like "steroids" above, remember that in an acutely anxious individual, he/she is making cortisol, which increases WBC count)
- ***Low*** *= Leukopenia*
    - Viral infection
    - Aplastic anemia (all cells are decreased)
    - Chemotherapy/radiation therapy
    - Drug reaction (causing aplastic anemia; sulfa is most common)

The Normal WBC Differential

- *Segmented neutrophils (polymorphonucleocytes= PMNs) = 70%*
    - increase % in bacterial infection
- *Lymphocytes = 20%*
    - increase % in viral infection
- *Monocytes = 5%*
    - increase % in autoimmune disease
- *Eosinophils = 2%*
    - increase % in allergies & worms
- *Basophils = 1%*
    - basophilic "stippling" suggests lead poisoning

PEARL: About the WBC:

- **Left Shift** is seen in a bacterial infection. The WBC will increase (leukocytosis), and immature form of the WBC (band) will appear. Because the "differential" is a percentage of cells, obviously the lymphocyte count will decrease.

- **BANDS** are significant but do not suggest a leukemia – the appearance of bands suggests a bacterial infection---- it means the bone marrow is working overtime to try to make more segs (which are dying in battle) – in this attempt to help, the marrow sends out these slightly immature forms.

- **BLASTS** are never ok
  - Myeloblasts = *acute* myelogenous leukemia
  - Lymphoblasts = *acute* lymphoblastic leukemia
  - Monoblasts = *acute* monoblastic leukemia

- **Viral infections** (like mono) typically cause a leukopenia (low WBC) and an increase in the percentage of lymphocytes (usually 50% segs and 50% lymphocytes) but remember – never bands and never blasts!

The Red Blood Cells

Normal RBC count = 4-6 million (higher in men than in women)

- *Elevated*
  - In severe dehydration and in polycythemia (primary or secondary)
- *Decreased*
  - In anemia, blood loss, or loss of cells by sequestration in the spleen
- *HGB (Hemoglobin)*
  - This is what carries oxygen.
  - Hemoglobinopathies are relatively common, inherited abnormalities.
  - Almost all cause a decrease in the red cell indices (looking like an iron deficiency anemia) --- use the ethnicity of the patient given to you to suggest this as a reason for a microcytic anemia.
- *HCT (Hematocrit)*
  - Percentage of RBC's in one ml. of blood.
  - Increased if dehydrated (because less fluid, therefore hemoconcentrated)
- *RDW (Red cell distribution width)*
  - This measures the size of the RBC's as they go through the machine
  - If there is only one size (be it large or small), the RDW will be normal
  - If there is more than one cell size or cell "population" as in RBC's and reticulocytes (which are larger cells), then the RDW will go up, (or be wide)
  - In an anemia where the cells are small, a normal RDW will tell you they are *all* small (i.e. no retics present); conversely, if the RDW is increased, it is telling you that some are normal, some small, and some large.

The Red Cell Indices

- **MCV – measures the size of the RBC – normal is 80-100**
    - *Decreased (<80)*
        - Iron deficiency
        - Thalassemia
        - Sideroblastic anemia
        - Anemia of chronic disease
    - *Increased (>100)*
        - Vit. B12 deficiency
        - Folic acid deficiency
        - The red cell is unable to make DNA due to no B12 or folate, mitosis is impaired, so instead of dividing into two cells, the single cell just gets larger
        - this leads to both anemia, and macrocytosis, or megaloblastic anemia
- **MCHC – measures Hgb concentration**
    - It is almost always normal or low (in anemia)
    - When MCHC is *high* = **spherocytosis**! You do not even have to read the rest of the choices!

PEARL: About the red blood cells:

- RBC's are anucleate cells that are biconcave and have a pale center.
    - This central pallor causes a reduction in Hgb concentration in the cell when measured by the machine.
- Reticulocytes are immature RBC's that are larger than normal and lack central pallor.
- Nucleated RBC's are even *more* immature cells and indicate that the marrow is working overtime to make new cells for some reason.

The Platelets

Platelet Count – normal 150,000-450,000

- *Increased (thrombocytosis)*
    - Essential thrombocytosis
    - Severe anemia (in the architecture of bone marrow, the erythroid cell line is "next door" to the megakaryocyte cell line) and so as marrow is working to make more RBC's, it makes more platelets.
- *Decreased (thrombocytopenia)*
    - Drugs (including alcohol)
    - ITP (idiopathic thrombocytopenic purpura)
    - TTP (thrombotic thrombocytopenic purpura)

Questions illustrating anemias, coagulation problems and WBC issues are found in the Hematology Chapter 23.

LIVER ENZYME AND BILIRUBIN EVALUATION

PEARL: About the liver panel:

- *Remember that the liver enzyme panel is not actually measuring function of the liver*
    - If you want to measure function; you need to measure
        - albumin
        - direct bilirubin
        - prothrombin time/INR

- *The "transaminases", AST and ALT, are enzymes that leak from damaged or diseased or diseased hepatocytes*
    - ALT is most specific for liver damage
    - AST comes from both liver and skeletal muscle

- *In end stage liver disease, these transaminases are not as useful as you would think:*
    - Mr. Jones is a "varsity drinker" and has very poor liver function, his hepatocytes are mostly dead; he has only 3 hepatocytes left
        - His ALT/AST are not going to be markedly elevated.
        - However, his liver's function is horrible.
    - Therefore, his serum albumin will be low, his INR will be high, and he will be jaundiced.
    - Because his albumin is low, he will "third space" his fluid to normalize oncotic pressure; more importantly, he has no albumin to make immunoglobulins; anticlotting proteins; etc.
    - Because his INR is high, he has increased risk of bleeding.

- *Alkaline phosphatase*
    - a biliary tree enzyme
    - but also present in bone
    - produced by the placenta in a pregnant female (normal mild elevation in pregnancy)

- *Two main things to pay attention to when a liver panel pops up*
    - Look for evidence that tells you that this is acute, or that this is a chronic problem.
    - Look at your choices for one that is acute or one that is chronic.

Specifics about the components of the liver panel:

- **ALT**
    - Specific for the liver
    - Leaks into serum from damaged/destroyed/inflamed hepatocytes
    - Marked elevation in *acute* liver damage
- **AST**
    - From liver, but also from heart, and skeletal muscle

   - Many reasons for increased AST as not very specific
   - *In alcohol – AST will be greater than ALT* (skeletal muscle wasting/damage)
- **Alkaline phosphatase (alk p'tase)**
   - More specific for the biliary tree
   - Also found in bone (increased in fracture; in both primary bone cancers and bone metastasis; in bone metabolic disorders)
   - In placenta (always increased in pregnancy);
- **T. Bilirubin**
   - Total amount of bilirubin in serum
   - Gets transported to liver for "conjugation" as a byproduct of RBC turn over
   - May be elevated for many reasons
   - Direct bilirubin
      - Bilirubin that has been "conjugated" by the liver and is now water soluble
      - Able to be excreted by the kidney, if need be (may appear on urine dip & cause brown urine)
   - Indirect bilirubin
      - Bilirubin that is not conjugated
      - Not water soluble
      - Not able to be excreted by kidney
      - Therefore, urine is yellow and dips negative for bilirubin (even if elevated)
- **LDH**
   - Is a very nonspecific marker (present on fluid panels from almost any fluid in the body)
   - Is a very general test that tells you cell membranes are being lysed. That's all.
- **INR**
   - Thought of as a coagulation test; but in liver failure it is a pretty good estimate of the prognosis of the disease (if this is high, it's a chronic and severe problem)
- **T. Protein**
   - Again a function of the liver (if this is low, it's a chronic and severe problem)
- **Albumin**
   - Again a function of the liver (if this is low, it's a chronic and severe problem)

Deciphering a liver panel problem:

1. *First, take a quick look at the level of elevation of the ALT and AST.*
   - Are they > 50-100 elevated? (probably an acute hepatitis of some type)
   - Are they only 2-10 times elevated? (probably a chronic hepatitis of some type or primarily a biliary problem)
2. *Next, take a quick look at the alkaline phosphatase.*
   - Is it 100 times elevated? (ALT/AST not so much?) then a biliary problem ---- look for a biliary disease in the choices
   - Is it 10 times elevated? (ALT/AST sky high?) then a hepatic problem --- look for a liver disease in the choices
3. *Finally, are the ALT and AST only mildly elevated, and the AST>ALT by about 2:1 --- alcohol*
   - In other primary liver diseases not due to alcohol, the ALT (specific for liver) will be higher than the AST (not so specific)

HEPATITIS SEROLOGY

Most importantly, when a question presents about Hepatitis serology, the key is to pay attention to whether the question is discussing the antigen (Ag) or the antibody to the antigen (IgM or IgG)

When you are tired, it is easy to get confused!

- **Hepatitis A**
    - Patient eats or drinks "feces" containing Hepatitis A virus (HAV) - (yuck!)
    - Patient develops an acute viral hepatitis --- HAV -Ag is present in his serum
    - His immune system makes IgM to the HAV antigen --- you have a positive IgM-HAV
    - Then, after 4-5 weeks or so, your immune system makes IgG to the HAV antigen – you now have a positive IgG to HAV and are immune!
    - You can go ahead and drink contaminated water and not get sick (from HAV, anyway)

- **Hepatitis B** is much trickier
    - *Recovered Hepatitis B*
        - Patient shares a needle or body fluids with a patient who has active Hep B
        - Patient develops acute viral hepatitis – HBsAg, HBcAg, HBeAg are present in his serum
        - His immune system (hopefully) makes IgM to all three particles
        - Then, his immune system makes IgG to all three particles
        - He is now immune (resolved Hepatitis B --- no increased risk for liver damage; or liver cancer; not contagious)
    - *Chronic Hepatitis B*
        - Patient shares a needle or body fluids with a patient who has active Hep B
        - Patient develops acute viral hepatitis – HBsAg, HBcAg, HBeAg are present in his serum
        - His immune system is not very good, and only makes antibody to the core (HBcAg) and the envelope (HBeAg)
        - He never makes antibody (neither IgM nor IgG to the surface antigen) and so has chronic HBsAg in his serum
        - He is now a chronic Hep B patient with increased risk for liver damage and liver cancer
        - If he has seroconverted (IgG to HBcAg and to HBeAg) he is minimally infective
    - *Chronic Active Hepatitis B*
        - This patient is just like the patient with chronic Hepatitis B, but he does not have any antibodies to the envelope (HBeAg)
        - He will likely have antibody to the core (but this does not do much in Hepatitis B in terms of infectivity).
        - If you see a patient with + HBs**Ag** and +HBe**Ag**, he is both at risk for liver problems and highly infectious

- *Vaccinated Hepatitis B serology*
  - So what would your serum look like?
    - You have seen only the HBsAg portion
    - You seroconvert and make IgM, and then IgG to HepBsAg --- you now have anti-HBsAg or HBsAg-IgG
    - You are good to go
- (However, if you have antibody to any of the other particles, you are not a vaccinated person, you saw the whole darn virus! ***Do not get tricked!***

Hepatitis B Serology

Clinical Status	HBsAg	Anti-HBs	Anti-HBc	HBeAg
Susceptible (never infected or vaccinated)	Negative	Negative	Negative	Negative
Immune (prior infection)	Negative	Positive	Positive	Negative
Immune (vaccination)	Negative	Positive	Negative	Negative
Acute infection	Positive	Negative	Positive	Positive
Chronic carrier (active carrier)	Positive	Negative	Positive	Positive
Chronic carrier (inactive carrier)	Positive	Negative	Positive	Negative

- **Hepatitis C** -Even scarier
  - *Transmission is blood borne, like Hepatitis B*
    - Most commonly IV drug use
    - Needle stick
    - Tattoos (especially "homemade")
    - Debate about sexual transmission
  - In HCV infection, even if you do seroconvert (and most patients do), it does not confer immunity
  - IgG to HCV does not mean the patient is immune
    - 80% of people continue to have disease, unfortunately
  - Viral load testing (measuring RNA replication) is the only way to know for sure

LABORATORY EVALUATION OF RENAL FUNCTION

Serum Creatinine

Creatinine is the only substance cleared entirely by the kidney – so it is the best test of renal function.

If you want a definitive GFR, you have to do 24-hour urine for creatinine clearance:

- Creatinine is a muscle breakdown product, i.e. it would be increased in a muscular man, and decreased in a thin, cachectic female.
- The Cockroft-Gault formula estimates the amount of creatinine a particular human should make from normal muscle turnover.
- The C-G formula accounts for differences in muscle mass, and therefore creatinine produced
    - Do not memorize the C-G formula (there's an app for that!)
- Lab compares amount estimated to be produced with what is excreted in 24 hours
    - If excretion of creatinine is impaired, or slowed due to renal dysfunction, the serum levels of creatinine will rise
- The 24 hours urine is imply too cumbersome to do daily in a hospitalized patient, so serum creatinine is used as a good indirect measure of creatinine clearance.

PEARL: Creatinine is most important in its change over time.

If the creatinine increases by 1.0, (say from 0.6 to 1.6) the patient has lost almost complete renal function in the past 24 hours.

Serum creatinine should be ordered daily on anyone inpatient. There is a 25% chance of causing renal failure in our hospitalized patients iatrogenically. Pay attention to any significant increase, even if still within the normal parameters on the pull down menu).

BUN (Blood Urea Nitrogen)

- BUN is excreted both by the kidney and by the gut; therefore, when the BUN is elevated think kidney or gut, i.e. renal failure or GI bleed.
- The most common reason for elevation of the BUN is *dehydration.*
    - When a body is dehydrated, the BUN will increase significantly more than the creatinine:
    - This may be called "an increase in the BUN to creatinine ratio", or be depicted as BUN: creatinine > 20:1.
- When a kidney is chronically failing, the BUN will not increase nearly as much (because the gut is able to get rid of it); therefore, the BUN: creatinine ratio will be < 20:1.
- So, when you see a BUN of 56; and creatinine of 1.5 = think acute renal failure or dehydration or GI bleed.
- And, when you see a BUN of 28 and creatinine of 4.8 = think chronic renal failure.

Mr. Jones is a 42-year-old diabetic with admittedly poor diabetic control who presents for generalized malaise and fatigue for the past two days associated with a productive cough. He has not been seen in the clinic in "several years".

He has been taking his medications as ordered, including lisinopril, glipizide, metformin, atorvastatin, and is also taking 800 mg ibuprofen every 8 hours for the past two days for his myalgias.

His physical examination shows that he is febrile, has bronchial breath sounds in the right base with rhonchi. He appears significantly dehydrated with dry mucous membranes, and poor skin turgor.

- **Labs: CBC with WBC 15,000 with 91% segs, 8% lymphs, 1% monos**
- **CMP with normal LFT's, normal albumin, normal electrolytes with normal anion gap of 10, glucose 234, creatinine 2.4, BUN 57**
- **Urinalysis shows no RBC's, no WBC's, negative nitrite, 1+ protein**
- **Imaging: CXR shows a consolidation in the right base without pleural effusion**

Of the following, which represents the most likely etiology of his elevated BUN and creatinine?

A. Septic shock
B. Membranous nephropathy
C. Diabetic nephropathy
D. Ibuprofen use
E. ACE induced decreased renal perfusion

Answer: D.

***Discussion*:** Ibuprofen is the most likely cause of the "pre-renal" azotemia (a perfusional decrease to the kidney due to lack of prostaglandin). While this patient is ill with pneumonia, the stem states that his PE is normal, and if they do not say he is hypotensive, then don't make him hypotensive! (Therefore, no sepsis) Membranous nephropathy is a chronic nephrotic syndrome and least likely of these causes. Diabetic nephropathy is certainly present (1+ proteinuria), but it is not the cause of his acute renal failure.

How do I know this is acute and not chronic?

Answer: Because –while the creatinine is high, the BUN is higher relative to it

Discussion: A high BUN suggests:

- Dehydration
- relatively acute renal insufficiency issues (since the gut would be able to help get rid of it in time)
- GI bleed – which is not in our differential here.

- His albumin is normal. (this is a function of the kidney, and if chronic would be low)
- His anion gap is normal, and he has normal electrolytes. (CO_2 normal suggests no significant acid-base abnormality)

What are the most common reasons for acute renal failure?

- Sepsis/shock
- Iodinated contrast dye
- Nephrotoxic drugs (tobramycin and gentamycin most commonly)
- ACEI (which can decrease perfusion to an already poorly perfused kidney)
- Ibuprofen, which does the same thing as ACEI
  - Since ibuprofen is what was started lately, this is the most likely cause

Mr. Jones is a 42-year-old diabetic with admittedly poor diabetic control who presents for generalized malaise and fatigue for the past two days associated with a productive cough. He has not been seen in the clinic in "several years".

He has been taking his medications as ordered, including lisinopril, glipizide, metformin, atorvastatin.

His physical examination shows that he is febrile, has bronchial breath sounds in the right base with rhonchi. He appears significantly dehydrated with dry mucous membranes, and poor skin turgor.

- **CBC with WBC 15,000 with 91% segs, 8% lymphs, 1% monos**
  - **H&H shows a marked anemia with Hgb 7 (nl 15-17), HCT 21% (nl 45-51)**
- **CMP with normal LFT's**
  - **S. albumin is very low at 1.8**
  - **K is elevated at 5.4**
  - **CO_2 is 13 (low)**
  - **anion gap of 22**
  - **glucose is 234**
  - **S. creatinine 5.7 (nl .06-1.4) , BUN 29 (nl 6-20)**
- **Urinalysis shows no rbc's, no wbc's, negative nitrite, 4+ protein**
- **IMAGING: CXR shows a consolidation in the right base without pleural effusion**

Of the following, which represents the most likely etiology of his elevated BUN and creatinine?

A. Septic shock
B. Membranous nephropathy
C. Diabetic nephropathy
D. Ibuprofen use
E. ACE induced decreased renal perfusion

Answer: C. Diabetic nephropathy

Discussion: Reread the explanation above – and note the abnormal kidney functions (anemia, hypoalbuminemia, metabolic acidosis, BUN: creatinine ratio). These findings suggest a chronic cause of his renal failure.

Please note that these two questions are almost identical; it is easy to take the same question, and rework it just a little to make it different, so do not be fooled if you see a question that you think is a "repeat". Stop and read it carefully to find the differences.

EVALUATING PROTEINURIA

- Proteinuria is an independent risk factor for chronic kidney disease and progressive atherosclerosis.
- Microalbuminuria is an early and sensitive way to test for dysfunction, and will identify those diabetics and hypertensive patients at risk for renal dysfunction.
  - A urine dip (performed in the clinic on voided urine) is too insensitive to be used to screen for proteinuria in its early stages. Microalbumin is defined as 30-300 mg/day of protein (urine dip is measuring 300 mg/dL not per day). If you use a urine dip to screen, you will miss proteinuria for several years, particularly in a diabetic or hypertensive
  - 24-hour urine is the best way to measure for microalbuminuria, but is cumbersome as discussed; so most often a spot urine is performed instead.
- *Recall DM is #1 and HTN is #2 cause of renal failure
- Protein (and specifically, for this section albumin), is important for many reasons (see Chapter 10 on the importance of albumin).
- The renal tubules have basement membrane pores too small for albumin to fit through (normally) and the basement membrane is negatively charged, as is albumin, which repels it back into the tubule, and therefore returns albumin back to the body.

Pathologic Proteinuria

Patients with pathologic causes of proteinuria will likely be presented in a question as presenting with hematuria and RBC casts (if nephritic syndrome), or with facial edema, hypertension and proteinuria (if nephrotic syndrome).

The most important testing to do is the 24-hour urine collection with measurement of total protein: by definition, nephrotic type proteinuria is defined as > 3.5 gm/day of proteinuria.

24-hour urine samples are difficult to do well; patients forget, do not comply, etc., so a spot urine protein: creatinine ratio can also be performed. In a normal patient, the protein should be low and creatinine should be normal (which is about 1.0 or less). The ratio is quite low at <0.2.

When proteinuria occurs, the protein will increase but creatinine, at least for the time being, will still be about 1 or less, so a protein : creatinine ratio of > 3.5 would be quite high.

Functional Proteinuria

There are functional causes of proteinuria, which can be benign and self-limited, but must be distinguished from the pathologic causes.

How is functional proteinuria (transient loss of protein which resolves without damage to the kidney) and orthostatic proteinuria (where the young tall thin patient loses protein when upright, but then returns to normal when supine) distinguished, then, from a pathologic cause on a test?

***Discussion*:**

- Functional causes would not have protein amounts > 3.5 gm/day (defined as nephrotic-type proteinuria)
- BUN and creatinine are normal in functional causes
- Microscopic urine is normal; without RBC's or casts
- The patient does not have edema, hypertension, in functional causes
- Patients identified as having functional or orthostatic proteinuria should continue to be followed every six months to a year with BP and urinalysis until all returns to normal.

The Electrolyte Panel

Na (Sodium)

- *Sodium is increased = Increase in sodium retention or loss of water*
    - Aldosterone release by the adrenal (hypoperfusion, or perceived hypoperfusion)
    - Dehydration
    - No ADH (diabetes insipidus – see endocrine chapter)

- *Sodium is decreased = loss of sodium by the kidneys or skin or increase in total body water*
    - Syndrome of increased ADH (SIADH)
    - Aldosterone receptor blockers (spironolactone)
    - Adrenal insufficiency (Addison's disease)

K (Potassium)

- *Potassium is increased = decreased ability of kidneys to excrete potassium or potassium is being exchanged for another anion*
    - Renal failure (#1)
    - Hyperglycemia

- Spironolactone & Addison's disease (see decreased sodium above)

- *Potassium is decreased = renal lose due to diuretic therapy, or loss of KCl*
    - Diuretic therapy (furosemide; thiazide)
    - Vomiting/ gastric lavage

Cl (Chloride)

- *Chloride is a negatively charged ion necessary for helping maintain the body's acid-base balance*
    - The kidney primarily controls chloride excretion and secretion in the process of acid-base balance – when bicarbonate is retained, chloride goes out; conversely, if bicarbonate is lost, chloride is retained
    - Therefore, when it goes up or down it is not a "true" change in chloride, but rather a "shifting" from one space to another

CO2/HCO3 (think of the CO2 and HCO3 as being interchangeable on an electrolyte panel)

- *The CO2 on an electrolyte panel is the total CO2 and when dissolved in body water, becomes HCO3 (bicarbonate).*
- *The CO2 discussed in a respiratory acidosis is the pCO2 (which is a weak acid)*
- *Increase in bicarbonate*
    - there are multiple reasons for increased bicarbonate and almost all are "zebras"(milk-alkali syndrome, Bartter's syndrome, etc... so I choose to get these wrong)
- *Decrease in CO2/bicarbonate = loss*
    - HCO3 loss is much more common clinically than excess bicarb
    - diarrhea is #1 cause; produced in the duodenal bulb to neutralize HCl acid

ELECTROLYTE ABNORMALITIES			
ABNORMALITY	**ETIOLOGIES**	**SIGNS & SYMPTOMS**	**CLINICAL INTERVENTION**
HYPONATREMIA Sodium < 135 Ref Ranges: 135 -145 mmol/L	•SIADH •Psychogenic polydipsia •GI fluid loss •Sweating	•AMS •Seizures • ↓ BP • ↑ ICP	•Monitor I & O •Limit fluids/ water •0.9% NS IV •Give Hypertonic IV fluids •Increase levels gradually
HYPERNATREMIA Sodium > 145 Ref Ranges: 135 -145 mmol/L	•Fluid deprivation •Diabetes insipidus	•AMS •Edema •Thirst •Tachycardia	•Monitor I & O •Encourage fluids •Limit sodium •Lower levels gradually •Give hypotonic IV, 1/4 or 1/2 NS solution
HYPOKALEMIA Potassium < 3.4 Ref Ranges: 3.4 - 4.9 mmol/L	•Diuretics •Alcoholism •Nasogastric suctioning •Vomiting •Eating Disorders	•Dysrhythmia •Leg cramps •Anorexia	•Cardiac monitor •Give Oral K+(K-Dur) 20mEq = 0.1↑K •Give IV K+ (dilute & give slowly) •Educate about K+ rich foods •√ Magnesium
HYPERKALEMIA Potassium > 5.0 Ref Ranges: 3.4 - 4.9 mmol/L	•Renal failure •Crush injuries •Potassium sparing diuretics	• ♥ Dysrhythmia • ♥ Arrest • ♥ Irregular pulse • ♥ Elevated T waves • Paresthesias	•Cardiac monitor •Monitor labs/ EKG •Give oral Kayexalate •Calcium Gluconate by IV •D50%+ 10 u. Reg Insulin IV/SQ •1HR continuous Albuterol nebs •Oral or rectal Kayexalate • Dialysis
HYPOCALCEMIA Calcium < 8.9 Ref Ranges: 8.9 - 10.3 mg/dL	•Renal failure • ↓ Vitamin D •Alcoholism •Hypoparathyroidism •Crohn's disease	•Chvostek's sign •Trousseau's sign •Tetany •V-Tach •Seizures •Long QT	•Calcium supplements/ vitamin D •Increase dietary calcium •Weight-bearing exercises
HYPERCALCEMIA Calcium > 10.3 Ref Ranges: 8.9 - 10.3 mg/dL	•Hyperparathyroidism •Malignancy	•Depressed DTR's •Mental status: lethargy, confusion, weakness • ♥ Dysrhythmia •Constipation	•Oral fluids (dilute urine) •Increase fiber •Limit dietary intake •IF NO kidney disease or heart failure- give diuretics & NS *IF THERE IS kidney disease or heart failure- give CALCITONIN
HYPOMAGNESEMIA Magnesium < 1.5 Ref Ranges: 1.2 - 2.2 mg/dL	•Alcoholism •Burns •Pancreatitis	• ↑ DTR's • ↑ HR, BP •Dysrhythmia •Vertigo •Seizures	•Provide safety for seizure risk •Increase dietary intake of Magnesium: whole grains, nuts, chocolate, seafood •MgSO4 4gm P.O or give IV •Monitor DTR's
HYPERMAGNESEMIA Magnesium > 2.5 Ref Ranges: 1.2 - 2.2 mg/dL	•Renal failure •Adrenal insufficiency	• ↓HR, BP •Coma •Lethargy •Muscle weakness	•Monitor vital signs •Monitor LOC •Provide dialysis if the level is critically high

Cardiac Biomarkers

Myoglobin

- *Myoglobin is released from muscle during injury*
    - It is always considered abnormal
    - It is a sensitive marker for muscle injury, but *not specific* to the heart – during an episode of chest pain, could be a sensitive early marker; CK-MB and Troponin are more useful after several hours
    - two hour peak (so earliest potential marker), but so nonspecific, not used much
- *Other causes of increased myoglobin include any kind of muscle damage*
    - Myoglobinuria may indicate rhabdomyolysis, which will then cause acute renal failure (toxic to tubules as the kidney tries to clear it); <treatment is hydration!!>

CK-MB

- *CK (or sometimes CPK) is an enzyme found in most muscle tissues*
    - Most of the CK (also called CPK) is in skeletal muscle , so if you order just CK, you are really "seeing" skeletal muscle damage if the CK-MM (muscle) is being released into the bloodstream
- CK is *fractionated into BB (brain) and MB (cardiac)*
    - CK-BB is not used clinically, only in research
    - CK-MB is used clinically to help distinguish cardiac muscle damage (CK may be elevated or normal, then look at the MB "fraction" in your pull down menu, if it is also elevated, think myocardial infarct)
- *Peak elevation at 10-24 hours with duration of 2-3 days*
- *Massive elevation of CK with a normal MB percentage = rhabdomyolysis*
- *Elevation of CK with a high MB percentage = myocardial infarction*

Troponin

- *Troponin I and T are found in cardiac muscle – much more specific than myoglobin or CK in acute myocardial infarction (AMI).*
    - Rise is slower than other enzymes, after 3-6 hours of myocardial muscle damage
    - But it stays elevated for several days (TropT for 7-10 days, Trop I for 5 days) this is useful, but sometimes not – see example questions below
- *Very sensitive and more specific than other tests, but may need to recheck after 4-6 hours to improve sensitivity (called "serial troponins")*
    - Remember - any cardiac damage can increase Troponin, i.e. myocarditis, pericarditis, recent surgery, recent stent
    - Also, may be increased in severe renal insufficiency
- *Peak elevation at 12-24 hours with duration of 7 days*

(?) **A 58-year-old man presents to the ED with complaint of chest pain that is somewhat pleuritic in nature. He is a smoking, hypertensive, diabetic male with poor glycemic control. EKG shows nonspecific ST-T wave changes. Cardiac enzyme panel is performed:**

CK (38-174 IU/L) **687 IU/L**

CK-MB (24-336 ng/mL) **343 ng/mL**

CK-MB% (< 4.0 ng/mL) **5.4**

Troponin I (0.0-0.15 ng/mL) **0.40 ng/mL**

What is the most likely diagnosis?

Answer: Non-STEMI is the most ikely diagnosis based on the lab values and history.

A 34-year-old female patient presents to the ED with complaint of chest pain which is somewhat pleuritic in nature. She is a healthy young female with no cardiac past medical history. She is on no medications. She has a mild fever (100.6) and has had recent URI. EKG shows nonspecific ST-T wave changes. Cardiac enzyme panel is performed:

CK (38-174 IU/L) **89 IU/L**

CK-MB (24-336 ng/mL) **34 ng/mL**

CK-MB% (< 4.0 ng/mL) **1.2**

Troponin I (0.0-0.15 ng/mL) **<0.02 ng/mL**

What is the most likely diagnosis?

Answer: Costochondritis, pleuritis, etc. are most likely, but less likely an AMI

A 38-year-old construction worker presents to the ED after a ten hour shift of heavy lifting with complaint of chest pain which is somewhat pleuritic in nature. He is a healthy male with no cardiac risk factors; with no history of hypertension, DM, he is a nonsmoker. EKG shows nonspecific ST-T wave changes. Cardiac enzyme panel is performed:

CK (38-174 IU/L) **687 IU/L**

CK-MB (24-336 ng/mL) **89 ng/mL**

CK-MB% (< 4.0 ng/mL) **1.2**

Troponin I (0.0-0.15 ng/mL) **<0.02 ng/mL**

What is the most likely diagnosis?

Answer: Skeletal muscle injury, costochondritis, but not likely an AMI.

A 62-year-old male presents 24 hours after discharge from the heart care unit after an inferior wall myocardial infarction with new onset of chest pain that is somewhat pleuritic in nature. He had cardiac stenting performed 4 days ago; left the hospital feeling well. He has no fever. EKG shows nonspecific ST-T wave changes and Q waves in II, III, and avF. Cardiac enzyme panel is performed:

CK (nl 38-174 IU/L)	**260 IU/L**
CK-MB (24-336 ng/mL)	**240 ng/mL**
CK-MB% (< 4.0 ng/mL)	**9 ng/mL**
Troponin I (0.0-0.15 ng/mL)	**0.7 ng/mL**

What is the most likely diagnosis?

Answer: Non-STEMI. While his numbers are not as striking as the first patient in this question list, it is, nonetheless consistent with MI, or at the very least warrants admission for ruleout.

A 78-year-old patient on dialysis presents to the ED with chest pain which is somewhat pleuritic in nature. He has risk factors for coronary artery disease including diabetes, hypertension, and end stage renal failure. EKG shows nonspecific ST-T wave changes. Cardiac enzyme panel is performed:

CK (nl 38-174 IU/L)	**67 IU/L**
CK-MB (24-336 ng/mL)	**30 ng/mL**
CK-MB% (< 4.0 ng/mL)	**2.0**
Troponin I (0.0-0.15 ng/mL)	**0.40 ng/mL**

What is the most likely diagnosis?

Answer: Renal insufficiency (CK, CK-MB and index are all normal; troponin is mildly elevated due to decreased renal clearance of troponin; however, AMI is always in the differential so this patient may warrant "serial" troponins to make sure it is not rising.

PEARL: ***Remember:*** Both troponin and CK /CK-MB will be elevated in patients with renal failure; especially those on dialysis (maybe due to chronic heart damage from renal failure and also failure of the kidneys to "clear" the enzymes from the body)

LABORATORY EVALUATION OF AUTOIMMUNE DISEASES

These laboratory tests are used in evaluating possible autoimmune diseases and are sensitive but not specific

- So sensitive that elevations may not be significant
- But not specific because, if elevated, you still have no idea why they are elevated
- These tests are most useful when they are negative

ESR (erythrocyte sedimentation rate)

- One hour test of whole blood to see how fast the red cells fall – "rouloux" is the principle, red cells which are in "inflamed" body fluid, fall faster

CRP (C-reactive protein)

- Much better test, but most importantly it is an acute phase reactant – not significantly elevated in a chronic condition

ANA (antinuclear antibody)

- May be positive in normal people (low titers)
- When negative, almost completely rules out SLE (lupus)

These tests are more specific in evaluation for autoimmune diseases:

Rheumatoid Arthritis

- *RF (Rheumatoid Factor)*
    - 80% sensitive and specific for Rheumatoid Arthritis (RA)
- *CCP (Cyclic Citrullinated Peptide Antibody)*
    - 96% sensitive and specific for RA

These tests, while useful to a Rheumatologist in evaluation of autoimmune disease are decidedly not useful to you on a test like this. Assume that if there are multiple autoantibodies listed in the stem of the question, that the patient has an autoimmune disease, so look for one in the list of choices.

- Anti-Rho
- Anti-Jo
- Anti-SSDNA
- Anti-DS-DNA
- ANCA
- Anti-whatever

Remember – Autoimmune diseases are *clinical* diagnoses, lab tests do not completely rule in or rule out any autoimmune disease

---

IMAGING STUDIES

It is important to add a few words about imaging studies here.

There are three things to keep in mind when you select an imaging study:

- *Harm to the patient*
    - Always select the least invasive test, or least radiation when at all possible
- *Cost to the patient*
    - Always select the most cost effective study when at all possible
- *Availability of the modality*
    - If the test you want to do is not there in your list of five choices, remember that not all PAs work in the big city with big city MRI scanners and interventional cardiologists. Some work in rural communities where the patient would have to incur the expense of a plane ride, helicopter or snowmobile to get to the MRI scanner 400 miles away.
    - There was, in fact, a time when we practiced good medicine without all those expensive fancy machines. If your answer is not there, put on your ear muffs, get the dog sleds ready, and pretend you are in remote Alaska and select the "next best" test from your five detractors.

PLAIN FILM RADIOGRAPHY

PEARL: When a CXR pops up on the screen:

- Read the stem of the question first
- Look at your five choices next
- often you will know the answer before looking at the image

Plain Films of the Chest

Have a "method" for reading CXR's – an example of mine:

- *Start with the **trachea and air column***
    - Is it midline? if not, suspect tension pneumothorax

    - Is it "peaked"? if it forms a steeple think acute bacterial tracheitis (or sometimes croup)
- *Then the **heart***
    - Does it fit? (should fit in the hemi thorax)
    - Does it have a normal contour (or look like a balloon)?
    - Is the aortic knob visible?
    - Is it too long and skinny and too vertical (think COPD) due to hyperinflation
- *Then, I look at the **lungs** starting at the apex and going down to the diaphragms*
    - Are the upper airways more aerated?
        - If not, there is a mass, a consolidation, or increased vascular pressure
    - Are the lower airways more perfused? (should be due to gravity)
        - If not, there is increased vascular pressure
- *Then, look at the **diaphragms***
    - Should have very "pointy" costophrenic margins
    - If lateral, make sure you check for that pointy posterior costophrenic sulcus – *this is the most commonly missed place for an effusion*
    - Is the R higher? it should be – liver "pushes it up", on the left the heart "pushes it down"
        - *Elevated hemi diaphragm has several causes*
            - Above the diaphragm - decreased lung volume
                - Atelectasis / collapse
                - Lobectomy / pneumonectomy
                - Pulmonary hypoplasia
            - Diaphragm
                - Phrenic nerve palsy
                - Contralateral CVA : usually MCA distribution
            - Below the diaphragm
                - abdominal tumor
                - subphrenic abscess
                - distended stomach or colon
- Then, look at the **bones**
    - Clavicles
    - Vertebral column
    - Ribs (posterior seen most easily)

PLAIN FILMS OF BONE

- First look at your five choices (it will help you figure out what the heck this is an image of)
- Next, look at the contour of the bone, all the way around looking for a nick, bulge, defect in the cortex, especially pay attention to the articular surfaces in the joint
- Finally, if an elbow, pay attention to lucency (dark area) along the bone that suggests blood; in a kid probably a supracondylar humeral fracture; in an adult, probably a radial head fracture --- often missed, so do not miss it on the test! This is the fat pad sign! See image.
- If you see a little chip of bone "floating" in a joint space, think ligament avulsion.

CT SCAN

CT Abdomen

- Best used to rule out pathology within the GI system
- Best on obese patients
- Used with contrast when possible
    - For tumors
    - For vascular concerns
    - For solid organs
- *Do not* use iodinated contrast if creatinine is elevated
- Oral contrast is used in addition to IV contrast to look at lumen of gut as well

CT Chest

- *Indications*
    - To evaluate a solitary pulmonary nodule
    - To look at mediastinal widening seen on cxr to evaluate the cause
    - To evaluate for pulmonary embolism
    - To evaluate other mediastinal structures in the chest
- *Check creatinine before giving contrast*
    - If looking at vasculature (i.e. Pulmonary embolism), you need IV iodinated contrast
    - V/Q scan will have to be ordered then
- *Great debate exists in the most appropriate imaging for PE in a pregnant woman*
    - Some experts recommend CT with shielding, and some recommend V/Q
    - In all cases, image the legs first with US to see if you identify a DVT
        - If DVT, additional imaging of the lungs is not necessary since the management will be the same (and you will avoid irradiating a fetus)

CT Head

- *Indications:*
    - Best used to look for acute bleeds
        - iIndicated in head trauma in elderly patient on blood thinners
        - Any patient with significant LOC (loss of consciousness)
        - Any head trauma in an "altered" patient (alcohol, cognitive impairment)
        - Will not completely rule out subarachnoid bleed on its own – if high index, needs LP looking for RBC's and xanthochromia
    - Useful in emergent situation for ruling out significant tumors
        - In orthopedics; useful in imaging bony abnormalities (gives better detail on complicated fractures) but will not image cord, ligaments, etc.
    - good for general sinus, orbit or maxillofacial imaging
- *Will not diagnose multiple sclerosis; not best imaging for pituitary (although can be done)*

PEARL:

- ***Caution:***
  - Significant radiation to the head (be judicious in its use in a young person)
  - CT should almost always be avoided in pregnancy, **IODINE IS CATEGORY X** in pregnancy and nursing and *must never be used*
  - avoid overuse of CT in child or young adult to reduce lifetime radiation exposure

General and important information about intravenous iodinated contrast:

IV contrast is required for the following exams:

- All angiography (to evaluate vasculature)
- Chest (malignant lesions, pulmonary embolism)
- All abdominal work that emphasizes liver, pancreas, kidney and/or bladder
- To rule in/rule out an intraabdominal or chest abscess

No IV contrast is required for the following CT exams:

- Renal Stone Study (contrast may obscure the stone since it is white)
- Spine workups including C, T and L-spine
- Extremity work (i.e. ankles, knees, wrists, etc.)

Patients who are in renal failure (and are not on dialysis) must have a creatinine performed (and found to be wnl) before ordering CT with contrast.

What do you do if the patient has a true allergy to iodine?

There are two accepted regimens for prophylactic premedication for iodinated contrast injection. The published literature suggests equivalent efficacy for these protocols:

- 32 milligrams of methylprednisolone given orally 12 hours and 2 hours prior to the
  - administration of intravenous iodinated contrast material
- 50 milligrams of prednisone given orally 13, 7 and 1 hour prior to the administration of
  - intravenous iodinated contrast material plus 50 milligrams of diphenhydramine given PO one hour prior to exam

MRI (GENERAL)

- Best used to look for chronic or subacute bleed in the head
- Best for imaging the spinal cord
- Best for multiple sclerosis; multi infarct dementia; metastatic tumors; other primary tumors; most neurologic etiologies; AV malformations
- Best for joints, knees, shoulders, tendons and ligaments, etc.
- Better imaging for breast cancer; although not "standard screening"
- ACS now recommends women at high risk (>20% lifetime risk) get a mammogram and MRI every year – this is relatively new (USPTSF disagrees with this recommendation)

- No ionizing radiation

<u>When NOT to do an MRI?</u>

- metal in critical soft tissue areas of the body, i.e. metal foreign body in orbit, bullet fragment in brain or chest
- metal clips will cause "scatter" and make image rendered useless
- pacemakers
- patients with claustrophobia (although you can use a benzodiazepine for sedation)
- morbidly obese patients
- those unable to be still, i.e. movement disorders, cognitive impairment, etc.

Most radiologist prefer closed MRI scanners with better resolution, so I would just assume a closed tube MRI is what you are putting your patient into; therefore, hard to get them out of there quickly - do not put a hemodynamically unstable patient into the scanner!

PEARL: in the past, MRI with gadolinium was preferred over CT with iodinated contrast dye in testing patients with renal dysfunction. Now it should ***not*** be used in patients with abnormal creatinine as it can/will cause ***nephrogenic systemic fibrosis***- a debilitating sclerosis of skin over the entire body that is permanent and devastating.

MRA – MR angiography

- Used to look at vasculature
- Frequently done in evaluating peripheral vasculature (thoracic aorta to toes)
- Also done for brain vasculature
- Gives 3-D image and is replacing most invasive angiography (and certainly CT)
- Can be done with or without contrast
- Same contraindications as anyone needing MRI (above)
- Be careful with GFR <30, no gadolinium for fear of causing NSF (see pearl above)

NUCLEAR MEDICINE SCANS (GENERAL)

- *"Hot" does not necessarily mean benign and "cold" mean malignant (like I was taught years ago)*
    - that axiom pretty much only works for thyroid scans
    - in almost all other scans, hot is bad – so instead of memorizing a list, think about what radioisotope is being used, and if it were put into your body, would you want it to light up?
- *Thyroid scan looking for uptake of iodine in a solid tumor*
    - yes, I want it to light up – it means the tissue is behaving "normally"
- *Bone scan looking for metastatic tumors*
    - nope, I do not want spots to light up
- *RBC scan looking for a gastric ulcer perforation*
    - nope, I do not want RBC's to be found outside my gut lumen

- *WBC scan in the foot of a diabetic*
    - nope, again, not good
- *Sestamibi scan (Calcium) –*
    - in a parathyroid tumor, will light up (hot)– not good
    - In a cardiac stress test, normal perfusion will light up the muscle (hot) – that's good!
- *PET scan (glucose)*
    - cancer needs lots of glucose, so lighting up is not good
    - normal tissue uses normal glucose, so no hot spots

Basic Interpretation of ECG's

BASIC TENETS OF INTERPRETING AN ECG:

Vectors and Electrical Conduction

- You are measuring electricity not function (the ECG only tells you in what direction electricity is flowing – it does not tell you if there is blood actually being perfused.)

- The premise of the ECG is that we put leads primarily directed toward the left side of the body, because if your heart is where it belongs, electricity should be flowing that way – to the left.

- However, if we are looking at leads on the right side of the body (AVR and V1, V2) an S wave or negative deflection will be present since the impulse from the left ventricle is traveling away from the leads.

THE ELECTRICAL AXIS

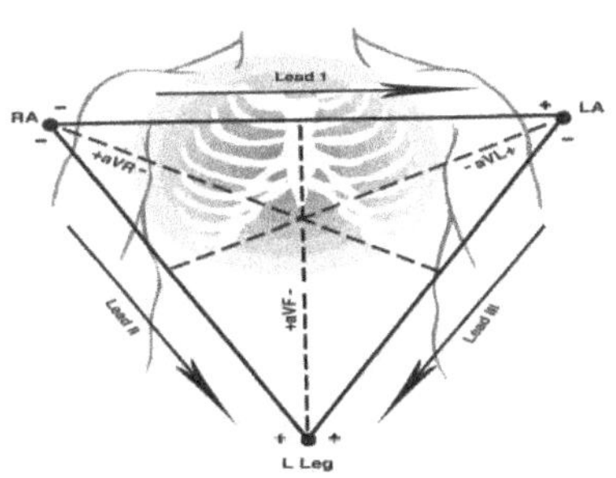

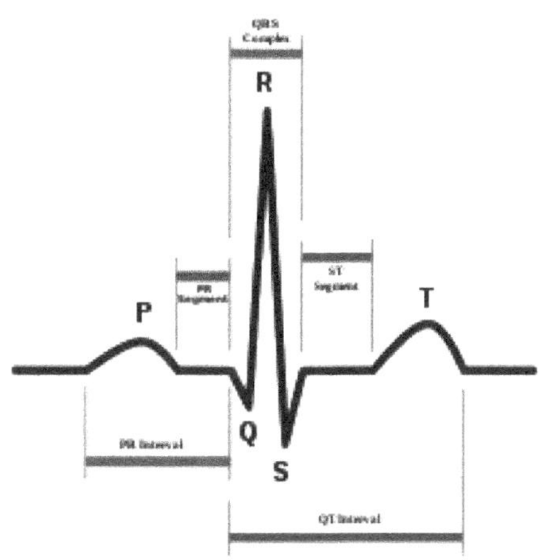

When trying to decide what the axis is (a very not-so-useful task), remember the triangle, which represents where leads are place on the body.

- Lead I measures electrical activity that goes from the right side of the body to the left side (which should be most of it, yes?)
- Lead avF measures electricity going toward the feet (which should be most of it, yes?)

When electricity is going toward an electrode it causes a positive deflection (above the baseline), when moving away, it goes below the baseling.

Normal Axis

- *Lead I should always be positive (electricity going toward the left)*
- *Lead avF should always be positive (electricity going toward the feet).*
- *If those two facts are true, you have a normal axis (probably 90% of all ECG's)*

LAD (left axis deviation)

- *Electricity is going leftward, and a little too far "north"*
    - causing a positive R wave in lead I (electricity going toward the left)
    - but a negative S wave in lead avF (going away from the feet).
- This is the next most common type of axis deviation that occurs.
- The most common reason for LAD is left ventricular hypertrophy (LVH).

RAD (right axis deviation)

- *Electricity is going rightward (very strange)*
    - so there is an S wave in lead I
    - but still heading toward the feet with a resultant R wave in avF.
- *The most common reason for a RAD is right ventricular hypertrophy (RVH).*
    - So, whenever you see it, look for a tall R wave in lead V1 and call it!
- *This is usually due to chronic increase in pulmonary pressures:*
    - COPD
    - Primary pulmonary hypertension
    - Restrictive pulmonary diseases

PEARL: When you see a rightward axis (an S wave in lead I, instead of an R wave), always check lead avR. Make sure that the P wave is "upside down", or that there is an "upside down" T wave. If avR has all positive deflections, either then the patient's heart is on the R side of his body, or the tech accidentally put the leads on the wrong arms. Which is more common?

PEARL: If a patient had a massive pulmonary embolism, would you expect to see RVH?

No. It takes years to develop hypertrophy. A massive PE can, however, dramatically and suddenly increase pulmonary pressures causing a change in electrical vectors. We call this an S1 Q3 T3 pattern (S wave in lead I, Q wave in lead III and inverted T wave in lead III). A zebra, for sure, but occasionally very useful!

THE ELECTRICAL CONDUCTION SYSTEM (in terms of rhythm: SA node, AV node, Bundle of His)

- **The *Sinus Node* is the normal and intrinsic pacemaker of the heart**
  - It fires at 60-100 bpm
  - If it fires, there will be a P wave
- **The electrical impulse leaves the SA node and travels to the *Atrioventricular (AV) node***
  - The time it takes to get there is the PR interval
- **If the sinus node failure to function, the *AV node* will take over**
  - It fires at a rate of 40-60 bpm. Usually, there will not be a P wave if the impulse is originating directly from the AV node
  - If the AV node takes over the rhythm, the rhythm will be regular
- **If the sinus node and AV node are both wiped out, hopefully, the *ventricular myocyte* will fire, and an impulse will occur.**
  - Ventricular myocytes themselves have intrinsic pacemakers
  - There will be no P wave as the impulse is originating below the atria
  - The intrinsic ventricular response rate is 20-40 bpm.
  - If the ventricle becomes the new pacemaker, the rhythm will be regular
- **The Bundle of His is there to make electricity coming to it travel rapidly through the conduction systems of both ventricles, and almost simultaneously depolarize both ventricles**
  - If this happens as it should, the QRS will be narrow and a single upright impulse (R wave) will be present in leads I and II, and the left sided precordial leads (V4, V5, and V6 illustrating electricity traveling leftward down the bundle.
  - If the impulse travels normally down the bundle of HIS, the duration of the QRS will be short, and the QRS will be a narrow complex
    - *this is measured on the horizontal axis, and should be <0.10 sec or two and a half teeny boxes.*
- **If there is a bundle branch block (BBB), or if the impulse originates somewhere within the ventricle and conduction is not normal down the bundle of HIS, it will take longer to depolarize the ventricles and the QRS duration will be >0.12 (three teeny boxes)**

What distinguishes an atrial fibrillation rhythm and an AV nodal rhythm? (Both would have no P waves, both would have normal narrow QRS complexes, so both of these rhythms will look very similar)

Answer: AV nodal rhythm will be regular; atrial fibrillation will be irregularly irregular

What distinguishes an idioventricular rhythm from a bundle branch block (BBB)? (Both have wide QRS complexes since ventricular depolarization is abnormal; both are regular rhythms.)

Answer: Idioventricular rhythms have no P waves (the atria aren't doing anything); BBB's will have P waves since the rhythm originates in the SA node, goes through the AV node, but then gets blocked in the bundle.

NORMAL SINUS RHYTHM

<u>If the rhythm originates in the SA node and is normal:</u>

- *There will be a P wave*
- *All P waves in the rhythm strip will look the same*
  - Come from the same spot in the atria
- *It will be upright in leads I, and II*
  - In the direction of flow from SA to AV node in the heart
- *There will be a QRS after every P*
  - conduction made it through the AV node like it should
- *The PR interval will be normal*
  - Conduction from the SA to AV node is normal & quick
  - Less than one large box (< 0.20 sec or 200 msec)
- ***Remember –***
  - If a normal P wave is present, the atrium has depolarized and SA nodal conduction is normal
  - If the PR interval is normal, it suggests that the SA to AV nodal conduction is normal
  - If the P is present, but PR interval is long, there is slowing at the AVN (more later)
  - This has nothing whatsoever to do with the QRS (more about the QRS later)

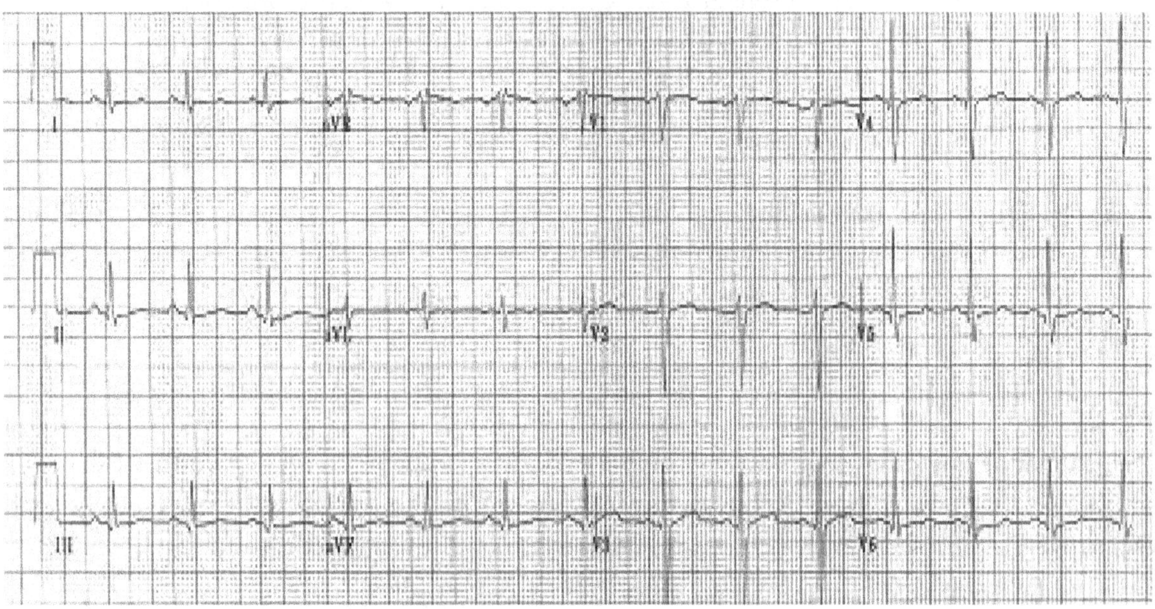

Normal sinus rhythm on a 12-lead ECG

THE *RATE* OF THE HEART

Each pacemaker in the heart has its own intrinsic rate (normal for that pacemaker):

- Sinus (SA) node = 60-100 bpm
- AV/junctional node = 40-60 bpm
- Ventricular myocyte = 20-40 bpm

PEARL: It is important to realize that if this really was what happened, and your SA and AV node were not working, and your ventricle took over as the pacemaker at 30 bpm, you would not be perfusing your brain very well. The body can try to fix that poor cardiac output by increasing the heart rate (the sympathetic nervous system through beta adrenergic activity will do this for you), and you will, hopefully, develop an "accelerated" idioventricular rhythm, or even, perhaps, a ventricular tachycardia. Recall the formula here: (cardiac output = stroke volume x heart rate)

Which patient has the "sicker" heart?

A. The one with the rate of 30 in an idioventricular rhythm? Or,

B. The one with an accelerated idioventricular rhythm?

Answer: The slower one, because his body is not helping him maintain his cardiac output.

THE "NORMAL" RHYTHMS OF THE HEART

NSR (normal sinus rhythm) 60-100 bpm

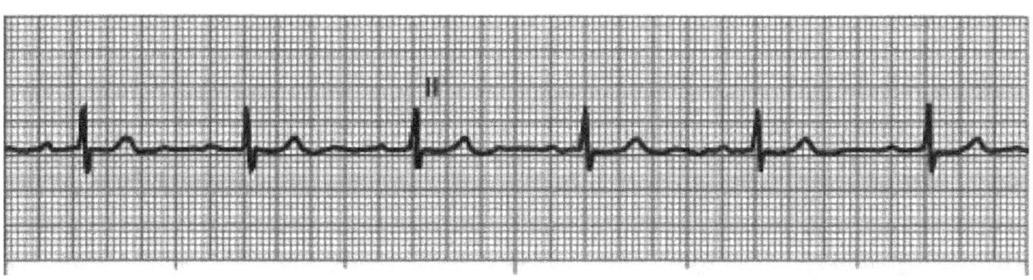

Sinus tachycardia >100 bpm

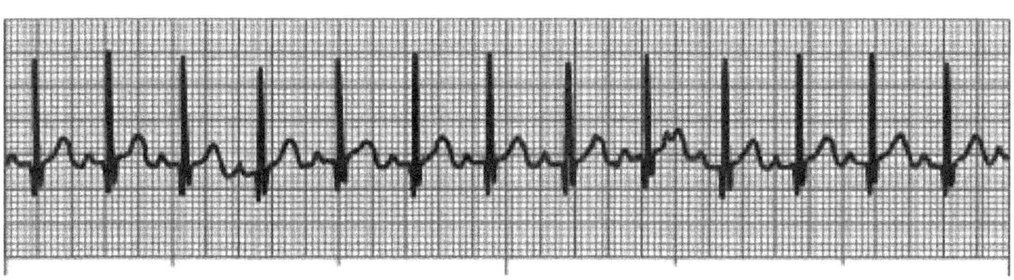

Sinus bradycardia < 60 bpm

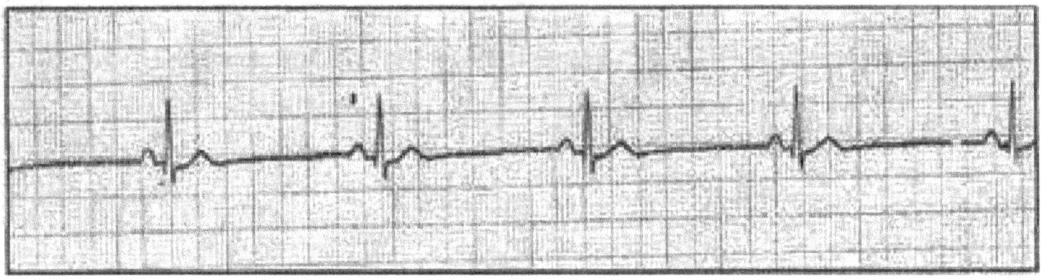

THE *"OTHER"* RYTHMS OF THE HEART

AV Nodal Rhythm (Junctional Rhythm)

- If the SA node is no longer functioning, the AV node (or junction) will take over:
- If the rhythm is regular, but there is no P wave, it is either a junctional or ventricular rhythm
- Look at the QRS complex --- is it narrow?
    - *Then the rhythm is "supra" ventricular and going down the Bundle of His normally*
        - if the rhythm is regular, you likely have a junctional (AV nodal) rhythm
        - if the rhythm is irregularly irregular, you likely have atrial fibrillation
        - there are multiple other reasons, but these are most likely

Ventricular Rhythm (Idioventricular Rhythm)

- If both the SA and AV node are no longer functioning, the ventricle will take over:
- If the rhythm is regular & there is no P wave, look at the QRS complex - is it wide? (> .12 sec)
    - *Then select idioventricular (or ventricular) rhythm*
        - Or accelerated ventricular rhythm (if HR> 40 but less than 100)
        - Or ventricular tachycardia (if HR > 100)

Junctional rhythm (Nodal Rhythm)

- AV node becomes the pacemaker
- Regular rhythm
- 40-60 bpm
- No P waves (or retrograde)
- QRS is narrow

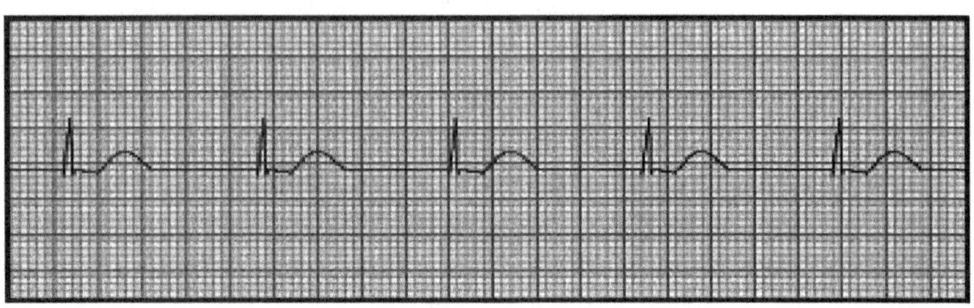

Why do you think a nodal rhythm (no P wave, normal regular narrow QRS) is usually faster than 40-60?

Answer: Humans do not perfuse their brains very well at 40 bpm. The beta adrenergic system will speeds things up if the brain is not well perfused. We call that an "accelerated" nodal rhythm.

Accelerated Junctional (Nodal) Rhythm

- Due to sympathetic tone, HR is "accelerated"
- HR 60-100 bpm
- Provides better cardiac output (CO = SV xHR)

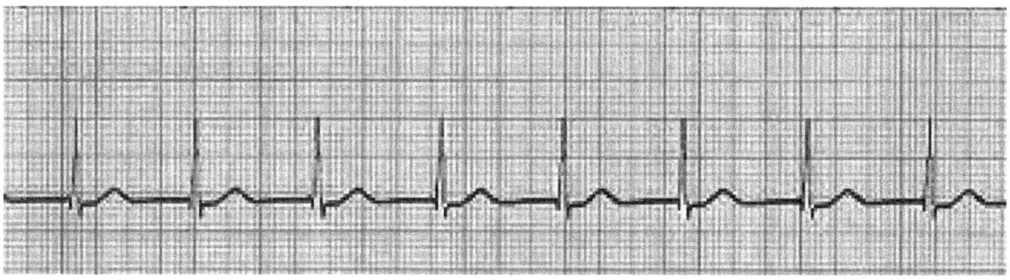

Junctional Tachycardia

- Same as accelerated, but even a little faster
- HR > 100 bpm
- Recall that it doesn't get driven as fast as SVT, i.e., if > 180 without P waves, call it SVT!

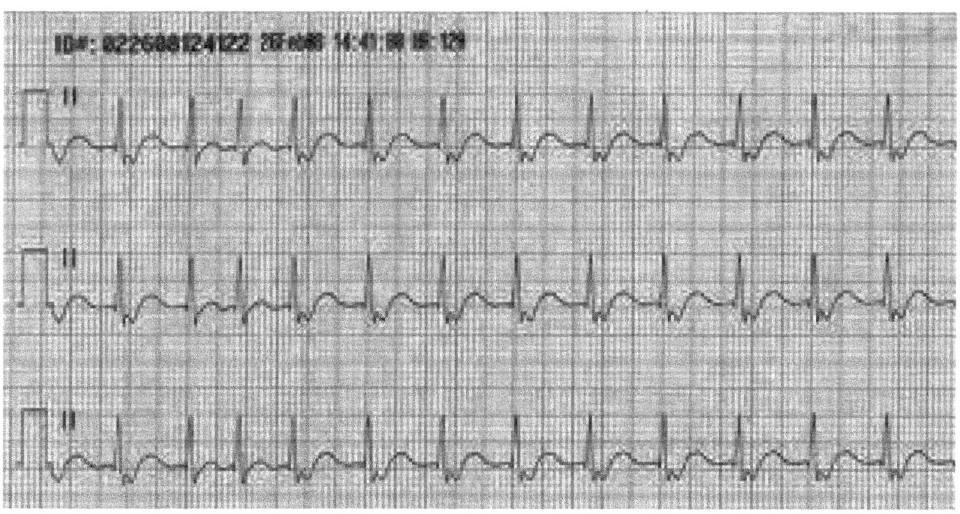

VENTRICULAR RHYTHMS

Idioventricular Rhythm

- Ventricular myocyte takes over as pacer for the heart
- Regular rhythm
- Rate 20-40 BPM
- No P waves (impulse originates in ventricle)
- QRS is wide (travels "backward" through the bundle)

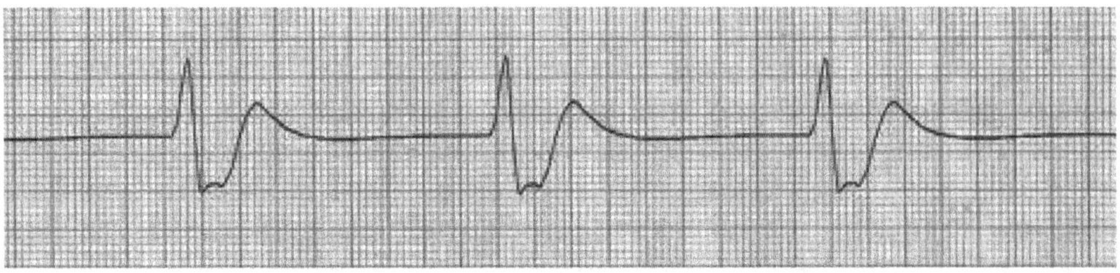

PEARL: So, what do you think you call an idioventricular rhythm in which the Beta-adrenergic system has been stimulated due to low cardiac output, and the rate is now 60-100 bpm?

Answer: An *accelerated* idioventricular rhythm

Accelerated Idioventricular Rhythm

- Regular rhythm
- Rate 40-100 bpm
- No P waves
- QRS is wide

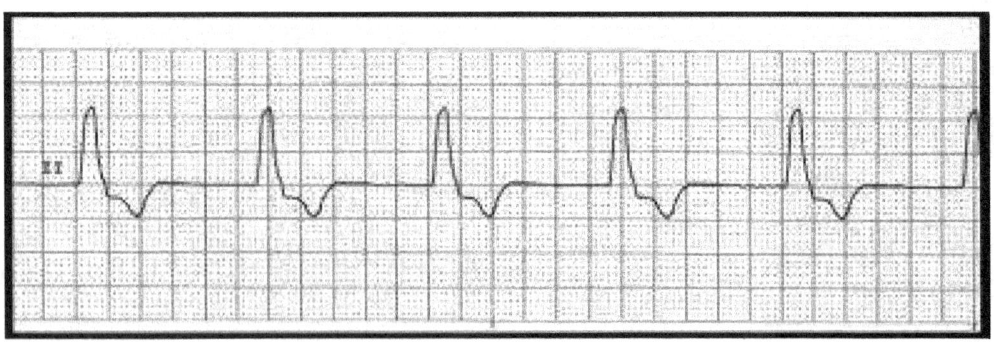

Ventricular Tachycardia

- Regular rhythm
- Rate >100 bpm
- No P waves
- QRS is wide

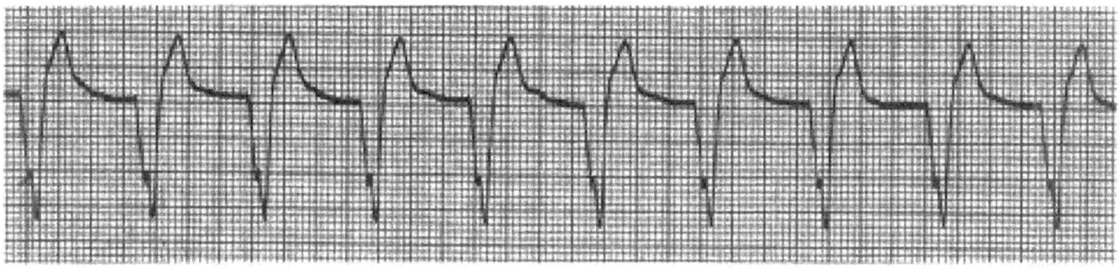

THE P WAVE (AND RHYTHM)

FAST REGULAR RHYTHMS (From the atrium, or "supraventricular")

Sinus Tachycardia – Typically 100- 140 bpm (rarely above 140 bpm)

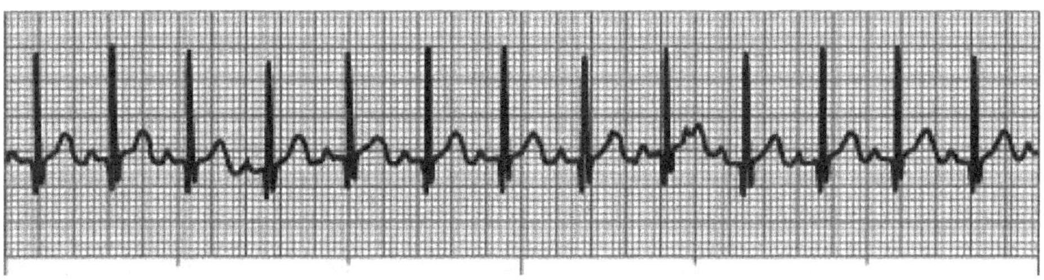

Atrial Flutter

- 300 is the "typical" atrial rate
- 2:1 @ exactly 150 bpm -- P waves not visible
- 3:1 @ 100 bpm – flutter waves (sawtooth P waves) are now visible
- 4:1 @ 75 bpm – flutter waves easily seen

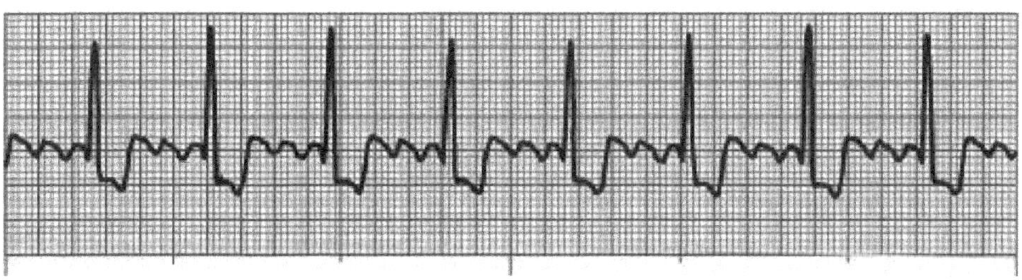

Supraventricular Tachycardia

Very fast! - Narrow – regular, typically > 180 bpm

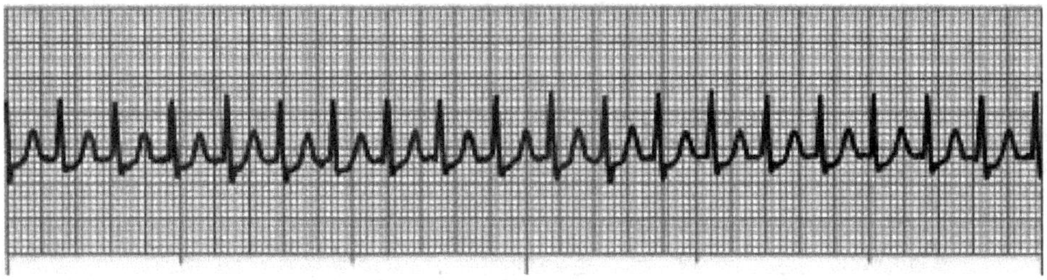

What kinds of things can cause tachycardic supraventricular rhythms?

Answer:

- Fever
- Anemia/hypovolemia
- Anxiety/Panic
- Pulmonary embolism
- Amphetamines/stimulants
- Alcohol withdrawal/opiate withdrawal

IRREGULAR RHYTHMS

Sinus Arrhythmia

- *Etiology*
  - Usually in young healthy patients
- *ECG findings*
  - **Regularly irregular** rhythm
  - Always a P followed by a QRS
  - Rate increases with inhalation, and decreases with exhalation
- *Reassurance – no intervention needed*

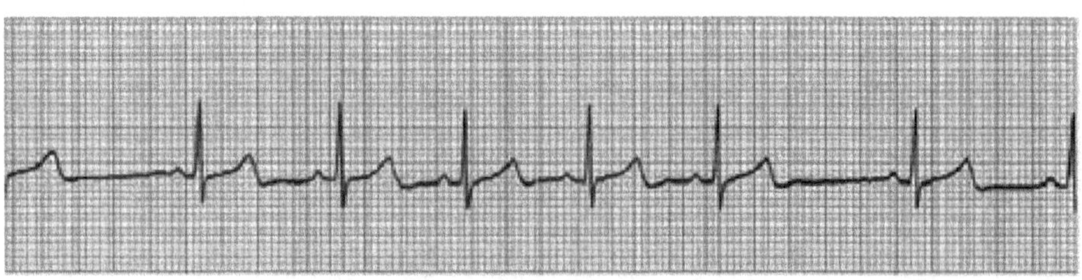

Atrial fibrillation

- *Etiologies*
  - Most common sustained arrhythmia
  - Structural heart problem
  - Ischemic heart problem
  - Elderly
  - Grave's disease – if patient is young and female
- *ECG findings*
  - **Irregularly irregular** rhythm
  - Narrow QRS

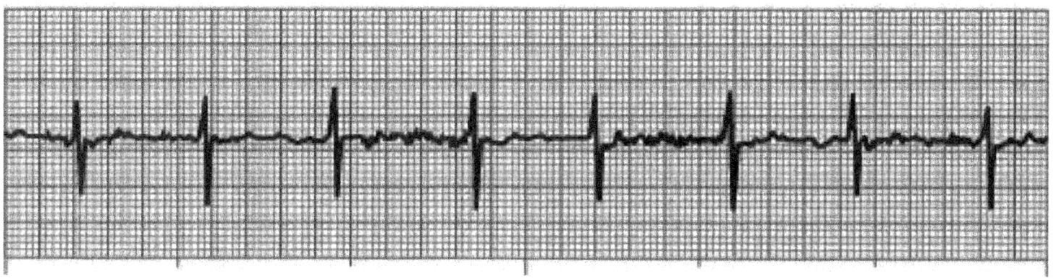

with normal ventricular response rate (8 complexes/strip = 80 bpm)

Multifocal atrial tachycardia

- *Etiology*
  - Occurs in an atrium which is hypoxic or has increased atrial pressure
  - I.e., most common in COPD
  - Occurs from theophylline (which few patients are taking)
- ECG findings
  - P's are present
    - By definition, *three* abnormal P waves are necessary for the diagnosis

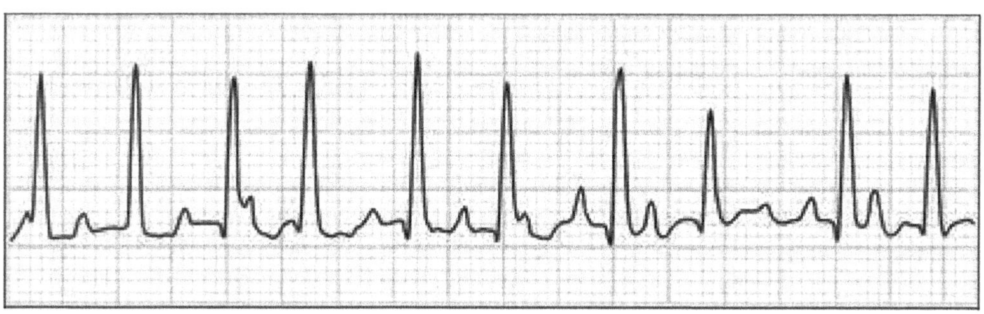

AV NODAL BLOCKS

- *Etiologies*
  - Conduction abnormality through the AV node
    - Medications
    - Lyme disease
- *All of these drugs slow conduction at the AV node; and may, in fact, be the cause of the blockade, but you certainly would not want to give someone with an AV block one of them!*
  - Beta blockers
  - Calcium channel blockers (verapamil and diltiazem)
  - Digoxin (digitalis)
  - Lyme disease
- *In general, who needs a pacemaker?*
  - Second degree Mobitz II AV block
  - Third degree AV block
  - Others who are symptomatic/hemodynamically unstable

PEARL: AV blocks will usually present on a rhythm strip, do things in this order and they will be easy:

- Look to be sure that every P wave is followed by a QRS
- *If it is,* then find a QRS that is on a dark line, and see if the P wave in front of it fits nicely in the big box in front of the QRS (that big box measures 0.20 sec)
- *If not,* call it first degree AVB
- If a P wave does not make it through the AV node, there will be no QRS, and instead another P wave
  - This is either second degree Mobitz I, second degree Mobitz II, or third degree block
- **Mobitz II and Third degree AVB need pacemakers!!**
- So, rule out Mobitz II first!
  - Patient needs a pacer, and it is the easiest one to r/o first
  - Find some PR intervals that exist on the strip, and see if they are all the same
    - If they are, it's a Mobitz II!
  - Now let's say they are not:
    - Then look to see if they are getting longer, longer, longest and then P dropped
    - Then it is a Mobitz I (Wenckebach), and likely needs no intervention
  - If there are QRS's "missing" or P's following P's and the above two criteria are not met:
    - I.e. PR intervals are not all the same (Mobitz II)
    - I.e. PR intervals are not getting longer, then dropped P (Mobitz I)
    - Call it a third degree AVB and get the patient a pacemaker!

First Degree AV block

- Looks exactly like NSR
- P for every QRS
- But ---PR > 0.20 sec

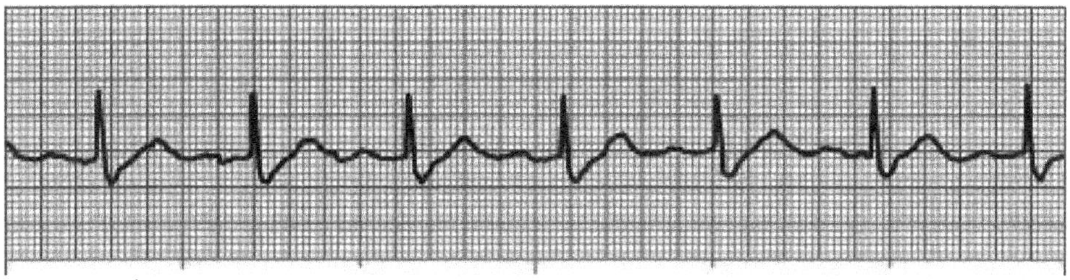

Look at 5th QRS complex – does the P wave fit nicely in the big box in front of it? No!

Second Degree – Mobitz II

Note a P with no QRS after, check the PR interval
If every PR interval is the same, Mobitz 2

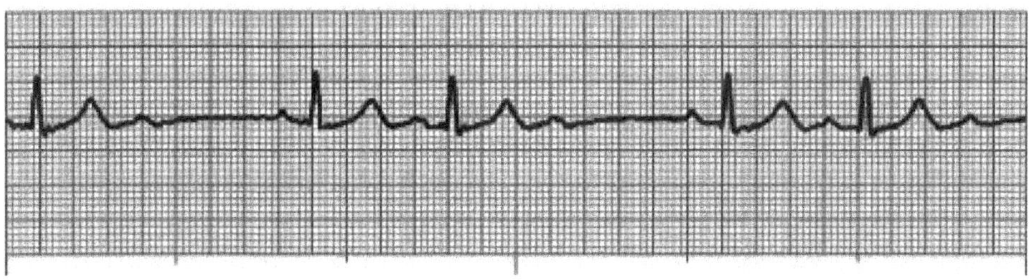

Second degree – Mobitz I, Wenckebach
Longer, longer, longest, ……dropped QRS

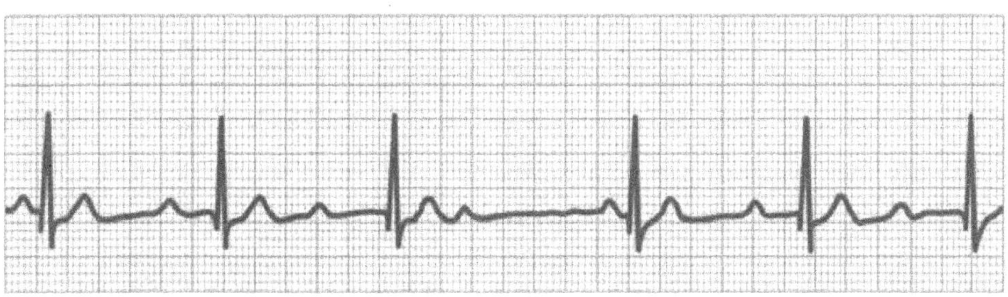

3rd Degree AV block

- P followed by P, no pattern to PR intervals ----
  {pacemaker needed}
- This one is very difficult without calipers, so use the two rules above for Mobitz second degree blocks, and if not either one of those, then pick this one!

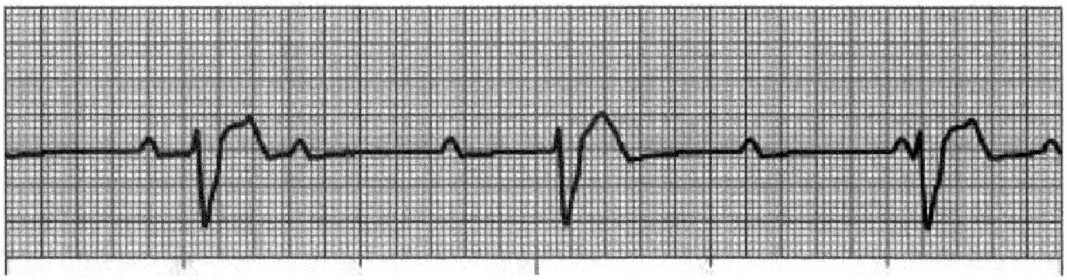

"SHORT PR INTERVAL"

- *Delta waves = WPW syndrome (Wolff-Parkinson-White)*
- Due to an accessory bundle (congenital)
  - Called the Bundle of Kent
  - It is situated closer to the AV node than the SA node is
  - This can cause pre-excitation (or early depolarization of the ventricle)
- Patient is predisposed to SVT
- *Do not use Diltiazem – can precipitate VT!!*

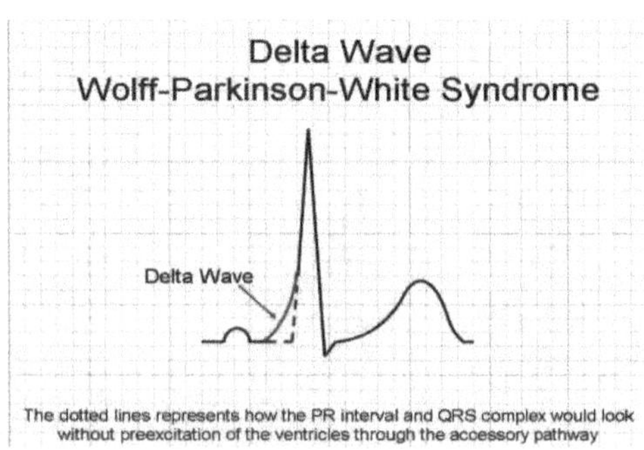

The QRS

__Wide QRS- Recognize these!__

V Tach

- No P waves
- QRS duration > 0.12 sec
- Fast rate
- Visible complexes (patient may or may not have a pulse)

See image next page (and compare it to the BBB illustrated!)

The patient with ventricular tachycardia (and other tachyarrhythmias) may have a pulse, may not have a pulse or may have "pulse deficit"; i.e. Apical pulse 180, radial pulse 60, why?

Answer: The radial pulse is just how much blood is in the wrist that you can feel with your finger, yes? If there is decent filling of the ventricle only every third contraction, you may not feel a pulse with every beat

Where is the best place to evaluate the pulse on a patient during the physical exam?

Answer: Either the apical pulse with stethoscope or the carotid pulse with palpation

PEARL: Treat the patient not the rhythm (pay attention to the vital signs and description of the patient's status)

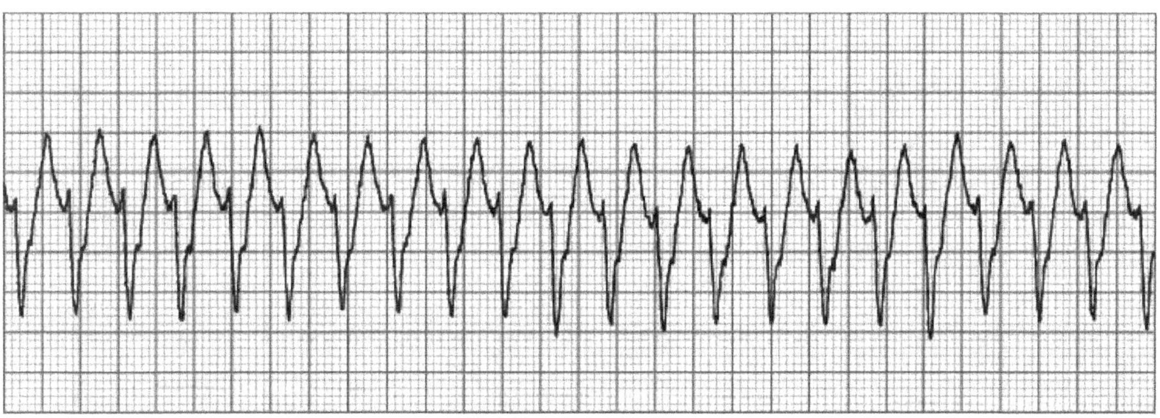

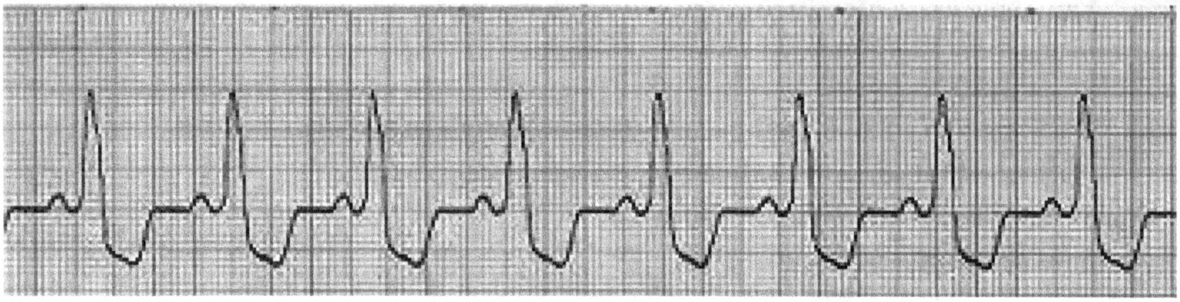

What distinguishes Ventricular Tachycardia from a tachycardic Bundle Branch block?

Answer: P waves!

Discussion: Recall that both will have wide and bizarre QRS's, since they are conducting "backwards" from the ventricle through the bundle.)

It would be quite rude to DC cardiovert Mr. Jones who is sitting up watching TV because you thought he was in V tach, and in fact, there were P waves in front of each wide and bizarre QRS --- it was just a BBB!

What is it called when a patient is in V Tach, and the apical (and carotid) pulse is 180, but the radial pulse is only 60 (because not enough blood gets pumped in a single ineffective contraction of V tach to make it palpable to you at the radius?

Answer: Pulse deficit

V FIB

- No pulse
- Defibrillate STAT

PEARL: If the test question states that the patient is alert, check the gains and the leads, do not defibrillate

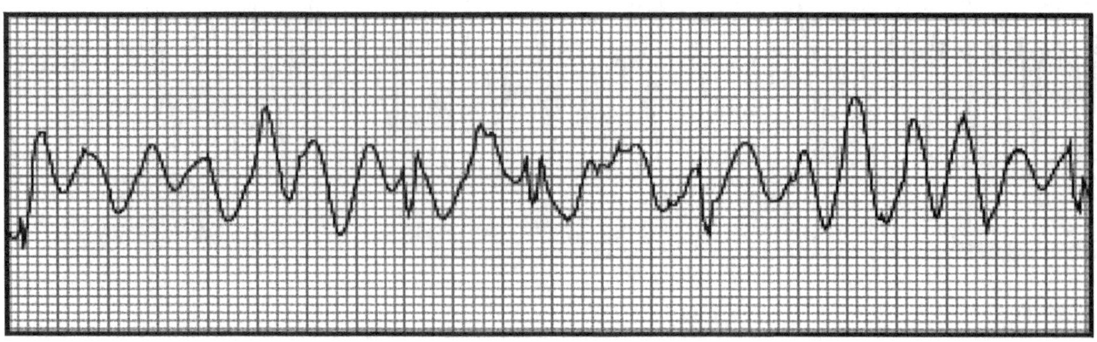

BUNDLE BRANCH BLOCKS

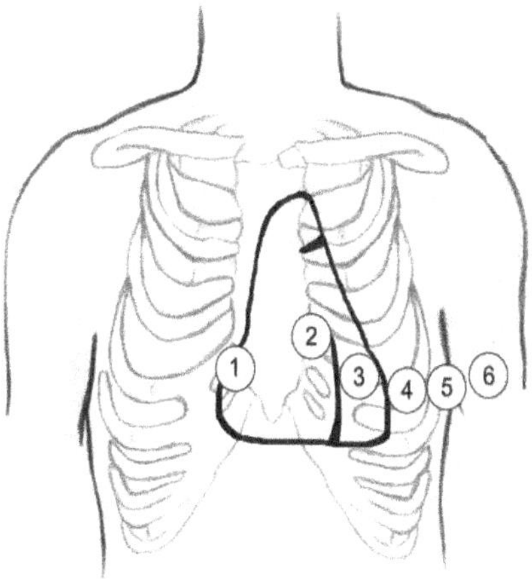

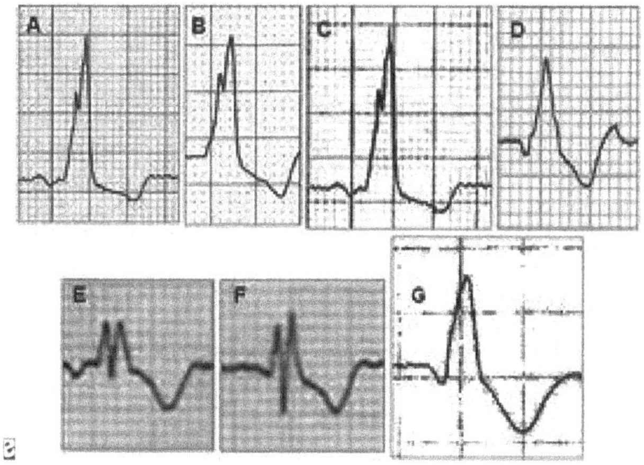

PEARL: Because they kind of look like rabbit ears, the rule is "rabbit ears in right leads = RBBB, and rabbit ears in left leads = LBBB" – the right sided precordial leads are V1 & V2 (on the right side of the chest) and the left sided precordial leads are V5 & V6.

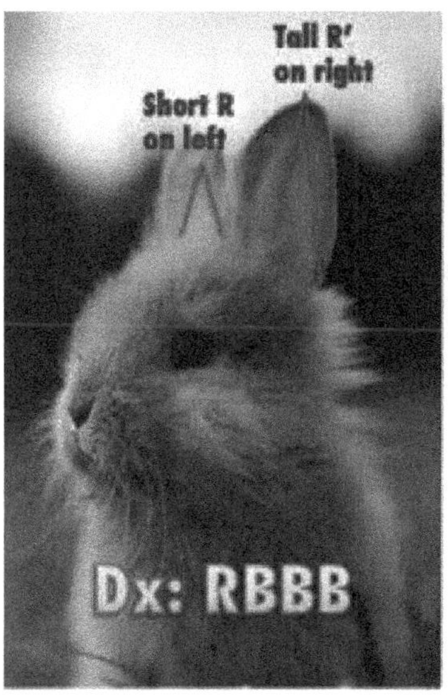

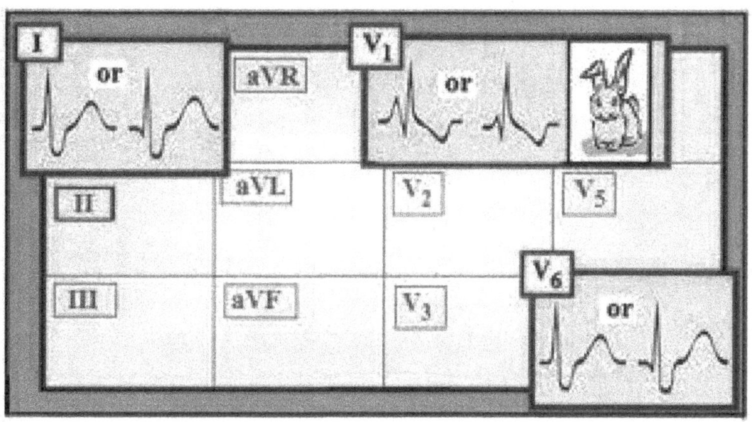

Left Bundle Branch Block

- Is an acute myocardial infarction (AMI) in a patient with chest pain until proven otherwise
- "Rabbit ears" are present in the left precordial leads
    - V5 & V6

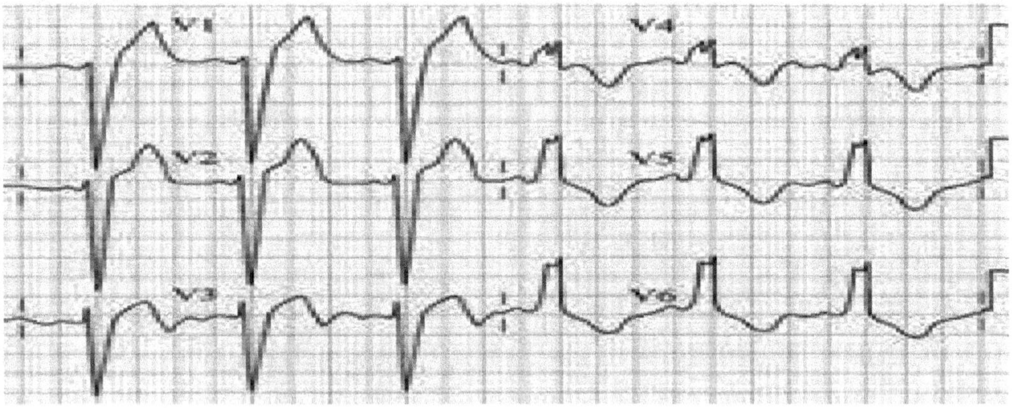

PEARL: A *new* left bundle branch block (LBBB) should always raise the suspicion for a myocardial infarction!

Right Bundle Branch Block

- Mainly self-limited, can be "normal variant"
- "Rabbit ears" in right precordial leads
    - V1 & V2

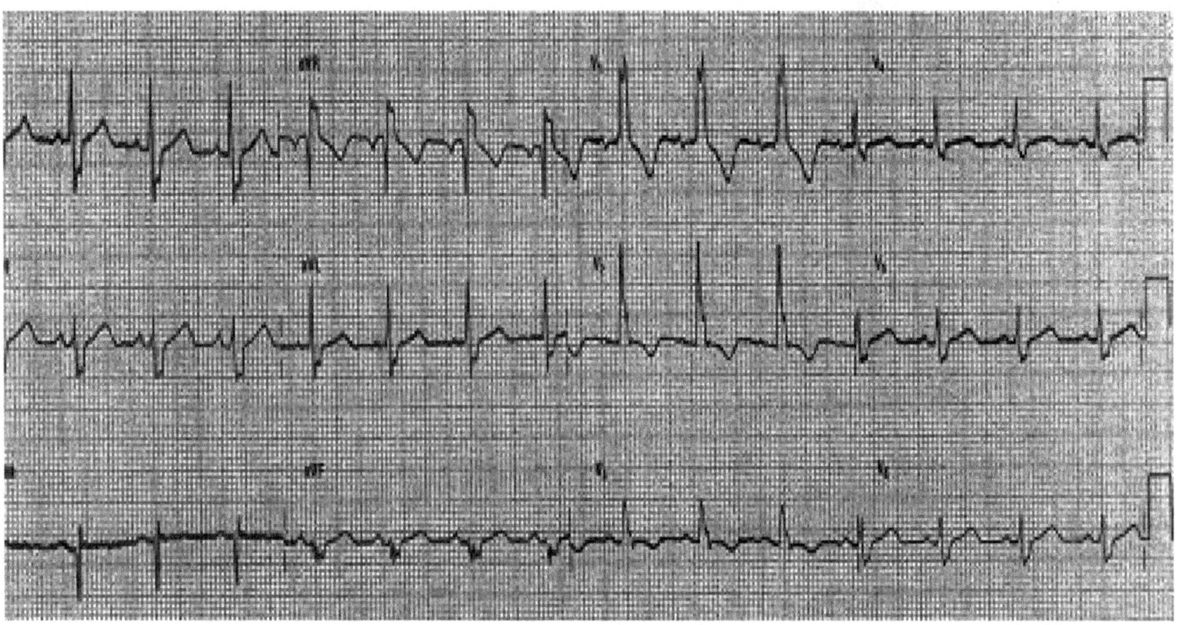

THE ST SEGMENT

Various change in the ST segment

- *Depression* = ischemia
    - Seen most commonly during an abnormal ECG stress test

- *Elevation* = injury = STEMI
    - Seen during acute infarct
    - This will result in a Q wave as well

- *Nonspecific* = nonspecific = NSTEMI
    - Hyperacute T's
    - T wave inversion
    - Flattening of the T waves

PEARL: The coronary arteries:

The left main comes off the aortic root on the left and is responsible for providing oxygenated blood to the entire anterior wall, the high lateral wall and most of the septum. Therefore, the left main bifurcates into other vessels: the septal branch, the circumflex branch (high lateral wall) and the LAD (left anterior descending). If you had to lose a coronary artery, you don't want it to be THIS one!

- The right coronary artery (RCA) comes off the aortic root on the right side and can be small or "dominant". It can feed just the right ventricle and inferior wall of the left ventricle, or can go all the way around the posterior wall of the heart and feed the posterior wall and low lateral wall as it wraps around the heart.
- The RCA supplies the AV node and SA node in about 85% and 65% of patients, respectively.
- The inferior wall of the heart lies just on top of the diaphragm.
- The vagal nerve and phrenic nerve run near the inferior wall, and are often "stimulated" during an inferior wall infarct.

Using this information, tell me what symptoms you might expect from a patient who presents with chest discomfort if his ECG shows ST elevation in leads II, III, and avF (which is a RCA occlusion effecting the inferior wall of the LV)?

Answer: The patient could have any of the following: hiccups (phrenic nerve), bradycardia, hypotension, nausea, diaphoresis (vagal nerve), AV blocks or SA nodal dysfunction

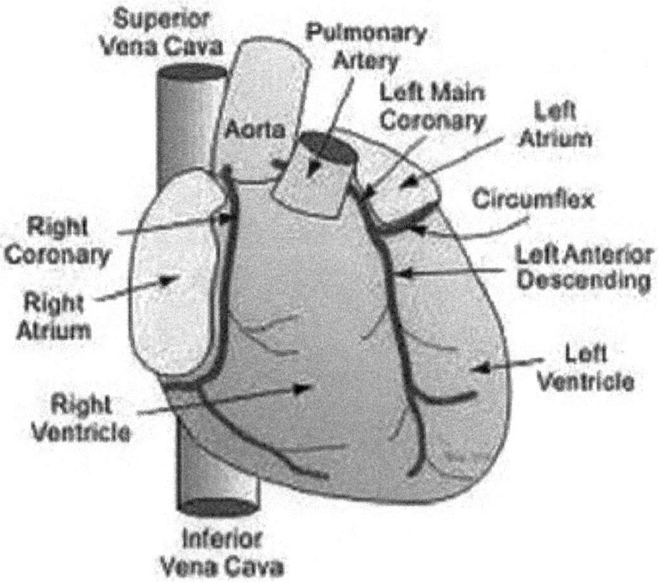

ECG correlation with MI

- ST elevation in the corresponding leads below suggest injury or infarct in the corresponding coronary artery (STEMI)
- Often, during a STEMI, Q waves are already forming. Recall (and this is discuss below), Q waves will remain after the ST elevation has resolved and be your "clue" that the patient has had an infarct (though it will not tell you *when*).
- In Non-STEMI, there will be ST and T wave changes in the same corresponding leads
- Reciprocal ST depression in the opposite wall leads increases S & S to almost 95%!
    - The inferior wall (II, III, avF) is reciprocal to the high lateral wall (I, avL)
    - The anterior wall is reciprocal to the posterior wall
    - Do not be fooled and call the reciprocal ST depression the site of the infarct.
    - ST ELEVATION denotes the infarct leads; reciprocal depression in the opposite wall leads just "nails" the diagnosis!
    - ST depression is what we look for when walking a patient on the treadmill trying to identify ISCHEMIA. Don't get them mixed up!

PEARL: These are the leads to look in to identify where the infarct is occurring.

MEMORIZE THESE:

Inferior wall MI (RCA occlusion)
- II, III, aVF

Left main occlusion
- I, avL, V1-V6 (everything BUT II, III, and avF!)

Septal wall (branch off the LAD)
- V1, +/- V2

Anterior wall MI (LAD occlusion)
- V2, V3, V4

Lateral wall (circumflex branch, but can be RCA as well)
- I, avL (+/- V5, V6)
    - A faculty member taught us to remember "**L**ateral **I**nfarct" as ST elevation in **L** and **I** (i.e. avL and lead I

Use the information above to identify the acute infarct in each of the following 12-lead ECG's:

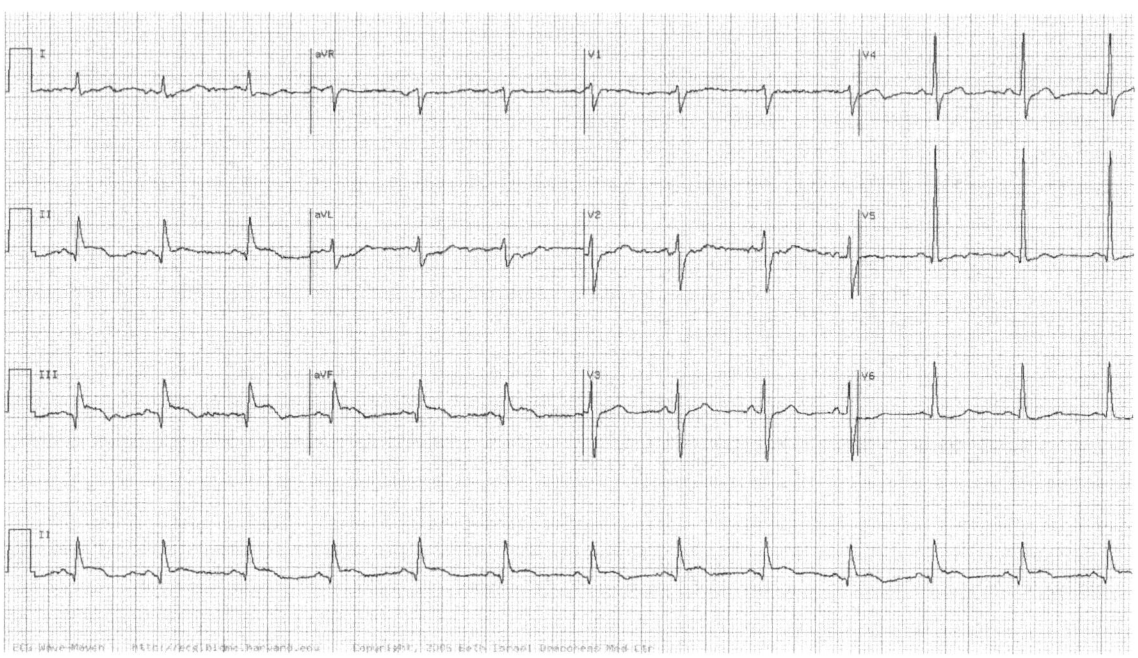

Acute Inferior wall MI

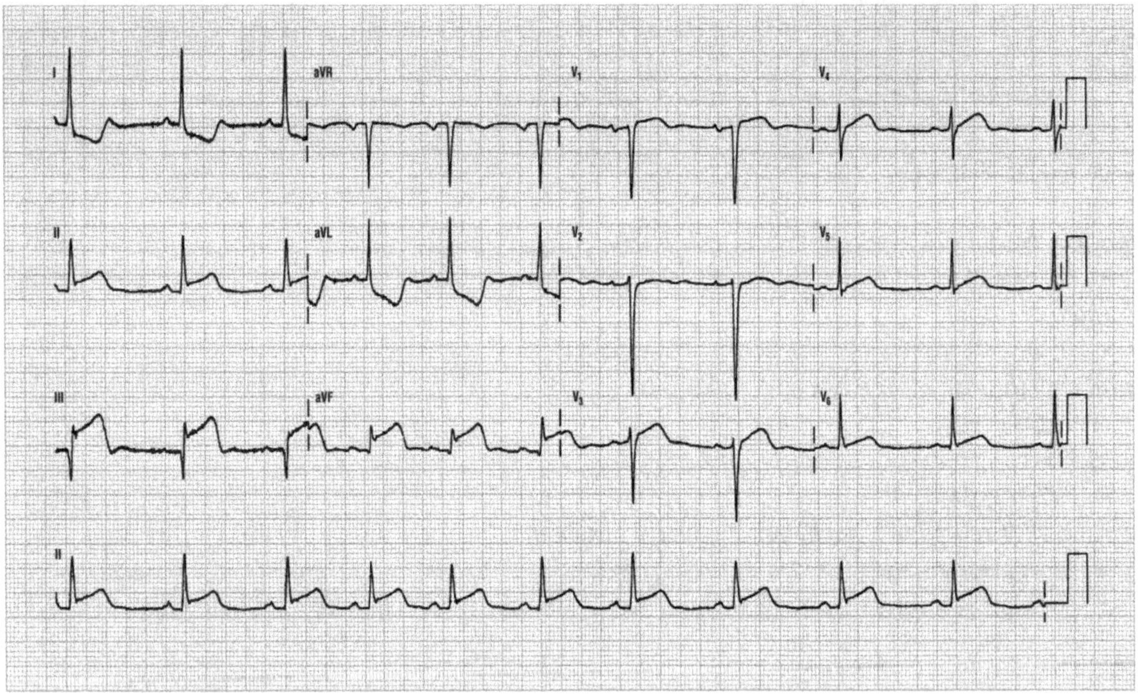

Acute Inferior Wall MI with reciprocal changes in leads I & avL

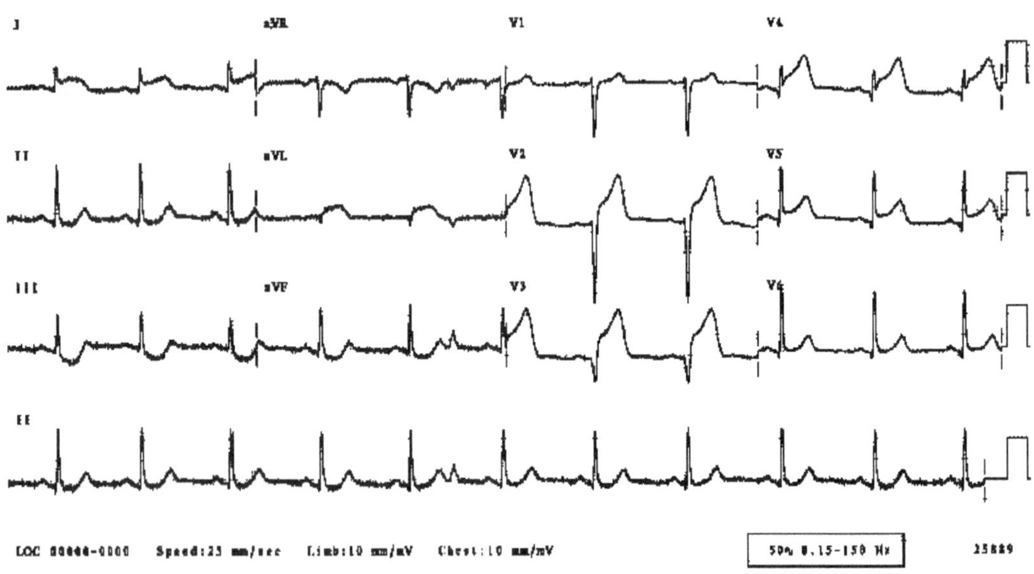

Acute anterolateral wall infarct with reciprocal changes in leads II, III, and avF

Q WAVES

- **"Physiologic Q's"**
    - Represent depolarization of the septum
    - Normal Lead I, II if very tiny and narrow
- **"Pathologic Q's"**
    - In same corresponding leads as ST elevation for AMI
    - Only occur following STEMI (no Q waves in a Non-STEMI infarct)
    - Greater than one small box wide
    - Greater than 1/3 the height of the R wave
    - Indicates *old infarct* (necrotic tissue)

PEARL: now go back to the infarct ECG's above and find the Q waves that are developing. Eventually, the ST elevation (tombstones) will go away, and the Q waves will persist to mark the old infarction for us! (in the anterolateral wall MI there are deep Q waves in V2,3,4, and a smaller one in V5. In the inferior wall MI scan there are Q waves developing in lead III). These Q waves will persist after the tombstones "resolve". They signify an "old" (but no one can tell how old) MI.

Long QT Interval

- *Defined as QT longer than 0.5 second (500 ms)*
    - Congenital (Brugada syndrome)
    - Acquired (most common)
        - Secondary to medications-
            - Procainamide/quinidine
            - Erythromycin/azithromycin/clarithromycin
            - Droperidol
            - Ketocanazole (and other antifungals)
            - Epileptic drugs
            - Antidepressants-MAOI
        - Secondary to seizures and CNS abnormalities
        - Secondary to electrolyte abnormalities
- *Complication of long QT interval*
    - Torsades de Pointes
    - Results in sudden cardiac death
- *Treat with magnesium (MgSO4, 2 – 4 gm. IV), not cardioversion!*

Torsades de Pointes ECG:

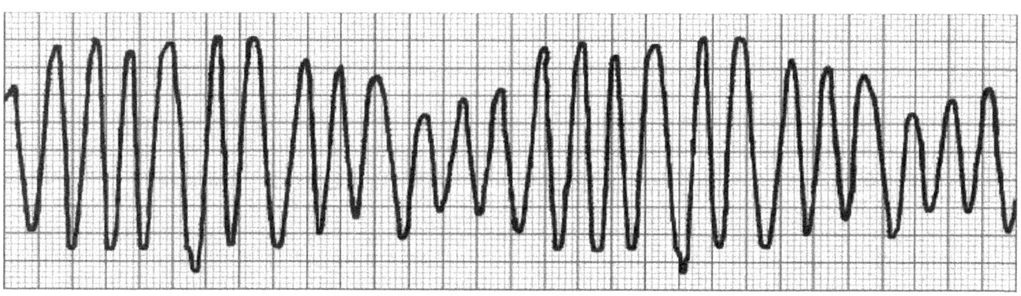

VOLTAGE

LVH – Left Ventricular Hypertrophy

- There are multiple "criteria" for the suggestion on an ECG that voltage is too hig
    - *There is no good reason to memorize all these criteria, as it does not make the diagnosis*
    - *Measure the voltage in the deepest S wave and add to the voltage in the tallest R wave in the precordial leads; >35 mm = suggestion of LVH*
    - *In the example below, V2 has a voltage of 23 below the baseline, and V5 has a volt age of about 23 - that equals 46 which suggests LVH.*
    - *For those who want an 800 on the exam (get a life!), note the "biphasic" P wave in lead V1, this suggests left atrial enlargement (LAE), often seen with LVH*
- The paper of the ECG is designed so that all complexes should fit nicely within each of their receptive areas, i.e. all the QRS's in lead I should fit nicely in that space, should not run off the ECG paper or run into the lead II QRS's below it. If this happens, it suggests too high a voltage.
- If there are instances where there are overlaps of the typical QRS's into the others, that suggests LVH
- *The diagnosis of LVH is made only with echocardiogram*

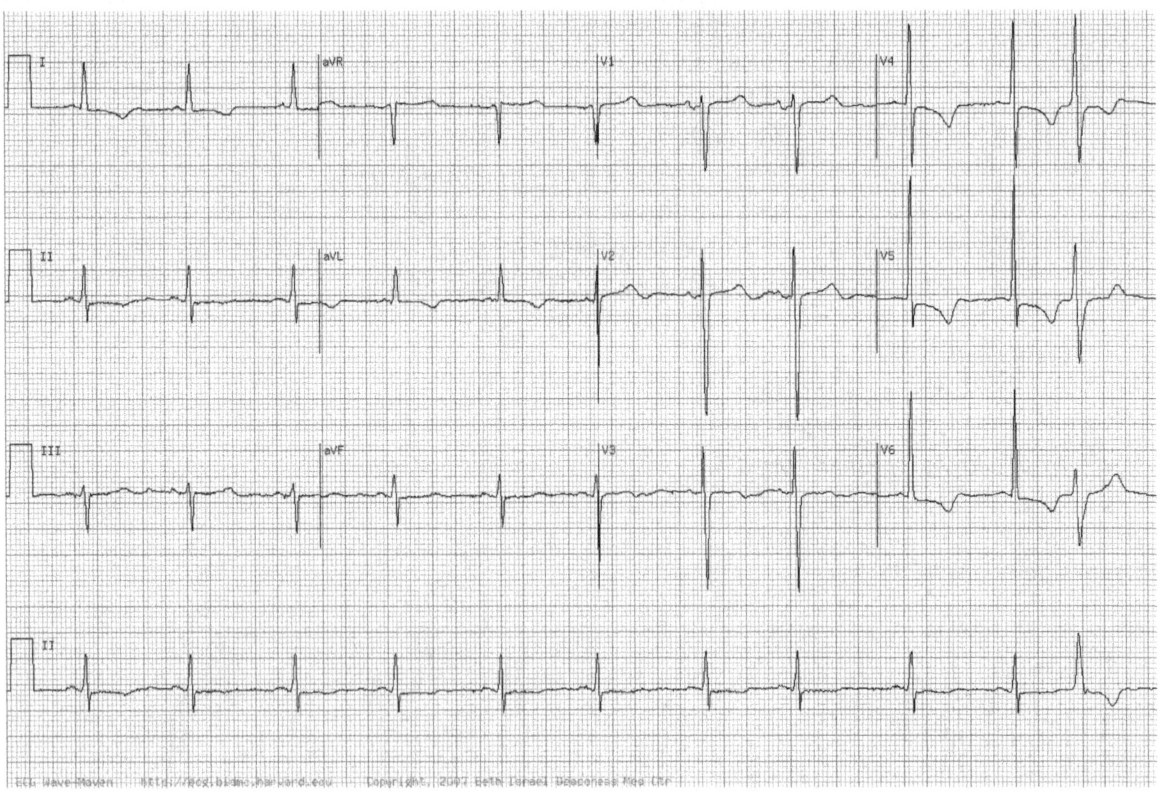

Causes of LVH:

- Uncontrolled hypertension #1
- Hypertrophic cardiomyopathy
- Aortic stenosis
- Can be normal in young athletic patients – need echo to r/o LVH (and these are the same kids prone to HCM), so if on PE you hear a murmur, and on ECG there is LVH – get an ECHO before signing any athletic release for sports!!!!!

RVH – Right Ventricular Hypertrophy

- In RVH the main lead to look at is lead V1.
- In a normal ECG, lead V1 (which is a right-sided lead on the right sternal border of the chest) should have a teeny tiny R wave (this R wave represents the electrical energy heading toward the V1 lead --- since it is a R sided lead, there should not be much going that way, yes?)
- So, if you see a tall R wave in precordial lead V1, it is unusual. (see below)
  - *There should not be that much electricity heading to the R --- so that suggests RVH (along with right axis deviation, it is most certainly RVH)*
- Notice that most RVH is due to pulmonary problems
  - *The right ventricle is not accustomed to pumping against high pressures.*
  - *The R side of the heart is a low pressure system with pressures coming into the RVH from the pulmonary vascular bed which is a low pressure system.*
  - *If exposed to increased pressures over time, the right ventricle will hypertrophy*

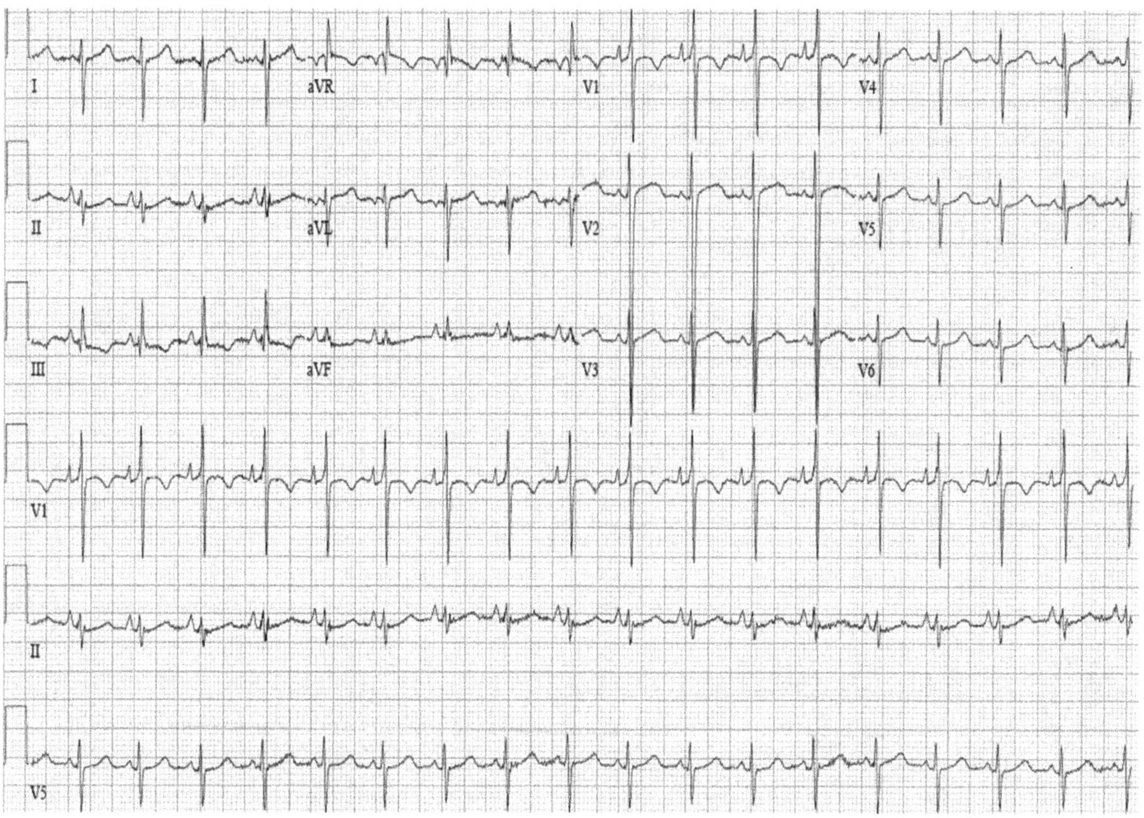

Causes of RVH:

- *Chronic*
    - Pulmonary hypertension
        - COPD
        - Primary pulmonary hypertension
        - Cystic fibrosis
    - Ventricular septal defect

- *Acute*
    - Large (or saddle) pulmonary embolism
    - Right sided valve endocarditis
    - Tetralogy of fallot (neonate with cyanosis)
    - Pulmonary valve stenosis

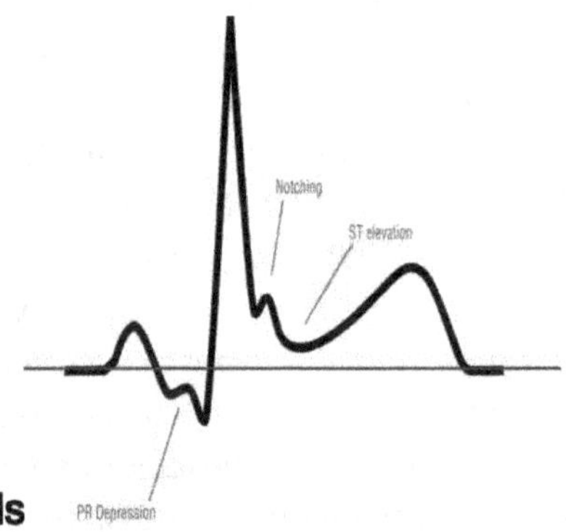

Pericarditis on ECG, changes seen in all leads

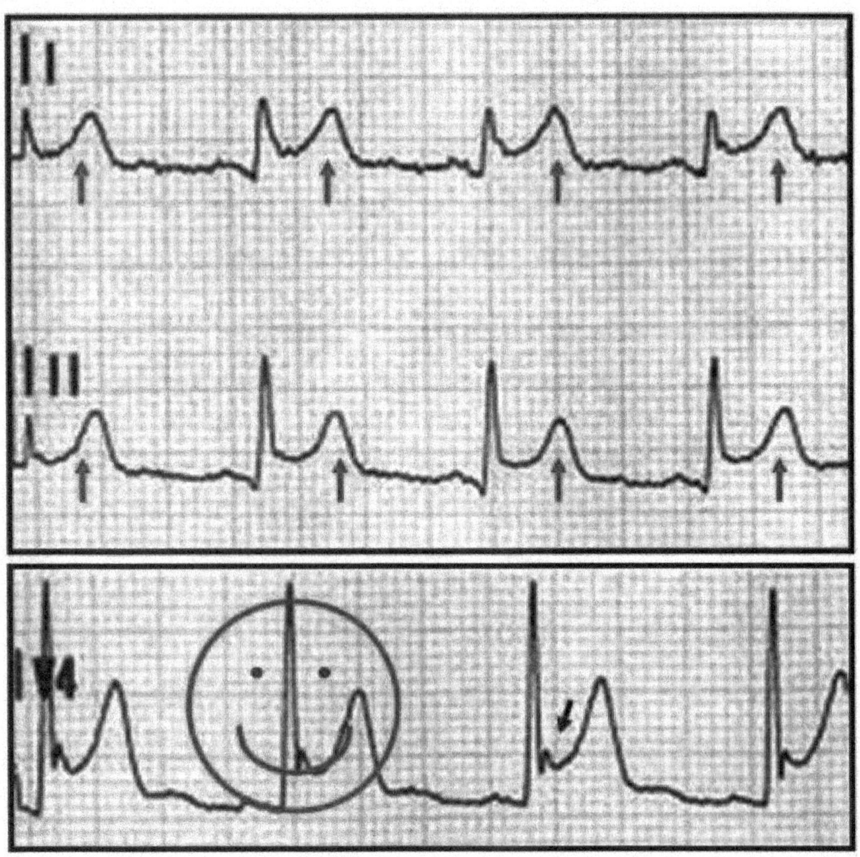

PACEMAKER MALFUNCTION

Failure to Capture

- This occurs when a pacer spike 'should have happened, but did not'.
- Either no firing at all, or an impulse too low may not depolarize the ventricle
- Frequently due to a broken or misplaced wire
- Clinical intervention
    - *Monitor patient's vital signs*
    - *Contact pacer rep to interrogate*
- If wire broken or misplaced, consult cardiology

Failure to Sense

- The pacemakers fails to sense the patient's own intrinsic beat and generates a spike on top of the patient's QRS – this can create a Q on T phenomenon and cause "Torsades de Pointes"
- Clinical intervention is needed to have the pacer "interrogated" by a rep from the company, likely sensitivities on the pacer need to be increased.

Cardiac Stress Testing

Basic tenets of stress testing:

- The best way to "stress" the heart is by walking the patient on the treadmill
    - *Best sensitivity and specificity*
- But, the ECG alone is not the most sensitive and specific way to look for ischemia
- So, use the treadmill to stress the heart
    - and a radio-nucleotide to actually *look* for perfusion (see myocardial perfusion testing below)

Hold the following drugs 24 hours before stress test (or perform pharmacologic stress test if unable to hold the medication:

- Increases resting heart rate (achieves target too soon)
    - *Theophylline*
    - *Caffeine*
- Lowers threshold heart rate (blunts HR response)
    - *Calcium channel blockers (verapamil & diltiazem)*
    - *Beta blockers*
- Can cause hypotension
    - *Nitrates*

There are three basic stress tests (all discussed in more detail below):

Exercise treadmill test (ECG exam)
- Walk the patient to 85% predicted max HR
- Observe BP, pulse, and ECG
  - *ECG changes of J-point and ST **depression** suggests ischemia*
  - *Must occur in appropriate leads corresponding with artery occlusion*
  - *Sensitivity and specificity is modest*

Myocardial perfusion test (NM = nuclear medicine exam)
- Walk the patient on the treadmill to 85% predicted max HR
- Inject radioactive substance at peak and 4 hours later at rest
- Look for perfusion
  - *Fixed defect*
  - *Reversible defect*
  - *Normal perfusion throughout both at rest and peak exercise*

Pharmacologic stress test (can be with echocardiogram, or NM test)
- Lay the patient in a bed, and use a drug to raise the HR to 85% predicted max HR
- Use an echocardiogram to look for wall motion abnormality

In addition, there is stress echocardiogram for select patients, and a variety of different combined methods utilizing both a NM nucleotide and echo.

EXERCISE STRESS TESTING

- *Indications:*
  - Establish diagnosis of CAD in patient with angina
  - Assess functional capacity in patients post-MI
  - Evaluate exercise –induced arrhythmias
  - Assess patient for ischemia after revascularization procedure or on medical therapy
- *Interpretation is based on the following:*
  - Exercise capacity
  - Patient must reach at least 70-85% pre-determined heart rate to be a "good" test
    - In other words, if Mr. Jones gets on the treadmill but can only go 5 minutes and does not achieve his predicted max heart rate; has no ST depression; this would *not* constitute a negative test.
    - Your clinical intervention will be to repeat a stress test using a pharmacologic agent to increase his heart rate.
- *Clinical response*
  - Angina constitutes a positive test
  - BP response
    - If the BP drops, positive test; if it skyrockets, positive test
  - ECG response
    - J point and ST80 depression of 1 mm. or more (2 mm. most sensitive)
- *Interpretation*
  - Patients who have more severe ST changes at lower workloads or hypotension have a poorer prognosis

- *African Americans, females, hypertensives are more likely to have a false positive result*

Choose a different method if:

- *If the ST segment is abnormal on the resting ECG, such as:*
    - BBB
    - LVH with strain
    - WPW
    - Digoxin (digitalis) therapy
- *Patient unable to walk*
    - Patients unable to achieve exercise capacity
- *Too high a false positive rate*
    - Women
- *Those where your clinical suspicion is high (you want the best sensitivity/specificity, yes?)*
    - Elderly
    - Diabetic

Absolute Indications for Termination

- Drop in SBP of > 10 mm Hg with evidence of ischemia
- Moderate to severe angina
- Near-syncope
- Ventricular tachycardia
- ST elevation (get him to the cath lab!)

PEARL: I am not a fan of memorizing lists because they are forgotten as quickly as they are learned; critical thinking is necessary here. The contraindication is the one that, if chosen it, will do harm to the patient – use the detractors to help you answer the question. For example:

Would I stop the treadmill stress test if:

A. the BP drops?
B. the patient develops angina?
C. the patient collapses?

Would I give this drug if:

A. the patient has a brain tumor?
B. the patient is pregnant?
C. the heart rate is < 60 bpm?

Myocardial Perfusion Imaging with single photon emission CT (SPECT)

- Improved S & S over treadmill ECG testing alone
- Estimates LV function
- Radioactive cardiac specific tracer
    - *Sestamibi/Thallium/Cardiolyte*
    - *Injection at peak exercise – image*
    - *Image again after 4 hours at rest*

- Interpretation
    - *Normal at peak and rest*
    - *Underperfused at peak, normal perfusion at rest (reversible defect)*
    - *Underperfused both at peak and at rest (fixed defect)*

This method (MPI with SPECT) can be done either with the treadmill, or with a pharmacologic agent to increase myocardial oxygen demand. When possible, exercise the patient on the treadmill. A recent report discussed the fact that too many pharmacologic tests were being done for "convenience" and is not, in fact, the most sensitive approach to achieving good cardiac myocardial oxygen demand.

PHARMACOLOGIC STRESS TEST

- *Use in patients who are unable to perform exercise test:*
    - Aortic stenosis (syncope can occur during exercise)
    - LBBB (due to resting ECG abnormalities)
    - Pacemaker (due to resting ECG abnormalities)
    - Severe hypertension (due to resting ECG abnormalities)
    - Patients on medications that blunt HR (BB, CCB's)
- *Procedure:*
    - Patient at rest
    - Heart's response to drug is measured
        - *Dipyridimole (Persantine) or adenosine*
            - Do not use in asthma/COPD
            - Do not use in > first degree AV block unless paced
        - *Dobutamine*
            - Can induce arrhythmias
            - OK in asthma/COPD
        - *Regadensan (Lexiscan)*
            - New, approved by FDA in 2008
            - Induces increased coronary artery flow (rapid in onset and termination)
            - Main indication in patient unable to exercise due to morbid obesity
            - OK in asthma/COPD
    - Pharmacologic agent increases myocardial oxygen demand
    - Ischemia is measured in the same ways:
        - As stress echo (wall motion akinesia)
        - As NM test or SPECT

Coronary vasodilators open up the "good" vessels, and areas that are stenotic do not have this "increased perfusion". The muscle is relatively ischemic and demonstrates wall motion abnormality. Normal pharmacologic test confers a 1-2% per year cardiac event rate (<1% with exercise test)

STRESS ECHOCARDIOGRAM

- *Looks for wall motion abnormality at peak exercise*

  - Can be done as exercise test on treadmill
  - Most useful in young females
  - Must have a skilled technican
  - Most commonly with pharmacologic "stress" due to difficulties in getting patient from treadmill to cot and imaging done within 90 seconds of peak exercise
- *Interpretation*
  - Stress-induced decrease in regional wall motion on echocardiogram
    - In areas that do not receive enough oxygen (presumably due to plaque in the artery decreasing perfusion), the muscle that needs the oxygen will be ischemic and will decrease movement (i.e., wall motion abnormality in the inferior wall of the heart implies a plaque in the right coronary artery).
- *Advantages*
  - No need for delayed images
  - No radiation exposure
  - Less expensive than nuclear med test
  - More sensitive and specific than treadmill alone
- *Limitations*
  - Echo tech dependent
  - Obesity, lung disease and tachycardia limit image quality (10% have inadequate quality)

STRESS TESTING IN WOMEN

- Different response to cardiac testing than men
- More likely to have single vessel of non-obstructive disease (decreased diagnostic accuracy)
- Treadmill -- 61% sens, 70% spec (men 72/77)
- Calcium scoring- mortality 5x higher than men with same score
- Best test = MPI with SPECT

Pulmonary Function Studies (PFT's)

- PFT's are not peak flows.
- PFT's are performed in a clinic or hospital as a scheduled test, usually on a "best" day - not during an acute exacerbation

Indications for PFT's include:

- Preoperative evaluation (i.e. In a COPD patient who needs hip replacement)
- Assessment of impairment
- Evaluation of efficacy of therapies
- Diagnosis of disease in symptomatic individual
- Assessment of heavy smokers (for early intervention)
- Occupational evaluation in patients at risk

Measurements taken:

- *Total lung capacity = amount of air in lungs at maximal inhalation*
    - This will be reduced in a restrictive disease
        - Lungs are noncompliant and stiff
    - This will be increased in obstructive disease
        - Air is "trapped" and increases lung volumes
- *Vital capacity = volume you can exhale with forceful effort, (long as it takes)*
    - This will be increased with air trapping, as in COPD and asthma or all obstructive diseases
    - This may be decreased in patients with restrictive diseases who have more trouble inflating their lungs
- *Functional residual capacity = what remains in lung after exhalation*
    - Increased in obstructive disease (in air trapping)
- *FEV1= amount of air exhaled in one second*
    - Reduced in COPD and asthma (basis of peak flow measurements)

Pulmonary Function Studies

Obstructive	Restrictive
FEV 1 is decreased	FEV1 is normal (or slightly decreased)
FEV1/FVC ratio is decreased	FEV1/FVC ratio is increased
FVC is normal or increased (chronic)	FVC decreased (more than FEV1)
TLC is normal or increased (chronic)	TLC is decreased

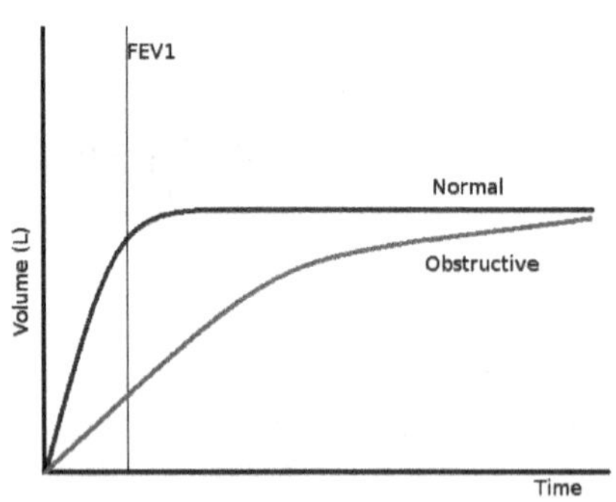

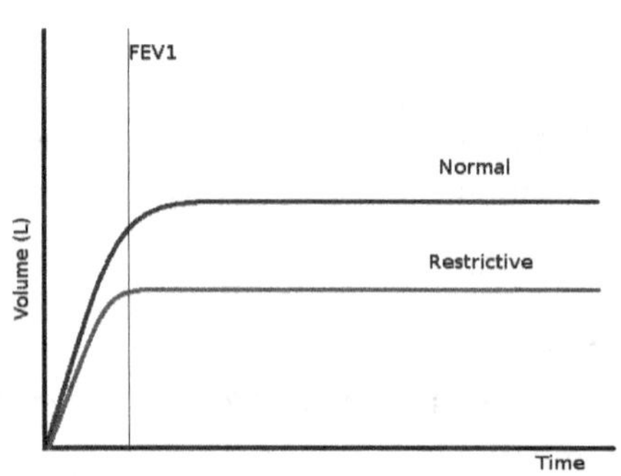

When looking at the flow loops above on a spirometry (PFT exam), note that in the obstructive process it takes much longer for the lower line to reach normal due to outflow obstruction.

In the restrictive problem, the lung capacity throughout is decreased compared to normal but the TIME is almost identical in taking about a second to exhale most of the lung capacity.

PFT'S IN ASTHMA AND COPD

- Increased TLC & VC (air is "trapped" and causes expansion)
- The diagnosis of asthma is made when PFT's are done and show completely (or almost completely) reversible obstruction
    - *FEV1 improves >12% or increases by 200 ml after albuterol*
- The diagnosis of COPD is made when PFT's are done and show incomplete response to albuterol
    - *<12% improvement or <200mL increase FEV1 after albuterol*

PFT'S IN RESTRICTED AIRWAY DISEASES

- Decreased TLC & VC
    - *Due to noncompliant tissue, infiltrated with "stuff"*
- Typically would have normal FEV1 (and normal peak flows)
    - *I.e. there is **no** obstruction to flow OUT of the lungs*
- Problem is that the lung is not able to fill easily or well

PEAK FLOWS IN ASTHMA (NOT DONE IN RESTRICTIVE OR COPD)

- This is not a PFT - it is a quick (and flawed, but good) estimation of the bronchospasm of the bronchioles
    - *Measures how quickly the patient can move air out*
- If acute bronchospasm, the obstruction causes a decrease in the amount of air that can be exhaled in 1 second.
    - *The patient can breathe in just fine, but has to "push" air out instead of it being "effortless", therefore it takes longer and less is exhaled in a second.*
- On good days, the patient performs peak flows to establish his own baseline.
    - *This is the number he compares against during an acute exacerbation, expressed as a percentage of his "personal best".*

ABG's are covered in acid-base discussion (Chapter 6, Labs & Diagnostics)

DERMATOLOGIC TESTING

KOH

- Skin scrapings are placed on slide, with drop of KOH (warming is sometimes done)
- KOH destroys the squamous cells and leaves the fungus behind
- It is used to diagnose *yeast* and *fungal* infections
    - *Hyphae, pseudohyphae and "budding yeast" = candida*
    - *Spaghetti & meatballs = tinea versicolor*

Wet Prep (Saline Prep)

- Leaves epidermal cells, white cells, red cells intact
- Used to look for live critters, like trichomonas
- In other words, doing a KOH to look for trichomonas would be incorrect, as it would kill the organism.

Mineral Oil Prep

- Used for scabies scrapings
- Take the scraping at the end of the burrow
- Place in drop of mineral oil and look under 40x

Diascopy

- Similar to a large microscope with lower power magnification
- Used to identify larger things
    - For skin, to look for telangiectasias (basal cell cancer)
    - For critters, used to distinguish markings on ticks, etc.

Excisional Biopsy

- Removing the entire lesion
    - Used for cancer diagnosis

Punch Biopsy

- Used to get a portion of a lesion when you just want a diagnosis
    - *Do not do a punch biopsy of a lesion suggestive for melanoma*

Shave Biopsy

- Just the epidermis
    - less invasive
    - no need for suture
    - do not do shave biopsy if concern for cancer!

CHAPTER 7

Clinical Intervention – 12%

Topics in this section as described in the NCCPA Blueprint:

- Management and treatment of selected medical conditions
- Indications, contraindications, complications, risks, benefits and techniques for selected procedures
- Standard precautions and special isolation conditions
- Sterile technique
- Follow-up and monitoring of therapeutic regimens - covered in Therapeutic Chapter
- Conditions that constitute medical emergencies
- Indications for admission to or discharge from hospitals or other facilities
- Discharge planning
- Available community resources
- Appropriate community resources
- Appropriate patient education
- Roles of other health professionals
- End-of-life issues
- Risks and benefits of alternative medicine
- Formulating and implementing treatment plans
- Recognizing and initiating treatment for life-threatening emergencies
- Demonstrating technical expertise related to performing specific procedures
- Communicating effectively; using counseling techniques
- Facilitating patient adherence and active participation in treatment
- Interacting effectively in multidisciplinary teams

Introduction to Clinical Intervention

Clinical intervention is covered in each content topic chapter in this book. When a specific clinical intervention is important, it will be specifically identified.

Clinical intervention means: what do you do NOW with this patient?

- Do you do an invasive study next?
- Do you admit to the hospital?
- Do you admit to the ICU?
- Do you send him home with reassurance?
- Do you give a drug?

- Do you give advice about lifestyle modification?
- Do you screen him for a disease?
- Do you refer for elective surgery?
- Do you refer for immediate surgery?
- Do you have the patient follow up in one hour? One day? One week? One month? Next year?

EXAMPLES TO ILLUSTRATE CLINICAL INTERVENTION QUESTIONS:

1. **A 17-year-old male presents with painless testicular mass. US confirms solid mass. What is the most appropriate clinical intervention in this clinical setting?**

2. **A 17-year-old male presents with painful L testicle. US confirms loss of blood flow to left testicle. What is the most appropriate clinical intervention in this clinical setting?**

3. **A 17-year-old male presents with painful L scrotum. He is febrile; has pain with palpation of the epididymis; testicle is nontender. What is the most appropriate clinical intervention in this clinical setting?**

4. **A 17-year-old female presents with irritative voiding symptoms, no fever. Urinalysis suggests UTI; culture is pending. What is the most appropriate clinical intervention in this clinical setting?**

5. **A 17-year-old pregnant female presents with irritative voiding symptoms, no fever. Urinalysis suggests UTI; culture is pending. What is the most appropriate clinical intervention in this clinical setting?**

6. **A 17-year-old female presents with irritative voiding symptoms and fever. Urinalysis suggests UTI; culture is pending. What is the most appropriate clinical intervention in this clinical setting?**

7. **A 57-year-old male presents with irritative voiding symptoms; without fever. Urinalysis suggests UTI; (>50 RBC's, > 50 WBC's, + LE, + nitrite); culture positive for E. Coli. What is the most appropriate clinical intervention in this clinical setting?**

8. **A 57-year-old male presents with irritative voiding symptoms; with fever and perineal pain. Urinalysis suggests infection. What is the most appropriate clinical intervention in this clinical setting?**

9. **A 57-year-old male presents with waxing and waning irritative voiding symptoms x 4-6 months; with no fever or perineal pain. Urinalysis is negative. What is the most appropriate clinical intervention in this clinical setting?**

10. **A 57-year-old male presents with obstructive voiding symptoms. Bladder scan confirms 50 cc of urine in the bladder. Serum creatinine is normal. What is the most appropriate clinical intervention in this clinical setting?**

11. **A 57-year-old male presents with obstructive voiding symptoms. Bladder scan confirms 1200 cc of urine in the bladder. Foley is placed. Serum creatinine is 6.4. What is the most appropriate clinical intervention in this clinical setting?**

12. **A 42-year-old patient presents with elevated BP on two occasions; rest of PE is normal; labs are all normal; he is obese and a smoker. BP 150's/90's. What is the most appropriate clinical intervention in this clinical setting?**

13. **A 42-year-old patient presents with elevated BP; history of Type 2 DM. BP150's/90's. What is the most appropriate clinical intervention in this clinical setting?**

14. **A 32-year-old female presents with RUQ pain several hours after fatty meal. She has Temp 99.8; + Murphy's sign; LFT's are elevated; Lipase 78 (nl <24). US confirms dilatation of common bile duct (CBD). What is the most appropriate clinical intervention in this clinical setting?**

15. **A 32-year-old female presents with RUQ pain several hours after fatty meal. She has no fever, LFT's are normal; lipase is normal. US confirms GB stones without wall thickening and normal bile duct. What is the most appropriate clinical intervention in this clinical setting?**

Answers:

1) Urgent referral to urology (same or next day)

2) Emergent consult (6 hours from onset of pain to relieve ischemia)

3) Ceftriaxone 250 mg IM plus Doxycycline BID x 10-14 days

4) 3 day short course of Bactrim/Cipro

5) 7 day course (no short course in pregnant women)

6) Admit, Rocephin IV

7) Repeat the urinalysis after treatment to ensure resolution of hematuria (could be bladder cancer!)

8) Treat with urinary fluoroquinolones (ciprofloxacin or ofloxacin) for 4-6 weeks;

9) Who knows? This is chronic bacterial prostatitis, no good treatment, eventual referral to urology; could obtain prostatic secretions and culture them (prostatic massage)

10) Treatment with either alpha-blocker (tamsulosin) or finasteride and follow up in 2-4 weeks

11) Urgent referral to urology for possible TURP

12) Start DASH plan; discuss smoking cessation; make appointment for recheck in 2-3 weeks.

13) Start DASH plan; begin therapy with ACE Inhibitor.

14) Make her NPO; admit to surgery for anticipated lap chole; duct exploration

15) Discharge on low fat diet; referral to surgery for elective lap cholecystectomy

RISKS AND BENEFITS OF ALTERNATIVE MEDICINES

Since there is a specific topic in Clinical Intervention related to alternative medicine that many of us do not specifically practice, I have decided to add a short section below with the most common practices and therapeutics. This is covered in a new chapter in the textbook, Current Medical Diagnosis and Treatment 2013.

Basics of CAM (complementary and alternative medicine) therapeutics:

Dietary Supplements

- Dietary supplement = vitamin, mineral, herb, botanical, amino acid, enzyme, organ tissue or glandular substance, metabolite, probiotic
- 20% of Americans take some sort of supplement

- The elderly take supplements with other prescription medications more often than any other age group
- Under-reported use in general among all patients
- Not regulated by the FDA
    - Herbal side effects and interactions are supposed to be reported to the FDA (online or by phone).
    - The only way the FDA can intervene in the manufacture of an herb or supplement is if there are reported issues.
- Homeopathic remedies are regulated separately

Main concern about supplement use with prescription drugs

- Impact on bleeding times
- Potentiation of effects of prescription drug
- Inhibition of effects of prescription drug
- Direct effect of supplement on the patient

Which are most important for clinical practice?

- *#1 St. John's Wort*
    - Many drug effects with multiple meds
- *#2 Garlic*
    - Antiplatelet; antithrombotic; fibrinolytic activity (post-op bleeding is common with use)
- *#3 Ginseng*
    - Decreases efficacy of warfarin
- *#4 Gingko*
    - Inhibits platelet activating factor (spontaneous bleeds and prolonged bleeding time have been reported)
- *#5 Goldenseal*
    - increases drug levels of SSRI's

PEARL:

Anything will likely interfere with warfarin and slightly less often, Digoxin (digitalis) --- just do not let your patient take any herbs if on either of these medications!

CHAPTER 8

Health Maintenance – 10%

Topics in this section as described in the NCCPA Blueprint:

- **Epidemiology of selected medical conditions**
  - i.e. TB occurs most commonly in prison populations; third world countries; lower socioeconomic populations
  - This information is covered in each topic where pertinent
- **Early detection and prevention of selected medical conditions**
  - This is covered in each content topic chapter where pertinent
- **Relative value of common screening tests**
  - See individual topics within the content chapters
- **Appropriate patient education regarding preventable conditions or lifestyle modifications**
  - Reviewed in each content section
  - Also specific preventive guidelines found in
    - Chapter 11 pertaining to endocarditis prophylaxis
    - Cancer screening guideline in Appendix A
- **Healthy lifestyles**
  - Review the risk factors for hypertension, diabetes, cancer, etc.
- **Prevention of communicable diseases**
  - Vaccination
  - Clean water & sanitation practices
  - Standard precautions for healthcare workers (Appendix B)
- **Immunization schedules and recommendations for infants, children, adults and foreign travelers**
  - Pediatric immunization schedule is in Chapter 24
  - Adult vaccines are covered in Appendix C
  - Travel vaccinations (most common) are covered in Appendix C
- **Risks and benefits of immunization**
  - This is discussed where appropriate in the particular disease discussion, i.e. HIB (hemophilus influenza B) infection is now rare since vaccination was begun; influenza is a common cause of death, risk is decreased with immunization, etc.
- **Human growth and development**
- **Human sexuality**
  - This is covered briefly in Urology Chapter 21, Women's health Chapter 15, and Endocrinology Ch. 20.

- **Occupational and environmental exposure**
- **Impact of stress on health**
    - Multiple somatic complaints
    - Disruption of personal relationships
    - Lack of sleep
- **Psychological manifestations of illness and injury**
    - Stress
    - Coping strategies for illness and stress
- **Effects of aging and changing family roles on health maintenance and disease prevention**
    - Aging population affects us all; be cognizant of geriatric issues
- **Signs of abuse and neglect**
    - *see Chapter 18*
- **Barriers to care (be aware!)**
    - Lack of insurance
    - Lack of funds
    - Lack of providers
- **Using counseling and patient education techniques**
    - Know that counseling improves patient compliance
    - Know that checking the blood sugars and blood pressures that the patient records improves patient compliance
    - Know that addressing obesity, smoking, lifestyle improves patient behavioral changes
- **Communicating effectively with patients to enhance health maintenance**
    - As above (in counseling patients)
- **Adapting health maintenance to the patient's context**
    - Cultural competence is what they are getting at here, i.e., nutritional guidance within the patient's cultural food preferences, etc.
- **Using informational databases**

Tackling The Health Maintenance Questions

Many of the topics listed here are "soft" and difficult to discuss, but are covered in PA school for new graduates, and are addressed on a daily basis in clinical practice for the seasoned clinicians.

In each chapter, I cover topics related to health maintenance in regards to screening for diseases, healthy practices and behaviors.

- Memorize the immunization schedule for children (see Chapter 24), as it changes every 25 minutes!

- Review screening guidelines for preventing cancer or diagnosing cancers early in Appendix A

- Pay attention to the known risk factors for the various diseases that are covered in each content chapter, and where I specifically mention health maintenance.

CHAPTER 9

Scientific Concepts – 10%

Topics in this section as described in the NCCPA Blueprint:

- Human **anatomy and physiology**
    - Anatomy covered in each chapter according to organ system
    - Physiology covered both in each chapter according to disease state
        - And in Chapter 10, Anatomy & Physiology

- Underlying **patho**physiology
    - Covered in Chapter 10, Anatomy & Physiology
    - Covered in each topic chapter as well

- **Microbiology** and biochemistry
    - Covered in Chapter 22, Infectious Disease
    - Covered in pharmacology bugs & drugs, Chapter 4
    - Covered in each topic area pertaining to typical pathogens

- Recognizing **normal and abnormal** anatomy and physiology
    - Covered in each topic area (as described above)

- Relating pathophysiologic principles to specific disease processes
    - Covered in each chapter according to disease state discussed

- Correlating **abnormal physical examination** findings to a given disease process
    - Covered in Chapter 5, History & Physical Exam

- Correlating **abnormal results of diagnostic tests** to a given disease process
    - Covered in Chapter 6, Labs & Diagnostics

SECTION THREE – PHYSIOLOGIC CONCEPTS

CHAPTER 10

Physiology and Pathophysiology Review

There is no topic list, per se, in this section. Anatomy is covered in each individual chapter as it pertains to disease states, and physical examination of the body is covered in Chapter 5, along with all pertinent anatomical discussions.

Most people try to memorize a list of topics and just learn as much as they can absorb for each individual disease state, including the myriad therapeutics that exist now.

A much more useful method is to review the anatomy and use it when analyzing a question, and review a few basic physiology pearls that you learned in PA school and utilize every day, but maybe have forgotten how they apply to patient presentation and therapeutic options for management on a test like this.

I am only going to review those anatomy & physiology topics that I find most useful in reviewing medical content. This is not a true physiology review...this is more like "physiology made ridiculously simple"... but it works!

BLOOD COMPOSITION

- *Blood is composed of plasma, RBC's , WBC's, platelets and dissolved gases, amino acids, proteins, carbohydrates, lipids, hormones, vitamins, electrolytes, hormones and waste products*
    - 55% of blood volume is plasma, 45% are the RBC's
        - 90% of plasma is water
    - Gases dissolved in blood = oxygen, carbon dioxide (as bicarbonateonate), and nitrogen
    - Proteins dissolved in plasma = albumin, globulin, and fibrinogen

Common Blood Products in Review

Whole Blood

- *Why is that we rarely give "whole" blood to our patients?*

- Whole blood is more likely a carrier of transfused infectious diseases than other products.
- Serious shortage of blood products necessitates using whole blood to make more specific blood products.
- Most patients only need one component of whole blood.
- Specific blood products (except RBC's) can be infused regardless of ABO blood group.

Packed Red Blood Cells

- Packed RBC's do not provide platelets, WBC's, or coagulation factors.
- *Indication:*
    - Symptomatic anemia (pay attention to the information given you, this patient will be short of breath, in congestive heart failure; markedly volume depleted, H&H typically < 7/21)
- One unit infused will increase hemoglobin by 1 gm/dl and hematocrit by 3%.
- All RBC transfusions must be ABO/Rh compatible with the recipient.

Fresh Frozen Plasma

- Plasma removed from a unit of whole blood; it contains all coagulation factors and has no RBC's, WBC's or platelets.
- *Indication:*
    - A patient with documented coagulation factor deficiencies who is actively bleeding or needs to undergo invasive procedure. (this could be your warfarin patient, liver failure patient or inherited coagulopathy like hemophilia-A)
    - A patient with supratherapeutic INR (from warfarin) too significant to "wait" for Vitamin K to work
- One ml. of FFP/kg will raise clotting factors by about 1%.
- This is not a concentrate
    - Concentrates are made from plasma, but each individual coagulation factor is then concentrated from as many as 120-140 units of plasma to get factor concentrate!

Cryoprecipitate

- *Indication:*
    - Patient with low fibrinogen levels who are bleeding or need invasive procedure
- Cryoprecipitate also contains 100 units of Factor VIII and vWF, as well as fibrinogen.

Platelets

- *Indication:*
    - Patients with bleeding due to thrombocytopenia and/or platelet dysfunction
        - Almost never used in idiopathic thrombocytopenic purpura (ITP)
        - The autoantibodies will rapidly remove the infused platelets from circulation anyway.
        - Therefore, only used in severe bleeding issue which almost never happens
- Platelet infusion also contains plasma; therefore coagulation factors, some RBC's, and some WBCs.

ABO/RH

The ABO blood system:

- **Red blood cells contain either proteins, antibodies or both:**
  - *Type A :* have A antigen and antibodies (IgM) to B antigen
  - *Type B :* have B antigen and antibodies (IgM) to A antigen
  - *Type AB :* have both A and B antigen but neither of the A or B antibodies
    - Type AB is called 'universal acceptor' because of the ability of patients with this blood group to receive blood from all other blood groups
      - *They have no antibodies; so they can receive any type blood*
  - *Type O :* have neither antigens but have both the A & B antibodies
    - Type O is called 'universal donor' because of the ability of people with this blood group to donate blood to all other blood groups respectively.
      - *They have both antibodies, so they cannot receive any other blood*
    - Type O patients can only receive Type O blood (because any other blood will have antigens which will cause an immune response by their body)

REMINDER ABOUT RH:

The Rh (rhesus <like the monkey>) blood group system is the most important after ABO (above).

While the D antigen (which is the most important antigen in the Rh system) is important for compatibility with transfused blood, it is much more important in isoimmunization during pregnancy.

- Rh-negative mom is a D antigen negative mom.
- She is pregnant with an Rh positive (D antigen positive) fetus.
- If any fetal cells cross into mom's bloodstream (as often does asymptomatically during pregnancy), that D antigen floating around in mom's blood will trigger an antibody response that will make her body produce IgM and then IgG to D antigen.
- This antibody is not much of an issue to *this* baby; but will cause "isoimmunization" in the mom.
- If she has another pregnancy where the fetus has D antigen, mom's IgG will cross the placenta (as does all her blood) and attack the D antigen on the Rh positive baby's RBC's.
- Isoimmunization of the Rh-negative mother may result in erythroblastosis fetalis in the fetus and in all subsequent pregnancies.
- Erythroblastosis causes fetal hydrops due to massive hemolysis.

To prevent isoimmunization, Rhogam is given (immunoglobulin that will bind any D antigen and prevent the mother from making IgG to D antigen). It should be given prophylactically during the pregnancy with any bleeding event, and after birth of an Rh-positive baby. It should be given after any miscarriage, ectopic, elective abortion, or significant bleeding in pregnancy.

Once isoimmunization has occurred in a patient, Rhogam is no longer indicated (it is too late for Rhogam or immunoglobulin at this point), and now we just follow titres, ultrasound frequently and hope for the best. Intra-umbilical blood transfusion can be given to the fetus for severe hydrops.

THE IMPORTANCE OF PLASMA PROTEINS

Albumin is the most abundant of the proteins.

- Albumin is used for binding to hormones, calcium, fatty acids, cholesterol and plays a huge role in plasma transport of these substances.
- Reductions in plasma albumin because of nutritional, liver and kidney disease will cause an osmotic loss of fluid from the blood and a "shifting" of fluid into the interstitial space.

Globulins, including high density (HDL)

- HDL functions in lipid transport carrying fats to cells for use in energy metabolism, membrane reconstruction and hormone function.
- HDLs also appear to prevent cholesterol from invading and settling in the walls of arteries.
- LDL carries cholesterol and fats to tissues for use in manufacturing steroid hormones and building cell membranes, but unfortunately deposits (if in excess) in arterial walls causing plaque.

THE AUTONOMIC NERVOUS SYSTEM

The autonomic nervous system consists of two parts:

The Sympathetic Nervous System

- *"Fight or flight" system*
    - Is stimulated by adrenalin released by the adrenal gland (like when you walk into the room to start your exam – that "fluttery" feeling is your sympathetic system doing its thing.
    - Is also stimulated in response to hypovolemia, hemorrhage, or any other reason that you need HR, BP, contractility and therefore, increased cardiac output.
    - Is comprised of alpha (α)stimulation and beta (β)stimulation
        - *The beta adrenergic system*
            - Increase HR, BP, contractility of the heart
            - This will increase the cardiac output (CO) of the heart
                - The good thing is, it increases CO (if that is what the patient needs)
                - The bad thing is, sometimes the patient does not actually need increased heart rate or BP; sometimes the problem is that the heart just cannot do it anymore, and this can then make matters worse.
        - *The alpha adrenergic system*
            - Causes peripheral vasoconstriction of arterioles
                - Through constriction of smooth muscles
            - "Moves" blood into central vascular system to increase vital organ perfusion

- The good thing is it increases BP (if you need more pressure)
- The bad thing is it increases BP (if you don't actually need more pressure and have a lousy cardiac pump)

The Parasympathetic Nervous System

- Once the dinosaur goes away, or the bleeding stops, or your exam begins and you realize you are going to pass this thing, the parasympathetic nervous system is activated.
- It brings you back to baseline:
  - Lowers HR, BP and contractility
  - Returns cardiac output to normal.

These two systems are in delicate balance; too much of either can cause problems. They are imperative to keep us alive, as I discuss several times throughout the book.

REVIEW OF CARDIOPULMONARY A&P

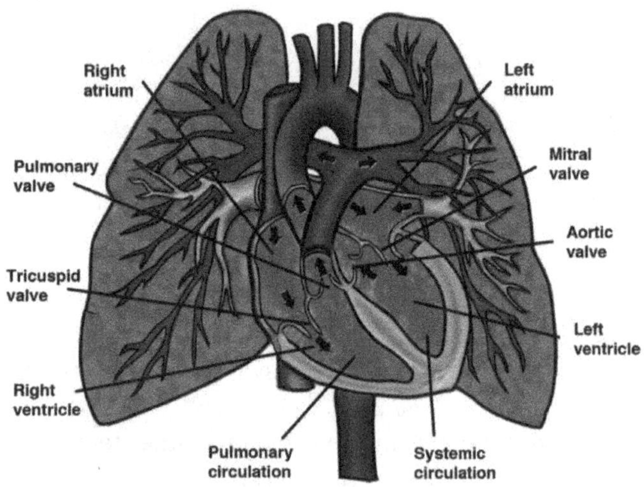

THE CARDIOPULMONARY ANATOMY

This is just a very brief review, with a picture. I do not mean to insult anyone, but this brief review of the anatomy will be referred to in the next section. Be able (in your mind) to imagine blood flow forward, and picture in your mind how pressure is transmitted "backward" in the system as well.

Let's start with blood going out of the left ventricle (recall, this is just a closed plumbing system):

Systole Begins

- Blood flows from the left ventricle through the aortic valve (which has three leaflets normally) without obstruction or increased pressure or any problem at all.
- It flows into the aortic root at high pressure (this is where the pressure is the highest in the vascular system).
- It continues throughout the entire peripheral system due to blood pressure.
  - Recall that BP is actually good for you. (We always think of BP as bad.)

  - If you have no BP, you have no perfusion.
- This blood will fill the aortic root and flow down the coronary arteries (left and right) during diastole to provide oxygen to the myocardium for the next contraction.
- The blood then continues around the aortic arch and fills the carotids with oxygenated blood.
- Blood then flows down the descending aorta, providing oxygenated blood to the upper extremities.
- This all occurs in the anterior mediastinal space.
- The aorta then enters the retroperitoneal space and oxygenated blood flows into the renal arteries.
- Immediately after the renal arteries, the aorta goes out into the abdominal space, slightly left sided in the abdomen.
- Oxygenated blood flows to the gut (superior mesenteric artery is most important to know), then bifurcates into the iliacs, and each iliac becomes the femoral and supplies oxygenated blood to the peripheral arteries of the lower extremities.
- The blood has now given up most of its oxygen during this trip, and now this blood enters the capillary beds. It flows across the capillary bed and enters the venous system of the lower extremities; and then enters the peripheral veins; flows back from the toes, and makes a 90 degree turn against gravity and flows up into the calf, thigh, and into the inferior vena cava (IVC).
- This is also occurring in the liver, the gut, etc., and blood from the head and neck and chest does the same thing but enters the superior vena cava (SVC).

We tend to ignore the right ventricle, but its role in providing blood to the left ventricle is hugely important as well.

Systole as occurs in the right heart:
- The R ventricle contracts, blood flows into the pulmonary veins, into the lungs, and crosses into the pulmonary arterial system.

Diastole Begins
- *On the right side of the heart, "venous" deoxygenated blood from the IVC and SVC fills the right atrium.*
  - When enough blood is present so that the pressure is higher in the RA than in the RV, the tricuspid valve opens and passive filling of blood from the RA to the RV occurs.
  - At the end of diastole, the RA contracts as the RV relaxes and 1/3 more blood enters the RV.
- *On the left side of the heart, oxygenated blood from the pulmonary arteries fills the LA.*
  - When enough blood is present so that pressure is higher in the LA than in the LV, the mitral valve opens and passive filling of blood from the LA to the LV occurs.
  - At the end of diastole, the LA contracts as the LV relaxes and 1/3 more blood enter the LV.
  - The coronary arteries will fill (just outside of the aortic valve, in the root)
  - At the end of diastole, the ventricle contains the most blood that it will ever contain; and the left ventricular end diastolic pressure (LVEDP) is at its highest as well.

Systole Occurs Again

- The left ventricle contracts and blood flows through the aortic valve into the aortic root.
- The right ventricle contracts and blood flows into the pulmonary vessels.

Review of Cardiopulmonary Physiology and Pathophysiology

Systemic Vascular Resistance

- The pressure in the peripheral vascular (arterial) system against which the left heart has to pump to get blood to the fingers and toes (and kidneys and brain)

Pulmonary Vascular Resistance

- The pressure in the pulmonary vascular system against which the right heart has to pump to get blood through the lungs and into the L heart

Increase in LV End Diastolic Volumes

- Increase in volumes (preload) will increase pressure within the ventricle
- Increase in volumes in the LV will cause dilatation of the ventricle
- This will cause displacement of the PMI and cardiomegaly on CXR

Increase in LV End Diastolic Pressures

- **Due to two likely causes:**
    - *Systemic vascular resistance*
        - Causing increased SBP
        - Hypertension within the vascular system
    - *Obstruction to flow out of the aortic valve*
        - Causes increase in pressure within the left ventricle
        - But not in the aortic root or the peripheral arterial system
        - Remember, SBP will not be elevated
            - Pressure in the LV itself will be elevated, causing hypertrophy

Left heart failure

- Failure of the left heart to provide arterial blood to the body
- Many causes, covered in the CV section
- LHF is the most common cause of RHF, but there are others – see below

Right heart failure

- **Most commonly due to the L heart failure**
    - Left heart becomes a lousy forward pump
    - Pulmonary pressures go up
    - Then the R heart has to pump against these high pressures
    - Causes R heart "strain"
    - Right ventricular hypertrophy occurs (RVH)
    - Right atrial enlargement occurs (RAE)
    - The right heart starts to fail

  - Decrease in blood presented to the lungs and left heart
- **Cor pulmonale**
  - Is due to a pure pulmonary problem – not a left heart problem
  - As a matter of fact, the left heart is "on vacation"
    - Low systolic pressures, low cardiac output
  - *Causes:*
    - *Acute* = pulmonary embolism; "flash" pulmonary edema
    - *Chronic* = COPD, primary pulmonary hypertension, pulmonary fibrosis, etc.

SYSTEMIC VS. PULMONARY PRESSURES WITHIN THE SYSTEM

- Systemic pressures in the peripheral vascular bed are quite high at systolic blood pressures exceeding 120 mm Hg.
- It is very important to remember that pulmonary pressures are *very* different from systemic pressures.
  - The mean arterial pressure in the pulmonary bed is only 12 mm Hg – and the lungs like it that way!

PULMONARY EDEMA

When pressures increase in the pulmonary bed, the lungs do not like it. They will do everything they can to "normalize" the pressures – which results in the following:

- Normally when standing - due to gravity - there will be increased perfusion in the inferior lung fields and increased aeration in the superior lung fields.
- Should the pulmonary pressures exceed 12 mm. Hg; the lungs will try to redistribute that blood into the entire pulmonary space.
- This *"revascularization"* will be seen on a PA chest film (performed upright) as an increase in blood flow to the upper lung fields occurs.
  - *This is also called*
    - Pulmonary revascularization or redistribution
    - Cephalization of the pulmonary vasculature
    - Pulmonary vascular congestion
      - All names for the same thing
  - *When pressures exceed 15 mm, and revascularization is not doing enough, the lungs will dump fluid out into the interstitial space.*
    - On CXR, this is seen as "Kerley B lines" (small peripheral lines in the bases) – impossible to see with the resolution of a computer monitor
    - When you see the words "Kerley B lines" it means increased pulmonary pressures/interstitial fluid
  - *When pressures exceed 20 mm, and revascularization and movement of fluid into the interstitium does not successfully lower pressures in the pulmonary bed, fluid will now move into the alveolar spaces:*
    - Now there is air bubbling through this alveolar fluid, and we hear rales (crackles) on auscultation of the lung fields.
  - If *that* does not work and pressures continue to rise, the lungs will dump fluid into the pleural space, and the patient will develop a pleural effusion.

The increase in pulmonary vascular pressures and the fluid in the lungs will cause the patient to develop shortness of breath and pulmonary edema.

DECREASE IN CARDIAC OUTPUT

As cardiac output goes down, the amount of blood flowing to the head and to the kidneys obviously goes down:

- The sympathetic nervous system will try to increase BP to maintain blood flow.
- If this fails to provide normal cardiac output, other systems will be activated:
  - The Renin-Angiotensin-Aldosterone system (RAAS)
  - Vasopressin/ADH from the brain
- These systems are described in detail below.

WHEN THINGS DO NOT WORK LIKE THEY SHOULD

The circulatory system is really just a plumbing system (per Dr. Richard Silberman, awesome cardiologist!). Just like any plumbing system, if water flows freely, all is good.
When there is a restriction to flow, two things happen:

- Flow through the restriction/obstruction becomes turbulent
- Pressure builds up behind the restriction

So, where can obstructions and restrictions to flow occur? Anywhere along the system, but from more common to less common:

Aortic Stenosis

- High pressures caused by having to pump against a stiff or bicuspid aortic valve will cause the ventricle to have to work harder.
- Pressure in the LV will go up.
- The LV will hypertrophy.
- Where will these LV pressures back up into now?
  - The left atrium

Mitral Stenosis

- High pressures caused by the left atrium having to push blood through a thick, stiff or abnormal mitral valve will cause the left atrium to work too hard.
- LA pressures will rise, and the atrium will dilate.
  - Recall that the atria do not hypertrophy, they dilate!
- These increased LA pressures will then back up into the pulmonary vascular bed causing pulmonary hypertension.

Pulmonary Hypertension

- High pressures in the pulmonary vasculature will back up into the RV, and eventually into the right atrium.
- If right atrial pressures are chronically high, where will this pressure back up?
  - into the superior and inferior vena cavae (JVD)
  - into the liver, the hepatic portal system (HJR)

So - make sure you completely understand circulatory flow forward and pressure buildup backward in the cardiopulmonary system.

MURMURS

- Simply a sound heard when blood flows
- Turbulent flow of that blood causes the "murmur"
- Sound travels in a straight line, so the murmur may be transmitted to a spot remote to the valve

Maneuvers Understood

- **Squat**
  - Increases amount of blood (from legs) into vena cava and, therefore, to the heart
  - This maneuver will increase preload, which will increase blood flow and cause turbulence (and the murmur) in an obstructive lesion.
  - Ironically, this maneuver also increases the murmur in a "functional" or normal murmur that can occur in a kid with good flow and a thin chest wall (see functional murmur in discussion below)
- **Valsalva**
  - Increases the intra-abdominal pressure to decrease venous return and therefore blood flow, thereby decreasing the turbulence (and the murmur) in an obstructive lesion.
  - Ironically, it also decreases the murmur in a "functional" or normal murmur that can occur in a kid with good flow and a thin chest wall (see functional murmur in discussion below)
  - *Note* – this is opposite of what happens in a hypertrophic myopathy patient whose murmur will increase with valsalva (see HCM murmur discussion below).
- **Hand Grip**
  - Increases the pressure just outside the aortic valve which will normalize a gradient across the valve (and decrease turbulence, thereby decreasing the murmur of an obstructive lesion)

Understanding Murmurs

All of these murmurs, their etiologies, clinical manifestations, and treatments are covered in the Cardiovascular Medicine Chapter 11. This section is intended to give you the "pearls" on how to quickly and easily make educated guesses, and get questions right as they relate to a murmur-type question.

First – it is important to remember that, once again, this is easier than clinical medicine; you will not have to wear earphones and describe the murmur; the description will be given to you. Pay careful attention to *only* the following descriptors to get the murmur correct:

Timing

- *Systole*
  - 90% of all murmurs occur in systole.
  - All functional (normal) murmurs occur in systole.

- *Diastole*
    - Diastolic murmurs are never "functional".
        - Get an echo!
- *Continuous (both systolic and diastolic)*
    - Patent ductus arteriosis vs. venous hum
        - PDA does not disappear with maneuvers
        - described as "machine-gun" type murmur
    - Venous hum
        - disappears when you lay the child down, turn his head

Location/Radiation

- *Base = aortic valve*
    - 2nd Intercostal space, right sternal border
        - *All* functional murmurs occur here (and are soft)!
    - loud AS murmurs will radiate into carotids
        - Functional murmurs would never radiate
- *Apex = mitral valve*
    - 5th intercostal space, mid-clavicular line (same as the PMI)
    - Radiates into axilla
- *Pulmonic area*
    - 2nd ICS, left sternal border
- Tricuspid area
    - 4th ICS, left sternal border

Intensity

- *Grade I – barely audible*
    - This is the typical intensity of a "functional" murmur
- *Grade II – audible but soft*
    - This is fairly common too; can be normal or may be valve problem
- ***Grade III – fairly loud (easy to hear)***
    - Abnormally loud – get echo
    - Most common intensity for aortic stenosis mumurs (systolic)
- ***Grade IV – same as III but with a "thrill"***
    - Abnormally loud – get echo
    - Most likely aortic stenosis murmur if systolic
- ***Grade V – heard by just touching edge of stethoscope to chest***
    - Uncommon (haven't heard one yet)
- ***Grade VI – heard just walking into the room***
    - Usually a mechanical valve (metal valve replacement)
- *Grades III through VI (**bolded**) are too loud to be "innocent or functional", deserves echo if undiagnosed or if patient is symptomatic

MOST IMPORTANT MURMURS

Functional murmur vs. Hypertrophic Cardiomyopathy

Functional Murmur (normal)	Hypertrophic Cardiomyopathy
Soft, grade I-II/VI systolic ejection murmur	Grade II or higher systolic ejection murmur
Murmur increases with squat (increased venous return) Since it is functional and due to blood flow, more flow = more sound	Murmur decreases with squat More blood (squat) = more blood in ventricle moves "obstruction" away from aortic orifice (decreases murmur)
Murmur decreases with valsalva (decreased venous return), less blood = less sound	Murmurs increases with valsalva Less blood = more obstruction = more sound
Normal ECG	LVH on ECG
Echo is normal (not indicated in normal flow murmur)	Echo shows septal thickening, LVH

<u>Mitral Stenosis vs. Aortic Stenosis</u>

Mitral Valve Stenosis	Aortic Valve Stenosis
Best heard at apex	Best heard at base
Diastolic murmur	Systolic murmur
Radiates into axilla	Radiates into carotids
Rumbling, low pitched (heard best with bell)	Harsh, high-pitched (heard best with diaphragm)
Rheumatic Fever	Bicuspid valve (young) or calcific valve (elderly)

Mitral Regurgitation vs. Aortic Regurgitation

Mitral Regurgitation/Insufficiency	Aortic Regurgitation/Insufficiency
Best heard at apex	Best heard at base; entire LSB
Systolic murmur	Diastolic murmur
Left atrium enlarges	Carotid volumes are large
Blowing, low pitched	"Austin-Flint" murmur in systole at apex
MVP	Rheumatic fever, Marfan syndrome, Infective endocarditis

Understanding Cyanotic Vs. Acyanotic Congenital Heart Defects

(covered in more detail in Pediatric Chapter 24)

- Defects in the heart will be either cyanotic or acyanotic depending on whether the defect makes blood flow from left to right (acyanotic), or right to left (cyanotic).
- When a defect (ASD, VSD) causes a left to right shunt --- oxygenated blood is flowing to the right heart and then going back through the lungs --- not efficient, but not cyanotic.
- When a defect (Tetralogy of Fallot (TOF), transposition) causes deoxygenated blood to flow into the left heart, the patient will be desaturated – that blood never gets to the lungs (or very little).
- Hypoplastic left heart is a special case where there is, essentially, no LV function at all, obviously causing cyanosis. This is usually evident immediately after birth or after PDA closure.

CYANOTIC LESIONS (IDENTIFIED BY CYANOSIS & NEONATE DISTRESS)

Tetralogy of Fallot – Most Common of Cyanotic Lesions

- *Tetralogy means "four" anomalies; they are:*
    - Pulmonary stenosis
    - Ventricular septal defect
    - Right ventricular hypertrophy (from the right sided circulation in utero)
    - Overriding aorta
- *Treatment = surgical*

Transposition of the Great Vessels

- *As it sounds, aorta comes off RV, and pulmonary artery off the LV*
- *Clinical intervention*
    - Prostaglandins; eventually surgical repair

- Keeps ductus arteriosus open so blood can mix
- Prostaglandin E1 (Alprostadil)

Hypoplastic Left Heart Syndrome

- Congenital absence or hypoplasia of the left ventricle
- Often die shortly after birth
- Treatment = heart transplant

These kids are in trouble – it is almost always evident fairly soon after birth with cyanosis being the initial concern. The clinical intervention is immediate intervention, surgery, resuscitation.

ACYANOTIC LESIONS (BABY SEEMS FINE)

Ventricular septal defect (VSD) – *most common*

Atrial Septal Defect (ASD)

Patent Ductus Arteriosis (PDA)

These kids can get into trouble, or be completely asymptomatic – what is evident after birth is a murmur, but you will recall that the ductus arteriosis can take a couple of days to close, and severe clinical manifestations may not present until PDA closure. Clinical intervention is close follow up; and if a loud murmur; or any pulmonary/cardiac symptoms – get an echocardiogram.

Manifestations of Renal Failure Explained

Cardio-Renal Physiology is complicated!

Kidney Function

- *Synthesis of erythropoietin*
  - If chronic renal failure, profound anemia results
- *Excretion of creatinine, uric acid, toxins*
- *Metabolism of Vitamin D to D3*
  - If chronic renal failure, hypocalcemia will result
- *Acid-base balance*
  - The proximal tubule secretes and excretes hydrogen ion.
    - If chronic renal failure, hydrogen ion not excreted = metabolic acidosis
  - The distal tubule makes bicarb, and retains bicarb to neutralize acid.
    - If chronic renal failure, no bicarb = metabolic acidosis
- *Synthesis of renin*
  - Synthesis of renin causes hypertension in most patients with renal issues.

Renal failure causes multiple issues all causing a constellation of events. Since renal failure is becoming an epidemic, it is important to recognize the pathophysiology caused by renal failure:

Decreased Renal Perfusion Activates the RAAS System:

- Renin is secreted in response to receptors that sense hypoperfusion.
- Renin secretion causes conversion of angiotensinogen (from liver) to angiotensin 1.
- Angiotensin 1 is converted to Angiotensin 2 by Angiotensin converting enzymes (ACE).
  - **A2 has two main effects**
    - *Peripheral vasoconstriction*
      - This moves blood from extremities into central vasculature
        - Increases BP/afterload
        - Increases preload
    - *Stimulates aldosterone secretion by adrenal*
      - Causes renal tubules to retain sodium
        - "Where sodium goes, so goes water"
        - Increases preload/volume
        - and with increased water, increases BP/afterload

Recall that CO = SV x HR (cardiac output = stroke volume x heart rate)
Stroke volume is dependent on:

- *preload*
- *afterload*
- *contractility of the heart*

When the kidney is underperfused, it will assume that cardiac output is decreased and will do what it can to increase preload, BP, and contractility. The sympathetic nervous system will take care of increasing the HR. All of this improves renal perfusion by increasing cardiac output.

Therefore, the renin-angiotensin-aldosterone system (RAAS) is:

- A good compensatory mechanism during times of drought/dehydration/hypovolemia
- A bad compensatory mechanism in a patient who has normal extracellular volume but poor cardiac output (*perceived* hypovolemia).

Consequences of Decreased GFR (Glomerular Filtration Rate)

- *Decreased excretion of creatinine*
  - Our most sensitive marker of renal failure
- *Decreased excretion of urea (elevated BUN)*
  - Causing generalized pruritis, anorexia, nausea
- *Decreased excretion of uric acid*
  - Causing gout and uric acid stones
- *Abnormal acid-base balance (typically, metabolic acidosis)*
  - We take in a high daily acid load; the kidney is responsible for buffering it.
  - Decreased excretion of hydrogen and potassium **and**
  - Decreased ability to make bicarbonate
    - Will result, therefore, in metabolic acidosis
- *Loss of albumin*
  - Decreased albumin for hormonal transport

    - Decreased albumin to make immunoglobulins
    - Decreased albumin for osmotic balance
        - All of this results in immunocompromised status, coagulopathy, third-spacing of fluid
- *Abnormal water balance*
    - Retention from all above
    - The loop functions late into failure, so furosemide works after thiazides no longer work at the renal tubule.

Vasopressin/ADH

- ADH is synthesized in the hypothalamus, and is stored in the posterior pituitary gland.
- The posterior pituitary gland secretes Antidiuretic Hormone (ADH), also known as vasopressin, in response to hypoperfusion
- *It causes the kidneys to :*
    - As ADH, it causes water retention to increase preload
    - As Vasopression, it causes peripheral vasoconstriction of the arteriolar system of the body to increase afterload
    - Increasing preload and afterload will increase the stroke volume and cardiac output.

Recall that this is great for the volume depleted patient, but not-so-great for the guy in the recliner eating hamburgers, fries, and beer with the lousy cardiac pump.

Are ACEI's good or bad?

Answer: Good – for the most part.

Discussion: The renal protective effects of ACE inhibition are proven. However, recall that ACE is there so that our kidneys help increase perfusion to themselves. When we block ACE to a pair of kidneys that are already under-perfused, the kidneys will be in trouble. Always remember to check a S. creatinine within a week to make sure that the kidneys are tolerating ACE inhibition.

What about NSAIDs?

Answer: If you are an ortho PA, they are good. If you are a nephrology PA, they are bad.

Discussion: Recall that prostaglandin is there to keep vessels open. (We use prostaglandin in cyanotic congenital heart diseases to keep the ductus arteriosis open so that blood can mix). If you block prostaglandin in a patient who has decreased renal perfusion, that perfusion will worsen. Many of the patients that I see in renal failure are taking NSAID's, and the treatment is to stop the NSAID, perfuse the kidney, and hopefully let the kidney recover. Be very careful in whom you given an NSAID to on this exam, and be on the lookout for the patient who should *not* be given an NSAID (aspirin or Tylenol would be a better choice in your renally insufficient patient).

WATER BALANCE, OSMOLALITY

Key Principles:

- 60% of body weight is water
- 2/3 of that water is intracellular (blood cells and tissue)
- 1/3 of that water is extracellular (plasma and interstitial fluid)

- Sodium (Na+) is most important extracellular cation
- Potassium (K+) is most important intracellular anion

- Decrease in blood volume activates RAAS system (see renal chapter)
- Decrease in body water activates ADH/vasopressin

Osmotic Pressure

- Pressure within the vascular system (extracellular) controls the distribution of body water among the "compartments"
- Osmolality = number of dissolved particles in the fluid (these are measured = NA+, K+, Cl-, HCO3-, Ca++, Mg, urea)
- Sodium is the most important cation effecting osmotic pressure
    - If sodium goes down, osmotic pressure goes down
    - If sodium goes up, osmotic pressure goes up
- If there is an "osmolal gap" – something is there that isn't measured (glucose, lipids, proteins amyloid, myeloma, toxins)

Can you think of something that could cause a patient to have low sodium, but have a high osmolality?

Answer: hyperglycemia

Discussion: Normally sodium determines the osmolality/osmolarity of the extracellular fluid (ECF). However, if the patient has a glucose of 500 mg/dL, then those large particles of glucose are now in the ECF (instead of the cell); and it will "displace" the sodium that is there. If you move that glucose back into the cell, the sodium "returns to normal". We call this "pseudohyponatremia". Diabetic ketoacidosis is the most common cause of a hyperosmolar hyponatremia.

Other causes would be mannitol or acetazolamide given to lower CSF pressures, or in treatment of acute angle glaucoma. Which is more common: DM or mannitol administration? Yes, DM is the most likely cause.

ARTERIAL BLOOD GASES AND ACID BASE BALANCE

Normal ABG Values (these numbers are for reference in the next section, remember – you will have a lab pull down menu on the test!)

pH = 7.35-7.45

pO2 = 80-100 mm Hg

pCO2 = 35-45 mm Hg

HCO3 = 22-26 mEq

SaO2 = 97-100%

MOST IMPORTANT CONCEPTS

- Increase in hydrogen ions = pH↓
- Decrease in hydrogen ions = pH↑
- CO2 is a weak acid (see equilibrium equation below), but:
    - In an ABG, the pCO2 is the acid; HCO3 is the base (as in my ABG examples below).
    - When you get an electrolyte panel on a CMP (comprehensive metabolic panel), the CO2 is the total CO2 and actually represents bicarbonate (HCO3) in the serum, not pCO2.
- The pO2 and the SaO2 are about perfusion (low = hypoxemia)
- The pCO2 is an acid, and is about ventilation (high = acidosis; low = alkalosis;)

Acid-Base Balance

$$H2O + CO2 \longleftrightarrow H2CO3 \longleftrightarrow H + HCO3$$

When trying to figure out a patient's acid-base abnormality, it is important first to decide if it is primarily a respiratory problem:

- Is the patient having difficulty breathing?
- Does the patient have a PMH of asthma/copd?
- Does the patient have a metabolic problem instead (i.e., renal failure, endocrine disease)?

The equilibrium equation above illustrates both. The left side of the equation represents the respiratory part of the problem, and the right represents the metabolic part of the problem. In the middle (and effected by both respiratory and metabolic problems), is carbonic acid = a weak acid.

Since this is an equilibrium equation, it would make sense that carbonic acid (weak acid) must be "equal to" water (neutral) + $CO2$ (which, therefore must be a weak acid).

Therefore, CO2 is a weak acid.

The way the lungs adjust acid and base is by either blowing off this weak acid, or retaining it. Ventilation is the process that gets rid of acid (CO2). Now, it's important to recall that ventilation has little to do with perfusion. Ventilation = CO2 Perfusion = 02

If I were to put my hand over your nose and mouth for 3 ½ minutes, you would still be perfusing, but you would not be able to ventilate. Even if your "bellows" were moving --- even if your intercostal muscles were retracting to try to ventilate --- as long as my hand stays firmly over your nose and mouth, you will not be ventilating. Your body will retain CO2, and you will develop a respiratory acidosis.

If you are sitting outside the Pearson Vue testing center waiting to take your exam, and your respiratory rate increases to 38, you will be "blowing" CO2 into the air in the testing center,(i.e. blowing off CO2), and you would develop a respiratory alkalosis.

- So, let's think about what is similar to my hand over your nose and mouth...COPD, severe asthma (with mucus plugging preventing ventilation), a PNB (pulseless non-breather), a heroin overdose with a RR of 4. All these patients have an acute or chronic respiratory acidosis.

- Now, let's think about what is similar to hyperventilation: anything causing tachypnea (i.e., an early asthma attack, panic attack, pulmonary embolism)

Frequently, the exam will give you the patient's vital signs. Make sure you pay attention to the RR or the patient's past medical history (COPD, 100 pack-year smoker, risk factors for PE; dusky leg). Or, the information in the stem may tell you that the patient has a respiratory acidosis and ask you for the most common cause from a list. Make sure you understand this concept, and any way that it is asked, you will get the question correct!

Now, let's do the metabolic side of the equation: H^+ + $HCO3^-$

- **Hydrogen ion is a strong acid.**
  - Hydrogen ion is secreted by the renal distal convoluted tubule in response to the kidney's perceiving an acidosis. If the kidney sees too much acid, its job is to get rid of it.

- **What is the most common way that a patient loses hydrogen ion? Vomiting (loss of HCl)**
  - Therefore, excessive vomiting will cause a loss of H+, and the patient will develop a metabolic alkalosis.

- **The kidney also has the ability to either make new bicarbonate or reabsorb bicarbonate in the proximal convoluted tubule to buffer an acidosis.**

- **Bicarbonate is a weak base.**
  - What is the most common way that a patient loses bicarbonate?

        - Diarrhea (loss of HCO_3, from the duodenum – used to buffer HCl coming from the stomach)
    - Therefore, prolonged diarrhea will cause a loss of HCO_3, and the patient will develop a metabolic acidosis.

ANION GAP

The easiest way to remember how to figure out the AG two years from now:

- When given an electrolyte panel:
- Take the highest number (Na) and subtract the other numbers from it
- Normal AG should be 10.

Na (Sodium)	**140**
Cl (Chloride)	**100**
CO2 (aka HCO3)	**26**
K (Potassium	**4**

So, 140 - 130 = 10 (normal AG)

Sometimes, the patient has something present in his body that is "acidic" and it is not Na, Cl, or HCO3. When you do the math, you find that there is a gap in the anion "count". The AG is 35. Well, what in the world is creating that gap?

It is something either being produced by the body that is acidic (causing the anion gap acidosis) or is something taken by the patient that is acidic (causing the anion gap acidosis).

We have an acronym for AG, but it is old and not very useful anymore --- so far, I have not been able to come up with anything better so I still use it: **MUDPILES**

- *Methanol*
    - Alcoholics will drink methanol accidentally or intentionally (to prevent DT's)
- *Uremia*
    - Patients with renal failure can have either an anion gap acidosis or a non-anion gap acidosis, depending on the amount of waste products built up in their blood
- *Diabetic Ketoacidosis*
    - **This is #1!**
    - The unmeasured anion is ketotic acid (or serum ketones)
        - It is produced as the metabolic breakdown product of fat metabolism in the diabetic.
        - There is no insulin to carry glucose to the cell for fuel.
        - The body utilizes fat for fuel, and this produces ketones, which are acidic.
- *Paraldehyde*
    - Ignore this one – never used anymore – used to be a neuroleptic drug

- *Ischemia? Inorganic phosphates? Isoniazid? No one agrees.*
- *Lactic acidosis*
  - **This is #2!**
  - The most common causes of lactic acidosis are:
    - A PNB (anaerobic metabolism of muscle)
    - An elderly person who falls and is not found until the next day (anaerobic metabolism of muscle)
    - Excess exertion (particularly if dehydrated) causes advanced muscle breakdown
    - Metformin can cause a lactic acidosis (particular in underperfused kidneys)
      - Contraindicated in CRF, CHF, alcoholism, liver failure
- *Ethylene glycol (antifreeze)*
  - Alcoholics developing delirium tremens will drink whatever they have to in order to avoid death. Unfortunately, drinking antifreeze kills them too – look in the question for an ETOH history.
- *Salicylate overdose*
  - We still see patients every occasionally who take bottles of aspirin - look in the question for a psychiatric history.

Compensation for acid-base problems

- The lungs compensate quickly for a metabolic abnormality of either acid or base:
  - If the patient has a metabolic acidosis, the lungs will hyperventilate CO2 to try to blow off acid; this is what happens in a patient with DKA (diabetic ketoacidosis)
  - If the patient has a metabolic alkalosis, the lungs will retain CO2 to try to increase the acid in the body and the respiratory rate will be depressed.
- The kidneys compensate too for a respiratory abnormality, but it takes 48 to 72 hours for a significant buffering to occur:
  - If the patient has a respiratory acidosis, the renal tubules will excrete H^+ and will generate and reabsorb $HCO3^-$.
  - If the patient has a respiratory alkalosis, the renal tubules will reabsorb H^+ and will excrete $HCO3^-$.

Autoimmune Pathophysiology

The Inflammatory Process

- Inflammation is a protective attempt by the organism to remove a foreign substance and begin the healing process.

- Inflammation is *not the same* as infection, even in cases where inflammation is caused by infection. Infection is caused by a foreign pathogen, while inflammation is one of the responses of the organism to that pathogen.

- Without inflammation, wounds and infections would never heal. However, chronic inflammation can also lead to a host of diseases. It is for that reason that the normal body closely regulates inflammation.

There are two main types of immune defense

- *Innate* - that we are all born with
    - The innate defense system includes cytokines, phagocytic activity, secreting interleukin, interferon, and tnf-alpha (tumor necrosis factor).
- *Acquired* - after being exposed to things.

What happens in an inflammatory response to injury or infection?

- *At the onset of an infection or injury, immune cells (monocytes, macrophages) undergo activation and release the inflammatory mediators discussed above.*
    - Vasodilation and its resulting increased blood flow cause the redness and warmth.
    - Increased permeability of the blood vessels results in leakage of fluid into the tissue causing swelling and edema.
    - Bradykinin release increases sensitivity to pain.
    - The mediator molecules alter the blood vessels to make them more permeable to the migration of leukocytes outside of the blood vessels into the tissue.
- *In addition to cell-derived mediators, several cascade systems consisting of plasma proteins initiate and propagate the inflammatory response.*
- *These include:*
    - The complement system activated by bacteria and other pathogens
        - The complement system has the potential to be extremely damaging to host tissues, meaning its activation must be tightly regulated. In many autoimmune diseases, the "control mechanism" that stops the complement system is "faulty" causing chronic destruction of normal tissue.
    - The coagulation and fibrinolytic systems activated by necrosis
        - This is why patients after trauma are considered *"hypercoagulable"*.

PEARL: In normal conditions, inflammation ceases once the stimulus has been removed. The problem with autoimmune diseases is that the inflammation never ceases, and the patient's system is destroyed by the constant assault.

Coagulation Physiology

I recall having to learn the entire coagulation cascade including all factors and cofactors. How well has that served me? Unless you use it every day, no one can remember it after 30 years! The key to getting coagulation questions correct is to remember a few basic tenets (simplistic, for sure)

There are three pathways – they work in concert with one another:

- the intrinsic pathway (Factor VIII)
- the extrinsic pathway
- the common pathway (platelet function)

This section will explain the most important parts of the pathway, the most important factors to understand, and a very general understanding of why it all works, and then, hopefully, you can understand what happens when it doesn't work, and remember it for the next 30 years.

NORMAL HEMOSTASIS

The best way to think about normal hemostasis is that nature provided several different ways to get clotting done. However, it is a balancing act --- once clotting is activated, it cannot continue unchecked. As cave dwellers, injuries occurred and there were no PAs to suture things up.

So, when an injury occurred to a limb:

- The first step was platelets were activated
  - *The action of platelets caused a loose kind of plug (think your hand around a hole in a garden hose, slows the flow but does not stop it)*
- Following platelet activation, if enough tissue factor is released, the coagulation cascade will be activated (provides a good fibrin clot).
- There are two parts to that cascade as well, so if one is missing factors on one side, the other side still helps. All designed to keep the human alive.
  - *The extrinsic pathway*
  - *The intrinsic pathway*
- Once clot is formed, the "anti-clotting" pathway is activated to limit the activity; without which the entire vasculature would clot, and that would be bad.

PLATELET ACTIVATION- PRIMARY HEMOSTASIS

- Platelets are very dynamic, bouncing around until activated.
- Normal platelets in normal vessels will not stick to undamaged vessel walls.
- Primary hemostasis occurs causing platelets to attach to the vessel wall (platelet adhesion)
  - Then they release platelet granules which call in more platelets
  - And under the effects of von Willebrand factor (vWF), these platelets stick to each other (platelet aggregation)
  - Under the effects of released GIIb/IIIa that binds vWF, causing a loose clump of platelets to form to slow flow.
- Tissue factor is exposed after:
  - damage to the endothelium (trauma to a vessel)
  - gram negative bacteremia (monocytes induce expression when trying to kill bacteria)
  - retained products of conception, term still birth, necrotic tissue; disseminated cancers; some leukemias

Vessel wall constriction also occurs at the same time as the tissue factor and platelet process.

- Endothelial cells normally have prostacyclin that maintains normal contractile state of smooth muscle
- If the endothelial cells are damaged and are unable to make prostacyclin, constriction will occur
- There is also epinephrine (released by the body in trauma) that causes vasoconstriction

THE COAGULATION CASCADE- SECONDARY HEMOSTASIS

- activated at the same time as primary hemostasis
- The clotting cascade begins to form a more effective clot
- Activation of the coagulation factors finishes the hemostatic process

The role of vonWillebrand Factor

- Responsible for making platelets "stick"--- we all have some – but there is an autosomal disorder which causes *decrease* in the amount of vwf present
- vWF causes platelets to "stick", and slows the degradation of Factor VIII which is degraded rapidly without it
- With too little vWF, there will be decreased platelet aggregation, and too little Factor VIII.

PEARL: My students have given me a way to remember the pathways this way:

- The intrinsic pathway causes more intravascular bleeding (spontaneous joint bleeds/hemarthrosis) than the extrinsic or platelet pathway.
  - The intrinsic pathway is for inpatients, who are on heparin, measured by the aPTT – **Factor VIII** is in this pathway (know this!)
- The extrinsic and platelet pathways cause more purpura, petechia, mucosal membrane bleeding (epistaxis, gingival, menstrual bleeding)
  - The extrinsic pathway is for outpatients, who are on warfarin --- PT/INR
  - The platelet's ability to function has to do with both platelet number and platelet function. Even with normal platelet numbers, if they do not "stick" there is going to be a problem with mucosal/skin bleeding

So, if the exam question tells you that a patient has purpura and petechiae but no internal bleeding, you should be thinking of a **platelet** problem or **extrinsic** pathway issue.

If the question tells you that this patient has spontaneous bleeding into his gut, or his joint, then you are looking at an **intrinsic** pathway problem (aPTT would be measured) – **think Factor VIII**.

The truth is clinically, we usually order these two tests together, but that would not get at the "scientific concept" issue of a bleeding disorder. So, know this basic distinction, and it will serve you well on the exam.

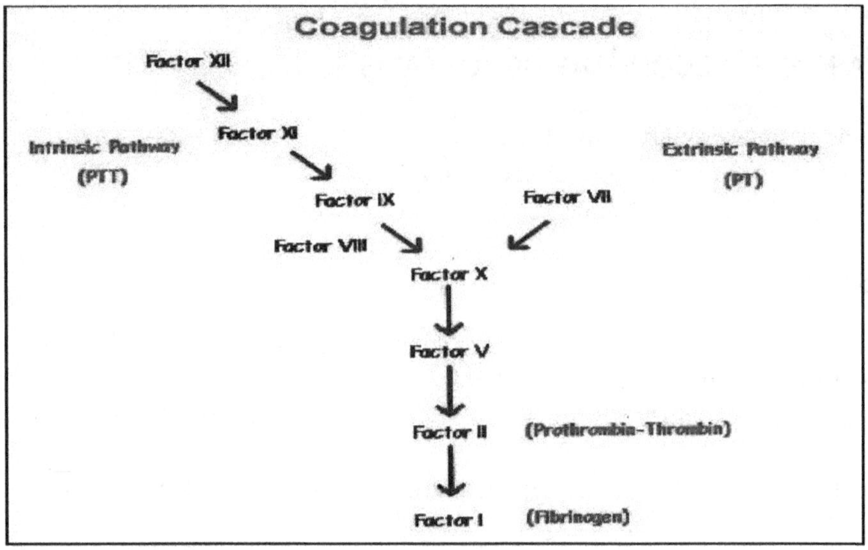

NOTE: Both pathways converge on the common pathway; activating Factor X, which results in prothrombin activation, and conversion of prothrombin to thrombin.

Now, the anti-clotting proteins (Antithrombin, Protein C, Protein S) start to work to limit the clot formation, and eventually remove the clot by breaking up fibrin (once the vessel is healed, no need for a big old clot), resulting in fibrin degradation products (also known as D-Dimer). *That's it!*

PEARL: Virchow's Triad = endothelial damage + stasis of blood + hypercoagulable state = clot!

PLATELET DISORDERS = COMMON PATHWAY

- ITP (Idiopathic thrombocytopenic purpura)
- TTP (Thrombotic thrombocytopenic purpura)
- vWD (vonWillebrand's Disease)

VITAMIN K DISORDERS= EXTRINSIC PATHWAY

- Liver disease
- Dietary deficiency/malabsorption

FACTOR DISORDERS= INTRINSIC PATHWAY

- Hemophilia A & B

All of these coagulation problems are covered in detail in Hematology Chapter 23.

Evaluating Bodily Fluids

(pleural, pericardial, synovial, peritoneal, CNS)

There are general concepts to understand whenever you get a question about evaluating the likely cause of a collection of fluid in the body.

The single exception to my general rule is when you evaluate CNS fluid, so that will be covered separately below.

In general, the main objective is to figure out if it is a "transudative" or "exudative" effusion:

- **Transudates are similar to water.**
  - Water has a low specific gravity (1.000), has no protein, would have no LDH, would have no cells; therefore would be transudative.

- **Exudates are similar to pus.**
  - Pus has a high specific gravity (due to particles in the fluid), has high protein, high LDH and increased white blood cells, and therefore would be exudative.

- **Glucose in the body fluid may vary** --- you compare the body fluid glucose to the serum glucose level. Think of glucose as being consumed by cells and bacteria in infections and exudative effusions, therefore, the body fluid glucose would be lower than that in the patient's serum.

PEARL: It is not about the body fluid glucose being "normal", it is about how much lower than the patient's serum glucose it is (so remember, in a diabetic patient):

- If serum glucose = 267 and pleural fluid glucose = 92
  - This is a *low* pleural fluid glucose for this patient (even though it is 92)!

Very generally then, when evaluating a list of laboratory results from a fluid specimen, look for these findings:

Clarity

- The cloudier the fluid, the more likely exudative
- Clear fluid is more likely transudative (straw color is normal except for CSF which should be completely colorless)

Specific Gravity

- The higher the specific gravity, the more likely exudative (>1.018)
- The lower the specific gravity the more likely transudative (< 1.005), i.e. like water

Cell Count

- The more segmented neutrophils present, the more likely it is bacterial (exudative)

- Lack of neutrophils, or just a few monocytes, the more likely it is transudative

Protein & LDH (also known as "Light's criteria for exudative effusion"

- The ratio of pleural fluid protein to serum protein is greater than 0.5
- The ratio of pleural fluid LDH and serum LDH is greater than 0.6

Glucose

- The lower the body fluid glucose compared to serum, the more likely an exudative effusion
- Fluid glucose and serum glucose are the same in a transudative effusion (it is just body water)

Most important to remember:

- The higher the LDH, the more likely malignant (cell lysis) –(increased pleural fluid: serum fluid LDH)
- The higher the protein, the more likely exudative (increased pleural fluid: serum fluid protein) – in other words the pleural fluid has more protein than the serum
- The lower the protein (or the ratio of pleural to serum protein), the more likely it is transudative (water does not have protein in it!)

Next step: know the most common causes of transudative effusions and exudative effusions:

Transudative effusions (water):

- Congestive heart failure – most common cause
- Renal failure (osmotic movement of fluid due to loss of albumin)
- Liver failure (similar to above)

Exudative effusions (pus/cells):

- Infection (bacterial, fungal, TB) – most common cause
- Malignancy
- Collagen vascular diseases (SLE, RA))
- Uremia

In Summary:

- ***Normal*** = low protein, normal glucose, no (<3) cells
- ***Bacterial infection*** = high protein, low glucose, >500 PMN's and monocytes
- ***Viral infection*** = high or normal protein, normal glucose, lymphocytes and monocytes

<u>CSF fluid is quite different:</u>

- Remember that the first thing that happens when the needle is inserted is "opening pressures" are measured – normal CSF opening pressure is 5-20. If > 30, there is a bacterial or viral infection.
- Unlike the rest of the body fluid, the CSF fluid should *not* be colored, it should be crystal clear.
- Unlike the rest of the body fluid, the CSF should contain no more than 3 (*three*) cells.
- In bacterial infection, cell count will be very high (> 500) with almost all of them PMN's (the bacteria white cells)
- In viral infection, cell count may be high but the cells should be monos and lymphs

CSF FLUID ANALYSIS

	Normal	**Viral**	**Fungal/TB**	**Bacterial**
Pressure (cmH20)	5-20	Normal /mildly increased		>30
Appearance	Normal	Clear	Fibrin web	Turbid
Protein (g/L)	<1	<1	0.1 - 0.5	>1
Glucose	Normal	Normal	Low	Low
Gram Stain	Negative	Negative	Negative	60-90% Positive
Glucose CSF:Serum Ratio	0.6	>0.6	<0.4	<0.4
WBC Count	<3	<1000	100-500	>500
Other		Monocytes/ 30% have >50% PMN	Monocytes	90% PMN

SECTION FOUR – THE CONTENT BLUEPRINT

CHAPTER 11

Cardiovascular Medicine – 16%

Introduction to the Cardiovascular Medicine Content

Cardiovascular medicine will constitute the majority of questions on the exam. It is the most common reason for presentation to a clinic or hospital, and ischemic heart disease is the number one cause of death worldwide.

Topics are not presented in alphabetical order as in the NCCPA Blueprint. Instead, I have organized the topics both in terms of importance, but also categorized together in a way to organize the learning.

The entire chapter is arranged so that the cardiovascular diseases that lead to congestive heart failure are discussed, and then congestive heart failure discussion follows. Life-threatening presentations are presented with more emphasis; and where a disease is very uncommon in clinical practice, this is noted as well.

In most instances, at the review course, attendees that did not score well on the exam were found to be lacking in their CV scores (which makes sense as this topic is weighted most heavily among all the topics in the Blueprint).

For this reason, this section should constitute the majority of your study, unless, of course, you practice Cardiology (lucky you!).

Ischemic Heart Disease

PEARL: *Ischemic Heart Disease:* As the most common cause of death in humans, ischemic heart disease causes acute myocardial infarction that eventually leads to congestive heart failure for most patients. The atherosclerotic disease that occurs in the coronary arterial system is the same disease that occurs in the aorta, carotid arteries, renal arteries, and peripheral arteries. All the plaques that develop are due to a constellation of risk factors including: dyslipidemia, hypertension, diabetes, smoking, family history, obesity and inactivity (look for these words in the stem as your "clue" that your patient may have plaque in an artery of the body)

ACUTE CORONARY SYNDROME

Angina Pectoris

Stable Angina

- Fixed threshold to pain ("x" amount of exertion produces pain, so patient keeps himself below that threshold)
- Always relieved quickly with nitroglycerin (NTG)
- Preventing future attacks
    - Beta-blocker

Unstable angina

- Either "new", or never experienced before, or
- Increase in frequency, or
- Lowered threshold of activity to produce discomfort, or
- More nitroglycerin required for anginal pain

ACUTE MYOCARDIAL INFARCTION (NSTEMI and STEMI)

- **Epidemiology**
    - Men > women prior to menopause, then incidence equalizes
    - Most common cause of death in humans on earth
- **Etiology**
    - Thrombosis - plaque rupture with platelet aggregation and occlusion of a coronary artery
    - Recall that historically (30 yrs ago) it was thought that this was an "embolic" phenomenon.
        - Of course, back then there was little understanding of the atherosclerotic plaque development problems.
- **Risk Factors**
    - Male gender
    - Female after menopause
    - Family history of premature coronary artery disease (CAD)
        - *The younger the onset of CAD in a first-degree relative, the greater the risk.*
        - *This is now felt to be a most important risk factor.*
    - Dyslipidemia
    - Hypertension
    - Diabetes
    - Smoking
    - Sedentary lifestyle; obesity
    - Increased "chronic" inflammation
        - Recent interest in measuring inflammatory markers
            - High-sensitivity CRP most commonly used
- **H&P Findings**
    - Chest pressure/squeezing/tightness/heaviness
    - Diaphoresis

- +/- Nausea/Vomiting
- S4 (due to myocardial "stunning")
- +/- rales;

- **Labs & Diagnostics** *(discussed in detail in Chapter 6)*
    - *Cardiac enzyme elevation*
        - CK-MB
        - Troponin
    - *ECG*
        - STEMI
            - ST elevation in corresponding leads
        - ST-T changes
            - Nonspecific, but in corresponding leads
- **Clinical Intervention**
    - ***<u>MONA B</u>***
        - **M**orphine
            - Not in SBP < 100 mm Hg
        - **O**xygen
            - Usually only needs 2 l. nasal cannula oxygen
            - If severely hypoxic, rethink diagnosis
            - More likely pulmonary (is it a PE?)
        - **N**itrates
            - Vasodilation
            - Will drop BP; do not use in SBP < 100 mm Hg.
        - **A**spirin (aspirin is first)
            - Only contraindication is anaphylaxis to aspirin in acute MI
        - **B**eta-blocker
            - After stable; within 24 hours, begin beta blocker if possible
                - Proven reduction in mortality if given within 24 hours
            - Not in HR < 60 bpm; SBP < 100 mmg Hg, AV nodal blockade, reactive airway disease
- **Health Maintenance**
    - Smoking cessation
    - Manage HTN
    - Manage lipids
    - 81 mg. ASA
        - Little advantage chronically between 81 mg. and 325 mg., and lower rate of bleeding with 81 mg. dose

PEARL: Beta-blockers are the only antianginal agents that have been demonstrated to prolong life in patients with coronary disease post-MI. CCB's do not; in fact, short-acting nifedipine *increases* the risk of death in the immediate post-MI period.

VARIANT ANGINA/PRINZMETAL'S ANGINA

- **Epidemiology**
    - Young women; minimal risk factors for CAD

- **H & P**
  - Chest pain, often at rest, during stress or without precipitant
- **Formulating Most Likely Diagnosis**
  - Nonexertional
  - Relieved with NTG
  - ECG evidence of ischemia during pain
  - Angiography shows no CAD
    - Shows coronary artery vasospasm
- **Clinical Intervention**
  - Responds to nifedipine/amlodipine
  - Avoid triptans if patient has migraine history, which many do

---

Cardiomyopathy

PEARL: *Cardiomyopathy:* Cardiomyopathy is an abnormality of the cardiac muscle itself (and not of the coronary arteries, per se.) which eventually leads to congestive heart failure. There are three main types of cardiomyopathies:

- Dilated
- Hypertrophic
- Restrictive

DILATED CARDIOMYOPATHY

- **Epidemiology**
  - Most common of the cardiomyopathies
  - Causes systolic dysfunction, ejection fraction (EF) < 40% is key!
- **Etiology**
  - Acute myocardial infarction (AMI)
    - Causing necrosis and poor muscle function
  - Alcohol = #1 poison
  - Viruses (Coxsackie most common)
  - Drugs (Doxorubicin most common – chemo for breast cancer)
- **H & P findings**
  - Dyspnea on exertion (DOE)
  - Jugular venous distension (JVD)
  - Hepatojugular reflex (HJR)
  - Peripheral edema
  - S3 (from volume overload)
  - Laterally displaced point of maximum impulse (PMI)
- **Labs & Diagnostics**
  - CXR showing cardiomegaly
  - Echocardiogram – dilatation of the left ventricle (LV)
- **Clinical Intervention**
  - Same as congestive heart failure chronic management (later in this chapter)
- **Therapeutics**

- Same as congestive heart failure (see below)

- **Health Maintenance**
  - Limit alcohol
  - Manage blood pressure
  - Manage lipids
  - Manage diabetes
  - Have patient exercise regularly
  - Prevention is key!

HYPERTROPHIC CARDIOMYOPATHY

- **Epidemiology**
  - Most common cause of diastolic dysfunction (EF>40%)
- **Pathophysiology**
  - Due to chronically increased LV pressures
  - Causes problems with filling (not with contraction)
- **Etiologies**
  - HTN (with resultant LVH)
  - Aortic Stenosis (with resultant LVH)
  - Septal hypertrophy (Hypertrophic Cardiomyopathy)
- **H&P findings**
  - Hyperdynamic PMI
  - S4 (pressure overload)
- **Labs & Diagnostics**
  - *ECG*
    - Increased voltage
  - *Echocardiogram*
    - Increased LV thickness
- **Clinical Intervention**
  - Medical management of hypertension
  - Surgical management of valve disease
- **Therapeutics**
  - Beta-blockers
- **Health Maintenance**
  - Make sure you recognize abnormal BP (>140 or >90) -and treat it!

RESTRICTIVE MYOPATHIES

- **Epidemiology**
  - Least common of the myopathies
- **Etiology**
  - *Infiltrative disease*
    - Multiple myeloma
    - Hemochromatosis
    - Wilson's disease (Cu overload)
    - Sarcoidosis

- **H& P findings**
  - May have pulmonary symptoms from restrictive pulmonary infiltrates
- **Labs & Diagnostics**
  - *ECG*
    - Low voltage (infiltrative proteins interfere with conduction of electricity)
    - AV conduction abnormalities
- **Clinical Intervention**
  - Treat as a diastolic dysfunction
    - By definition, EF >40%
  - Treat underlying disease
- **Therapeutics**
  - Beta blockers

Valvular Disease

PEARL: *Valvular Disease:* Valvular disease is another common cause of a patient eventually developing congestive heart failure. Some valve disorders occur acutely (papillary muscle rupture, endocarditis with vegetation on the valve) and cause acute and severe pulmonary edema; other valve disorders occur chronically over 30-40 years (bicuspid aortic valve, mitral stenosis) and cause more insidious onset of congestive heart failure symptoms. In general, if a valvular disorder causes increased LV diastolic volumes (aortic insufficiency (AI), mitral insufficiency); it will cause a dilated myopathy. If the valve disorder causes increased LV pressures, i.e., aortic stenosis, hypertrophic cardiomyopathy, it will eventually cause a hypertrophic myopathy.

A new murmur occurring in a "sick" patient with a fever is infectious endocarditis until proven otherwise.

- If the patient is an IV drug user, expect that the infected valve will be on the "venous" side of the heart, i.e. tricuspid vegetations most commonly, followed by pulmonic valve.
- If the patient has had his/her teeth cleaned recently, or at the very least is not an IV drug user, expect the infected valve to be on the "arterial" side of the heart, mitral and aortic valve vegetations.

Echocardiogram is the most important diagnostic test to order in a patient with new fever and new murmur – admit the patient – start IV to cover appropriate pathogens (staph) --- and consult cardiology and ID. This is covered in more detail in section below.

Murmurs are covered separately in Physiology, Chapter 10.

AORTIC STENOSIS

- **Two main causes:**
  - *Congenital*
    - Due to a bicuspid aortic valve
    - Initially asymptomatic until the ripe old age of 40 or so, when the valve becomes less compliant

        - Hypertrophy of the ventricle is a clue (without elevated systemic BP, remember pressures are not high in the patient's arms, they are high in the ventricle pushing against a smaller aortic valve orifice!)
    - *Old age (relatively speaking)*
        - Atherosclerotic/degenerative change to the valve
        - Causes similar noncompliance to above
        - Increase LV systolic pressures, causing LVH
        - No matter what the etiology, the rest is the same
- **H & P**
    - Slow uprise of carotid pulse, not bounding (that's AR/AI!)
    - Systolic murmur (loud, harsh, grade 2-4/6, heard at the base)
- **Labs & Diagnostics**
    - Echocardiogram
- **Clinical Intervention**
    - Once symptoms, the only treatment is valve replacement
- **Scientific concept**
    - If congenital bicuspid aortic valve--- high correlation with coarctation of the aorta (and vice versa)

PEARL: Symptoms of critical aortic stenosis (AS) = SAD (syncope, angina, dyspnea)

Keep this pearl in mind when you have a patient on the test with a murmur who presents with syncope, with angina (may not be coronary disease) or with dyspnea (may not be pulmonary) There is a reason they're telling you there is a systolic harsh murmur heard best at the base!

AORTIC INSUFFICIENCY (AORTIC REGURGITATION)

- **Etiologies**
    - *Acute aortic insufficiency*
        - Vegetations on the valve (bacterial endocarditis)
        - Thoracic aortic dissection
    - *Chronic aortic insufficiency*
        - Aortic root dilatation (idiopathic)
        - Marfan's Syndrome (or other connective tissue diseases)
        - Autoimmune vasculitic syndromes
- **Pathophysiology**
    - Huge blood flow (back and forth, dilates the ventricle)
    - *Remember* – acute presentation is not remotely like chronic presentation.
- **H & P**
    - *In acute*
        - Sudden onset dyspnea, exercise intolerance
        - Decreased contractility
        - Heart is not able to compensate (it becomes dilated beyond the Frank-Starling curve, discussed in Chapter 10).
    - *In chronic*
        - Dyspnea, fatigue, very vague symptoms
    - *In general*
        - Diastolic, soft, murmur heard at the LSB

        - S3 (increased preload)
        - Huge pulses
        - Quincke's pulsations (nailbeds)
        - DeMussett's sign (head "bobbing" due to huge carotid pulse)
        - Waterhammer pulse (bounding radial pulse)
        - Widened pulse pressure
            - SBP is normal (or slightly high due to sympathetic tone); DBP is low
- **Labs & Diagnostics**
    - Echocardiogram
- **Clinical Intervention**
    - Valve replacement when symptomatic

MITRAL STENOSIS

- **Etiology**
    - Rheumatic fever
- **H & P**
    - Diastolic, rumbling murmur, heard at the apex, opening snap
    - For many years, the patient is asymptomatic
        - Often first manifestation of symptoms is during pregnancy
    - Pulmonary symptoms due to increased LA pressures backing up into the lungs *(see cardiopulmonary physiology section)*
        - DOE (dyspnea on exertion)
        - Hemoptysis (pink, frothy sputum)
- **Diagnostics**
    - Echocardiogram
- **Clinical Intervention**
    - Valve replacement
- **Scientific Concept**
    - Common cause of atrial fibrillation (as is anything that dilates the left or right atria)
    - Once atrial fibrillation develops, patient becomes severely symptomatic.

MITRAL INSUFFICIENCY

- **Etiology**
    - *Chronic*
        - Mitral valve stenosis
        - Marfan's syndrome
        - Rheumatic fever
    - *Acute*
        - Papillary muscle rupture
        - Vegetations (bacterial endocarditis)
- **H & P**
    - Blood flowing backward into LA causes systolic murmur heard at the apex
    - *In acute*
        - Sudden increased flow backwards causes increased LA volumes which then causes increased LA pressures, which then is reflected "backward" into the pulmonary vasculature and causes pulmonary congestion (dyspnea)

- *In chronic*
  - May be asymptomatic; may have palpitations; may eventually develop AFib
- **Diagnostics**
  - Echocardiogram
- **Clinical Intervention**
  - When symptomatic, valve replacement
  - If minimally symptomatic; decrease afterload (ACE Inhibitor)

MITRAL VALVE PROLAPSE

- **Epidemiology**
  - Female predominant syndrome
  - Association with migraine, autoimmune disease (thyroid, SLE)
  - No known or accepted etiology (some think a normal variant)
    - Although much more common in Marfan's syndrome and Ehlers-Danlos syndrome
  - Only important if it develops into mitral regurgitation/insufficiency
  - Responsible for 90% of all cases of MVR (mitral valve regurgitation)
    - However, not all patients (few) develop MVR from MVP!
- **Presentation**
  - Click (sometimes with a late systolic murmur)
  - Arrhythmias
  - Atypical chest pain
  - Anxiety
- **Labs & Diagnostics**
  - Echocardiogram
- **Clinical Intervention**
  - If palpitations, Beta-blockers seem to work best
  - ***Prophylactic antibiotics for dental cleaning is no longer indicated***

TRICUSPID STENOSIS

- **Etiology**
  - Rheumatic fever (usually more than one valve involved)
- **Labs & diagnostics**
  - Echocardiogram (transesophageal echo (TEE) usually best)
- **Clinical Intervention**
  - Medical
  - Manage symptoms (congestive heart failure treatment)
  - Surgical replacement

TRICUSPID INSUFFICIENCY

- **Etiology**
  - *Acute*
    - Infectious endocarditis (think IV drug user; shooting in vein, staph goes to R side of heart, i.e. tricuspid valve)
  - *Chronic*
    - Rheumatic Fever

- **Labs & diagnostics**
    - Echocardiogram (TEE usually best)
- **Clinical intervention**
    - Medical – treat atrial fibrillation if it develops *(see end of chapter for management of atrial fibrillation)*
    - Surgical – annuloplasty or replacement

PULMONARY VALVE STENOSIS

- **Epidemiology**
    - Much more common than pulmonary insufficiency
    - 80% of all R ventricular outflow tract abnormalities
        - Usually congenital (familial)– causing murmur
- **Presentation**
    - Systolic murmur; heard at the LSB; with a click
    - In neonate with critical stenosis – *cyanosis!*
    - Without critical stenosis – asymptomatic for years; worsens with time
    - RHF symptoms (peripheral edema; RVH on ECG and echo)

PULMONARY INSUFFICIENCY

- **Epidemiology/Etiology**
    - Dilatation of the pulmonic valve annulus
    - Abnormality of the pulmonic valve leaflets (vegetations, Marfan's)
    - Congenital abnormality of the valve
- **H & P**
    - Diastolic murmur at LSB (Graham-Steell murmur)
    - *Only if severe:*
        - JVD (jugular venous distention)
        - As valve worsens; evidence of RV fluid overload
- **Clinical Intervention**
    - Usually none; if asymptomatic, just observe
- **Scientific Concept**
    - Present in almost all humans
    - considered a normal echo finding if mild and no murmur

PEARL: *For those who just cannot do valves!*

- 80% of all valve diseases involve the aortic and mitral, so only do those two
- Pay attention to whether the murmur is described as occuring:
    - In systole or diastole and
    - At the apex (mitral) or at the base(aortic) or LSB
- If you need to, spend 10 seconds drawing the heart in systole on your dry erase board, and remind yourself which valve should be open and which should be closed...
- Don't get hung up on the descriptions, (i.e. crescendo-decrescendo; early systolic, holosystolic, musical, etc)

- If a murmur is heard in a symptomatic patient, let's just get an echo!

PEARL: *For those who need an acronym to remember the valves:*

Most murmurs occur in systole. The acronym, Mr. AsTr (Mister Aster) identifies the valve disorders that cause systolic murmurs.

Systolic murmurs = Mr. ASTR, P.S.

- **Mr. = Mitral Regurgitation**
- **AS = Aortic Stenosis**
- **TR – Tricuspid Regurgitation**
- **The acronym needs a P.S. too (Pulmonic Stenosis).**

Jot down on your dry erase board: Systolic = Mr. Astr, P.S.

Then, if the question is about diastolic murmurs, you know that the opposite valve disorders would be involved. (Mitral stenosis, Aortic regurg, etc). My students have told me this acronym has helped them remember during very stressful situations, so maybe it will work for you too!

Atrial Fibrillation

- **Basic tenets of atrial fibrillation**
  - *Most common of the sustained arrhythmias in older patients*
  - *Most common cause of thromboembolic stroke*
  - Due to ischemic heart disease or valve disease
  - If occurs in a young patient with healthy heart think other causes
    - Alcohol intoxication; cocaine or amphetamine use, etc.
    - Grave's disease, etc.
- *Irregular irregular rhythm without P waves makes diagnosis on ECG*
- Can occur with a slow, normal or rapid ventricular response rate (RVR)
- Can cause atrial clots which can cause acute arterial occlusions peripherally
  - Middle cerebral artery (MCA) occlusion causing stroke, acute LE occlusion
  - Superior mesenteric artery (SMA) occlusion causing ischemic bowel

MANAGEMENT

Hemodynamically Stable Patient

- Asymptomatic, elderly typical patient
  - *Normal BP, normal ventricular response rate*
- Check thyroid; r/o other causes (AMI, CHF, renal insufficiency)
- Anticoagulation should be considered. (see CHADS2 discussion below)

Hemodynamically Unstable Patient

- Usually due to RVR
- If shock or severe hypotension
    - Urgent cardioversion
    - Increased risk of embolism if A fib present > 48 hours
- *If unstable but not severe*
    - Rate control
    - Beta-blockers preferred
        - But not in hypotension (see cardioversion above)
    - CCB's
        - Only diltiazem (verapamil is too negatively inotropic)
    - Digoxin
        - Very slow in onset (usually too slow) but improves contractility
- *If need for cardioversion, and patient is stable*
    - Trans-esophageal echocardiogram (TEE) to r/o left atrial (LA) clots should be performed first

CHRONIC MANAGEMENT – RATE CONTROL

- If relatively healthy, diltiazem or BB is indicated
- Avoid verapamil if CHF or EF < 40% for any reason
- If Class 4 failure digoxin is indicated
    - Does not prolong life
    - Does not control HR when patient is active

- Rhythm control
    - Pharmacologic or DC cardioversion
    - Anticoagulation for 3-4 weeks prior
    - If documented onset within 48 hours may cardiovert without anticoagulation
    - Risk of stroke is the same whether pharmacologic or DC cardioversion
- Anticoagulation
    - CHADS2 ≥ 2, anticoagulation recommended
    - CHF (1 pt)
    - HTN (1 pt)
    - AGE >75 (1 pt)
    - DM (1 pt)
    - STROKE/TIA (2 pts)
- If CHADS2 = 1, then employ newer Chads2-VASC recommendations and add 1 pt for each of these RF's: female; age 65-74; vascular disease
- If anticoagulation is indicated, what should you use?
    - Warfarin – reduces risk by about 32%; more than placebo or aspirin alone
        - Still the mainstay of therapy
        - Vit. K antagonist; must avoid Vit. K rich foods
        - Relatively easy to reverse (compared to the others)
        - Difficult to maintain adequate therapeutic levels

- Aspirin – better than nothing if patient refuses all else
- Clopidogrel – used with aspirin but increased risk of bleeding
- Dabigatran, rivaroxaban, apixaban (the trans and bans suffixes!)
  - Direct thrombin inhibitor
  - Not indicated in patients with valve replacements or decompensated valve disease or mitral stenosis or those who will need valve replacement.
  - Lots of folks with valve disease have A fib.

- No matter which anticoagulant you use, in a head injury, the patient needs head CT even if asymptomatic
- Increased risk of GI bleeds

PEARL: In other words, almost all the "typical" patients who get A fib already meet criteria because it is their CHF, hypertension, and vascular disease that caused it in the first place! It seems to me there is not much to memorize here, almost all my patients with A fib meet criteria at the onset. This is useful perhaps in the 28-year-old Grave's disease patient who will have a CHADs score of 0 (and does not warrant anticoagulation, but instead needs an endocrinologist)

Bacterial Endocarditis

- **Basic Tenets of Bacterial Endocarditis:**
  - Can be acute (presenting in 2-3 days with fever and congestive heart failure) or sub-acute (indolent several-month course)
  - Causes valvular insufficiency (look for murmur of regurgitation)
  - Causes acute or subacute congestive heart failure (pulmonary edema and failure)
  - Can cause both sterile and infected embolization to the body
  - Causes immunologic responses
    - *Roth spots* – retinal pinpoint hemorrhages
    - *Janeway lesions* – flat, painless, red-bluish spots on palms & soles
    - *Subungual hemorrhages* –splinter hemorrhages under fingernails/toenails
    - *Osler nodes* – painful nodules, red on pads of fingers and toes
- **Can occur as three main types**:
  - In native valves (NVE)
  - In prosthetic valves (PVE)
  - In IV drug users

NVE (NATIVE VALVE ENDOCARDITIS)

- **Etiologies**
  - #1 etiology = rheumatic fever (30% of all causes)
  - #2 etiology = congenital valve disease (25%)
  - #3 etiology = MVP (20%)
  - #4 etiologies = other = Marfan's, syphilis, calcified aortic stenosis
- **Prognosis (cure rates)**
  - For S viridans and S bovis infection, the cure rate is 98%.
  - For enterococci and S aureus infection in individuals who abuse intravenous drugs, the cure rate is 90%.

- For community-acquired S aureus infection in individuals who do not abuse intravenous drugs, the cure rate is 60-70%.
- For infection with aerobic gram-negative organisms, the cure rate is 40-60%.
- For infection with fungal organisms, the cure rate is lower than 50%.

- **Clinical presentation**
  - Fever
  - Murmur (of insufficiency)
  - Congestive heart failure/pulmonary edema
- **Labs & Diagnostics**
  - Blood cultures
  - Echocardiogram
  - CXR/EKG
- **Clinical Intervention**
  - Cardiology and CT surgery referral
- **Health Maintenance**
  - See New Guidelines for Endocarditis Prophylaxis below

PVE (PROSTHETIC VALVE ENDOCARDITIS)

- **Epidemiology**
  - Mechanical valve – presents within first 3 months after insertion
  - Bioprosthetic valve – presents > a year after insertion
- **Pathogens**
  - Staph aureus
  - Gram negative bacilli
  - candida albicans
- **Prognosis**
  - PVE patients were older, presented with more compromised clinical conditions, and had worse early and long-term outcomes than NVE patients.
  - PVE had a higher incidence of recurrence and worse prognosis, especially if the mitral valve was involved
- **IV drug users**
  - Tricuspid valve affected in 50% of cases
  - Staph aureus
  - Cure rates 90% as described above in NVE

NEW GUIDELINES *FOR DENTAL PROPHYLAXIS* TO PREVENT INFECTIVE ENDOCARDITIS

New recommendations now recommend prophylaxis only for the following patient populations:

- Artificial heart valves
- A history of infective endocarditis
- A cardiac transplant that develops a heart valve problem
- The following congenital heart conditions:
  - Unrepaired or incompletely repaired (residual defect) cyanotic congenital heart disease
  - A completely repaired congenital heart defect with prosthetic material or device during the first six months after the procedure

Patients who took prophylactic antibiotics in the past but no longer need to include those with:

- Mitral valve prolapse
- Rheumatic heart disease
- Bicuspid valve disease
- Calcified aortic stenosis
- Congenital (present from birth) heart conditions such as ventricular septal defect, atrial septal defect and hypertrophic cardiomyopathy

---

Hypertension

PEARL: *Hypertension:*

Hypertension causes chronically increased pressures within the left ventricle

- Which causes hypertrophy of the ventricle
- Which causes decreased relaxation or "compliance" and decreased lumen of the LV
- Eventually over time, these high pressures cause 'remodeling' of the ventricle.
- This causes dilatation of the ventricle and will lead to dilated cardiomyopathy
- Dilated cardiomyopathy is another common cause of congestive heart failure.

DEFINITION OF HYPERTENSION

Normal	<120 systolic	and	<80 diastolic
Pre-hypertension	>120-139 systolic	or	>80-89 diastolic
Stage 1 hypertension	>140-159 systolic	or	> 90-99 diastolic
Stage 2 hypertension	>160 systolic	or	>100 diastolic

There are two main types of hypertension recognized currently: ***Essential and Secondary***

- Essential hypertension has no distinct known cause; it is familial but causes just as much damage if untreated as hypertension with a known cause.

- Secondary causes of hypertension are important to recognize because the cause is often treatable, and then the hypertension is "cured". Pay careful attention to the section here on secondary causes, of which renal problems are most common; endocrinologic problems next most common.

A 38-year-old male is being seen by you in the clinic for a new patient routine physical examination. His BP today is 116/82. What is the most likely diagnosis?

A. Pre-hypertension
B. Stage 1 hypertension
C. Stage 2 hypertension
D. Malignant hypertension

Answer: A.

Discussion: I know that clinically I would think this is a good pressure, but in reality, this represents pre-hypertension (likewise, BP 122/68 constitutes pre-hypertension too!) Don't be fooled – this patient needs behavior modification, DASH eating plan, and follow up.

ESSENTIAL HYPERTENSION

- **Epidemiology**
    - Somewhat "genetic"; mainly occurs in the early 30's
- **Etiology – unknown**
- **H&P findings**
    - Exam should look for evidence of end organ damage or clues to secondary hypertension
        - Should be normal
- **Labs & Diagnostics**
    - CBC
    - BMP to include electrolytes and BUN/creatinine
        - Hypokalemia suggests hyperaldosteronism (see Endocrinology Ch. 20)
        - Potassium level may be affected by almost any drug given for hypertension
- **Clinical Intervention**
    - For pre-hypertension, behavior modification
    - For Stage 1, behavior modification and possibly thiazide
    - for Stage 2, likely two meds needed, one of them a thiazide (and behavior modification)
- **Therapeutics** – *Please see Chapter 4 for specifics on hypertension therapeutics*
    - Thiazide
    - ACEI/ARB
    - BB
    - CCB
    - Others

- **Health Maintenance**
    - Goal of therapy is < 140 sytolic and <90 diastolic
    - Unless any kidney problems or DM, then <130 systolic and < 80 diastolic

SECONDARY HYPERTENSION

- **Renovascular (1-2%)**
    - Renal artery stenosis (due to atheromatous plaquing in the renal artery)
    - Fibromuscular dysplasia – 50 y.o. women – genetic predisposition
        - ***Clue*** – ACEI causes marked elevation of creatinine --- stop ACEI and image renal arteries

- Any renal problem causing significant dysfunction
- **Endocrine** *(see Chapter 20)*
  - Primary hyperaldosteronism (Conn's tumor)
  - Grave's disease
  - Pheochromocytoma
- **Psychiatric disorders**
  - Anxiety, panic
- **Medications**
  - Birth control pills
  - Stimulant medications

HYPERTENSIVE CRISIS (Urgency/Emergency/Malignant) – 1% of hypertensive patients

PEARL: *Hypertensive Crisis:*

- Emergency and urgency are distinguished primarily by the presence or absence of end organ damage and not defined specifically by the actual numbers.
- It is usually not considered unless BP >180/100 mm Hg
- Recognizing which type (i.e., recognizing end organ damage) is the key to knowing how fast the BP should be lowered

HYPERTENSIVE URGENCY = No end organ damage (but may have symptoms)

- **Presentation**
  - Headache (but no AMS or papilledema)
  - Epistaxis
  - Vomiting/nausea
- **Clinical Intervention**
  - Outpatient discharge
  - Close follow up in 24-48 hours
  - PO medications
- **Treatment**
  - PO labetalol
  - PO furosemide (if JVD/peripheral edema/CHF)
  - PO ACE inhibitor (enalapril)
  - PO nifedipine/amlodipine
  - PO clonidine

HYPERTENSIVE EMERGENCY = End organ damage

- **Presentation**
  - Suspicion for end organ damage

        - Encephalopathy (altered mental status (AMS))
        - Papilledema
        - Renal failure/proteinuria
        - Acute MI (AMI)
        - Aortic dissection
        - Intracranial hemorrhage (ICH)
- **Clinical Intervention**
    - ICU admission
    - IV antihypertensives
    - Lower mean arterial pressure 25% in minutes to hour
    - Goal = 160/100 in 6 hours
- **Therapeutics**
    - IV Labetalol is preferred
    - Nicardipine is often used
    - IV Nitroprusside
        - Was most utilized years ago; not used often for this management
        - ICU; IV drip; do not use in intracranial hemorrhage
        - *can cause cyanide toxicity if renal or liver impairment*

MALIGNANT HYPERTENSION

- **Etiologies:**
    - Sudden cessation of beta-blockers/clonidine
    - MAOI with tyramine containing foods (i.e. aged cheeses, red wine)
- *Treatment as above (hypertensive emergency) depending on presentation*

PEARL: The general rule in the past has been to avoid beta-blocker in catecholamine-induced hypertension (cocaine, pheochromocytoma). This is now debated, and labetalol does have both beta-blocking and alpha-blocking properties, so it is sometimes used now. I do not know what the item writers believe at this point. If asked to choose, it is safest to go with Nitroprusside; however, this is used much less commonly than in the past. A scientific concept question could pertain to the idea that if you block only beta-receptors, you potentially create unopposed alpha stimulation. Another scientific concept question could be about the beta- and alpha- blocking properties of labetalol, which is a newer beta-blocker in the past 6 years (since your last recert)

Dyslipidemia - See Appendix A for NEW ACC guidelines - 2013

Fasting lipoprotein levels should be performed for screening for dyslipidemia.

The test is performed after a 9-12 hour fast because the LDL is "calculated" from the measured total cholesterol, HDL and triglycerides in the serum. If the patient has something to eat or drink, the triglycerides will be elevated and the calculated LDL will not be accurate.

Once you have the results of the patient's fasting lipoprotein levels, establish a goal of therapy based on whether or not the patient has a coronary heart disease risk equivalent:

- Known coronary disease
- Carotid disease
- Peripheral artery disease
- Abdominal aortic aneurysm
- HDL < 40
- Type 1 DM x 20 year
- Type 2 DM

If the patient has any of the above, the goal for LDL is < 70 (several textbooks still state < 100 as per the last ATP III guidelines, but accepted practice for several years now has been 70; so hopefully that will be there. If not, pick < 100 if it is the lowest available)

If the patient has no CHD, then look in the stem of the question for risk factors for coronary disease:

- Smoking
- Hypertension (even if treated)
- Family history for premature heart disease (father < 55 , mother < 65)
- Being a male > 45; being a female > 55
- If the patient has 2 or more RF's, then LDL goal of therapy should be < 130
- If the patient has 0-1 RF, then LDL goal of therapy should be < 160

There are many things that can raise lipid levels (secondary causes), including:

- *Hyperglycemia*
  - If you have a Type 2 diabetic who has an A1c of 14 and total cholesterol of 300; treat the glucose first and when at a reasonable A1c, repeat lipid evaluation
- *Corticosteroids*
  - If the patient must be on long term steroids, then you need to check and treat lipids
  - If the patient is on short-course steroid, then do not do lipid check until off steroids for 6-8 weeks
- *Hypothyroidism*
  - The thyroid affects liver function; the liver metabolizes cholesterol; therefore there will be elevated cholesterol in patients with hypothyroidism
  - Anabolic steroids
    - Think this in a high school or college athlete who has suddenly become much more muscular and has dyslipidemia

---

Congestive Heart Failure (CHF)

In order to understand the pathophysiology, H & P findings, and lab/diagnostic results and be able to treat congestive heart failure, you must understand the normal physiologic compensatory mechanisms that are working "against" the patient with a lousy heart.

To review the normal physiologic compensatory mechanisms please see Section Four, Chapter 6.

- **Epidemiology**
    - More Medicare dollars spent on CHF than any other diagnosis
    - Increasing in prevalence as patients live with cardiac disease of all kinds
- **Etiology**
    - Myocardial infarction (currently or in the past)
    - Valvular disorders
    - Cardiomyopathies (all types)
    - Hypertension
- **H&P findings**
    - Most common complaint is dyspnea on exertion (DOE)
    - Orthopnea, paroxysmal nocturnal dyspnea (PND)
    - Jugular venous distension (JVD) is present if fluid overload (in most)
    - Hepatojugular reflex (HJR) suggests right heart failure (due to the LV dysfunction)
    - Peripheral edema (evidence of volume overload)
- **Labs & Diagnostics**
    - *CBC (to rule out anemia as a cause)*
        - Anemia is a cause of high output failure.
        - The term high out put cardiac failure is a misnomer actually, because there is not a high cardiac output, there is a high metabolic demand on the heart.
    - *Creatinine (to evaluate renal function)*
        - The kidney takes a hit when cardiac output decreases
        - The decreased renal perfusion can cause renal ischemia
        - This activates the R-A-A-S system, worsening the failure
        - Many drugs are renally excreted; pay attention to the creatinine as an indirect measure of the kidney's function
    - *Electrolytes (Na, K most important)*
        - The electrolytes will change with treatment
        - Remember – using an aldosterone receptor blocker (spironolactone) will cause the body to lose sodium, so do not give it to a patient with hyponatremia!
        - Remember – ACEI's and spironolactone may cause on increase in potassium, so do not give it to a patient with hyperkalemia
        - Remember – furosemide will make the body lose potassium, so do not give it to a patient with hypokalemia

    - *TSH*
        - Both hyper- and hypo-thyroid function can cause CHF
    - *BNP (brain-type natriuretic peptide)*
        - Brain-type natriuretic peptide (BNP) is secreted by the cardiac ventricles in response to ventricular pressure overload and volume expansion.

- BNP level has been shown to be a useful adjunct to other clinical information for differentiating among the causes of dyspnea, proving more accurate than physical exam findings sometimes.
- In a patient with dyspnea, in whom the diagnosis is uncertain, a BNP > 200 (and frequently > 1000) suggests CHF; whereas, a BNP of 30 would suggest another cause (pulmonary, endocrine, hematologic?)

- *Diagnostics in CHF*
  - EKG to rule out MI as cause of heart failure
    - May be entirely normal
    - Could show signs of risk factors for CHF (like LVH from hypertension, Q waves from old infarct, arrhythmias, etc)
  - CXR
    - *Revascularization or cephalization or redistribution*
      - Blood is "redistributed" to the upper lung fields
    - *Kerley B lines from interstitial edema*
      - Tiny peripheral white lines in the lower lung fields
    - *Alveolar fluid*
      - Fluffy, patchy infiltrates (cause rales on physical exam)
      - "Bat wing" configuration in early edema
    - *Pleural effusions*
      - Blunting of the costophrenic sulcus
        - Make sure there is a sharp point laterally and posteriorly
  - Echocardiogram
    - The echocardiogram is the most important test in determining the prognosis of a patient with congestive heart failure, and discerns whether this is a diastolic failure or systolic failure.
      - EF < 40% -- Systolic failure (failure of the pump)
      - EF >40% -- Diastolic failure (failure of filling)

- **Clinical Intervention in CHF**
  - Many patients should be admitted to the hospital (remember, you will admit more patients "according to the book" on the exam than in typical clinical practice).
  - New onset congestive heart failure always deserves admission for a more complete workup. If the patient has been seen frequently and is in the process of "tweaking" medications, or has recently been given a beta-blocker or ACEI, it could be that the patient has simply developed some fluid overload and needs an adjustment of furosemide dose.
  - Carefully review the vital signs and any symptoms or signs of severe decompensation. Only if these do not exist, should you send the patient home.
- **Whether sending patient home or admitting the following should be done:**
  - *Reduce workload*
    - Rest, reduce anxiety/stress
  - *Reduce preload*
    - to improve "Frank-Starling" curve and improve contractility
  - *Reduce afterload*
    - Lower BP
  - *Improve contractility*
    - Use a positive inotropic agent to increase myocardial contractility.

- **Therapeutics (more details in Chapter 4, Clinical Therapeutics)**
    - **Diuretics** are the mainstay of therapy in the congestive heart failure patient with systolic failure and resultant volume (elevated BNP, JVD, peripheral edema).
        - Furosemide is the first drug of choice
            - Remember that furosemide will cause the patient to lose potassium in exchange for the sodium lost, so be sure to assess the patient's K status and monitor it during treatment.
- **After using furosemide to "remove" water from the patient, then drugs should be added in this order:**
    - **Nitrates** – nitroglycerin paste should be applied to cause "pooling" of fluid in the patient's legs until the furosemide is able to cause diuresis of this extra fluid. It provides quicker relief from too much fluid in the failing pump, and allows the pump to be on the "good side" of the Frank-Starling curve again.
        - *Reasons for not using nitrates include:*
            - Hypotension (SBP<100 mm Hg)
            - Erectile dysfunction drugs (tildenafil, sardenafil)

    - **Angiotensin Converting Enzyme Inhibitors** (ACEI's) – (this could also be angiotensin receptor blocker (ARB). *ACEI's should be used in all patients possible.*
        - *Reasons for not using an ACEI are:*
            - Hyperkalemia
            - End stage renal failure
            - Renal artery stenosis
            - Angioedema while on an ACEI

- **β-blockers** – should be used in all patients once fluid has been removed from the body. β-blockers block that sympathetic outflow that is beating the failing heart to death.
    - *Reasons not to use β-blockers include:*
        - Hypotension (SBP < 100)
        - Bradycardia (HR < 60)
        - AV blocks
        - Reactive airway disease

- **Aldosterone Receptor Blockers** – spironolactone can be added to patients with normal renal function (and normal Na and K levels) to block the sodium absorbing effects of aldosterone in the RAAS system. It will help the body get rid of excess sodium, but remember, it will increase the patient's potassium level (a very bad thing in a patient with renal dysfunction, as many patients with congestive heart failure have).
    - *Reasons not to use aldosterone receptor blockers:*
        - Hyponatremia
        - Hyperkalemia
        - Chronic renal failure

- **Health Maintenance in CHF**
    - Low salt diet
    - BP management
    - Lipid management
    - DM management (if diabetic)

PEARL: The classes of heart failure are useful in identifying "decompensation", i.e. if the test question states the patient was seen two weeks ago in clinic and had Class 2 failure, but today presents Class 4, something has happened.

Class 1 = Risk for CHF, but asymptomatic
Class 2 = DOE with vigorous exercise
Class 3 = DOE with ADLs
Class 4 = DOE at rest

PEARL: Remember that β-blockers are negative inotropic drugs and will reduce contractility (which is counter-intuitive to the problem). In fact, when I was a student many years ago, I was told never to use β-blockers in congestive heart failure patients, but studies have proven that they prolong life, and improve outcomes. Apparently, stopping the sympathetic "flogging" of the heart makes it last longer.

Peripheral Vascular Disease

ABDOMINAL AORTIC ANEURYSM

The whole point of the diagnosis is to suspect it and find it when it is asymptomatic. Aortic dissection and rupture are the consequences, often devastating, of an untreated or undiagnosed aneurysm of the aorta.

Risk Factors:

- Hypertension
- Smoking
- Dyslipidemia
- Age
- Male gender

Be on the lookout for questions that are leading you to suspect your patient may have an AAA.

- **H & P**
  - *Abdominal exam which shows:*
    - Abdominal bruits
    - Prominent aortic pulsation
    - A "widened aortic impulse" on palpation of the abdomen
- **Diagnostics**
  - *Ultrasound of the abdomen*
    - For screening
    - Diagnosis is made when the aorta measures > 3.0 cm
  - *Angiography*
    - Gold standard (prior to repair)
  - *CT with contrast*
  - *MRA*
    - not if hemodynamically unstable

    - no gadolinium in significant renal insufficiency!

- **Clinical Intervention**
    - therapy includes Beta Blockers to lower BP and slow expansion of the aneurysm
    - refer for repair when > 5.0 cm

A 78 year old male smoker presents for regular medication check and PE. He is on hydrochlorothiazide; enalapril; simvastatin. On PE, there is a prominent aortic abdominal impulse. What diagnostic imaging modality is recommended at this time?

A. CT of the abdomen
B. Abdominal angiography
C. Ultrasound of the abdomen
D. MRI of the abdomen
E. Pet scan

Answer: C.

Discussion: What I really want you to recognize are the key words in the stem of the question that leads you to the most likely diagnosis:

78 y.o.; male; smoker; HCTZ (htn); simvastatin (dyslipidemia) – these are all risk factors for ischemic disease in general; the abdominal aortic impulse narrows it to an aneurysm. Asymptomatic aneurysms just need ultrasound.

THORACIC AORTIC ANEURYSM

Much less common than abdominal aneurysms, and more commonly associated with connective tissue diseases (i.e., Marfan's syndrome, vasculitic syndromes (temporal arteritis) than with atherosclerotic disease. Lethal prognosis if rupture or dissection occurs.

- **Presentation:**
    - *Acute*
        - May present with any kind of chest pain; very nonspecific, but very severe
        - Abnormal pulses in upper extremities are a big clue!
        - Life-threatening emergency; CT of the chest
    - *Chronic*
        - Asymptomatic (most are found incidentally)
        - Have a high index of suspicion in Marfan's syndrome or Ehlers-Danlos syndrome
        - Pressure on anterior mediastinal structures
            - Dysphagia (esophagus)
            - Stridor (trachea)
            - Chronic hoarseness (recurrent laryngeal nerve)
- **Diagnosis**
    - CT angiography should be performed to establish definitive diagnosis and baseline for comparison for the future
- **Clinical Intervention**
    - referral to thoracic surgeon is likely indicated

    - lower BP
- **Therapeutics**
    - Beta adrenergic blockers (BB)
- **Scientific Concept – Risk of Rupture**
    - Size is biggest risk factor (>5cm)
    - If > 7cm, 40% risk and almost 50% death in 1 year if not repaired
        - COPD increases risk
        - Age increases risk.
        - Hypertension increases risk.
- **Complications of repair**
    - Embolization of debris
    - Spinal cord injury (paraplegia/paraparesis)
- **Have a high index of suspicion if the test question describes a "marfanoid" patient with these chronic non-cardiac sounding symptoms of dysphagia, hoarseness or sudden onset of severe chest pain.**

PERIPHERAL ARTERIAL DISEASE (PAD) VS. VENOUS INSUFFICIENCY

PEARL: *PVD:* It is important to remember that in this category, I am discussing two completely different diseases: arterial insufficiency and venous insufficiency. The concept of arterial vs. venous has confused my students over the years, so I am taking a moment to be clear about the pathophysiological differences and physical examination differences between venous and arterial issues.

The two are not even remotely similar, although they both comprise peripheral vascular diseases states. What makes them so different?

- Arterial diseases are caused by the same process as coronary artery disease: atherosclerotic plaques which decrease the lumen of the vessel and may rupture and cause platelet aggregation
- Venous diseases are caused by genetics and gravity (gravity is very unkind)

- Arterial diseases cause decreased oxygenated blood flow to the fingers and toes (and brain and kidneys, etc)
- Venous diseases cause decreased return of flow to the heart (no problem with oxygenated blood getting to the toes)

- Arterial diseases would cause decrease in pulses (recall that when we measure pulses, we are measuring arterial pulses, veins don't "pulse)
- Venous diseases would cause no problem at all with pulses

- On exam, arterial diseases, therefore, would cause decreased pulse, cool or cold, white or pale, hairless, painful legs/feet, with ulcers at the tips of the toes (often painless due to lack of nerve oxygenation)
- On exam, venous diseases, therefore, would cause normal pulses, warm burgundy feet, aching discomfort, with ulcers at the ankles (where blood has to make a 90° angle and go against gravity)

CHRONIC ARTERIAL INSUFFICIENCY

- **Pathophysiology**
    - Chronic occlusion causes chronic changes
- **H & P**
    - Claudication ("angina" of the lower extremities)
    - Loss of hair/ thin shiny skin
    - Cool extremities (although may be normal at rest)
    - Thick nails, ulcers at tips of toes
    - Gangrene
- **Clinical Intervention**
    - *ABI's (ankle-brachial index)*
        - Compare ankle systolic pressure with brachial systolic pressure
        - Ankle pressure should be > brachial
        - If ABI < 0.9, suggests claudication; insufficiency
    - *Medical management*
        - Clopidogrel; ASA
        - Exercise
        - Decrease risk factors
    - *Surgical management*
        - Angioplasty with stent placement
            - If large and discrete vessel
        - Femoral-popliteal bypass
            - For diffuse or smaller vessels
        - Amputation

ACUTE ARTERIAL OCCLUSION

- **Limb-threatening emergency**
- **May be due to embolism or thrombosis**
    - *Embolism* most commonly from atrial fibrillation with clot from left atrium traveling to lower extremity
        - Sudden onset is the clue
        - A-fib is the clue
    - *Thrombosis* has same risk factors as CAD – plaque rupture with platelet aggregation
        - RF's for ischemic disease is the clue
- **H & P (different findings than chronic insufficiency)**
    - No skin changes (particularly in a sudden embolic phenomenon, i.e. from atrial fibrillation)
    - *5 P's*

    - Pain
    - Pallor
    - Paralysis
    - Pulselessness
    - Poikilothermia (change in temperature from nonperfused to perfused part of leg)

VENOUS INSUFFICIENCY (CHRONIC)

- **Epidemiology/etiology**
  - Common – valve leaflets do not coapt or are scarred, thickened, or inadequate
  - Mainly due to increased abdominal pressure (putting pressure on venous return to the inferior vena cava); i.e. obesity, pregnancy.
  - Or due to standing for long periods (like at the O.R. table!)
- **H & P**
  - Peripheral edema
  - Stasis skin changes – brawny discoloration from hemosiderin leaking
  - Ulcerations will occur at the malleolus (this is where the venous blood has to return to the heart by making a 90-degree turn at the ankle against gravity).
  - These ulcers may become infected; but remember – gangrene occurs in arterial insufficiency due to lack of oxygenation; these ulcers will not be gangrenous.
- **Labs & Diagnostics**
  - If unilateral edema, Venous Ultrasound Doppler is indicated to r/o DVT.
  - This is a clinical diagnosis.
- **Clinical Intervention**
  - Wound care
  - Graduated ambulatory compression stockings
  - Elevation
  - Avoidance of prolonged sitting, standing
- **Health Maintenance**
  - Prevention is key
  - Weight loss; exercise

VENOUS THROMBOSIS (ACUTE)

Covered in detail in Chapter 12, Pulmonary Embolism

- **Risk Factors (Virchow's triad = stasis, endothelial damage, hypercoagulable state)**
  - Immobilization
  - Pelvic surgery; lower extremity injury/surgery
  - Estrogen
  - Cancer; CHF, trauma, hypercoagulable state
- **Presentation**
  - Unilateral leg edema, duskiness
  - Calf discomfort/groin discomfort
  - Homan's sign is unreliable
  - Palpable cord is noted in textbooks (but rarely actually felt clinically).
- **Labs**

- D-dimer
- Venous Doppler US
- Venogram/venography (gold standard though rarely used)

- **Treatment**
  - LMWH (heparin)
  - Warfarin x 6 months (at least)

PHLEBITIS/THROMBOPHLEBITIS

- **Etiology**
  - Inflammation (not necessarily infection) in a superficial varicose vein.
  - Inflammation in a vein used for IV access
- **H & P**
  - Erythema overlying the vein (not a diffuse cellulitis erythema of the skin)
  - Tenderness with palpation of the vein
- **Labs & Diagnostics**
  - Not needed (no ultrasound because it is not a unilateral leg swelling with calf or popliteal pain --- you can see the red vein – and superficial clots in the leg do not warrant ultrasound)
- **Clinical Intervention**
  - Warm moist compresses
  - No antibiotics are necessary

VARICOSE VEINS

- **Primary**
  - Inherited from a parent; acquired from pregnancy, obesity, standing too much
- **Secondary**
  - Acute occlusion of deep vein system (DVT or pelvic tumor) – sudden enlarged varicosities in someone who never had varicosities before

Which of the following vignettes represents a primary varicosity and which represents a secondary varicosity?

A. Mr. Jones woke up this morning and notes marked superficial varicosities in his left lower extremity. He has no prior h/o varicosities. He has h/o lymphoma, but is currently in remission.

B. Mr. Jones has had varicose veins in both lower extremities; noted first about 10 years ago. He has family history of varicosities. He presents today for chronic fatigue and aching in his legs at the end of his work day.

Answer:

A. is a secondary varicosity; he needs venous ultrasound imaging to r/o DVT; and may need additional imaging if that is negative looking for tumor, nodes, in the pelvis

B. is a primary varicosity; treatment with compression stockings; no need for diagnostic imaging

OTHER FORMS OF HEART DISEASE

ACUTE PERICARDITIS

- **Epidemiology**
    - Relatively uncommon (0.1%)
- **Etiology – many etiologies:**
    - Viruses
    - Inflammatory (lupus, RA, etc);
    - Post-op CABG
    - Post-MI

- **H&P findings**
    - Pleuritic chest pain, increased when supine, decreased when sitting and leaning forward
    - Friction rub (rarely heard in real clinical medicine, often described on an exam)
    - Distant heart sounds (water dampens the sound)
- **Labs & Diagnostics** *(see Chapter 6 for ECG examples)*
    - ST elevation in *all* the leads with "notching"
    - ECG= low voltage (if pericardial effusion)
    - Echocardiogram
- **Clinical Intervention**
    - Usually admission to the hospital
    - Consult by cardiothoracic surgery
    - Pericardiocentesis if exhibiting signs of pericardial tamponade (see below)

PERICARDIAL EFFUSION

- **Etiology**
    - Fluid collection due to pericarditis (usually)
    - Blood after surgery
    - Trauma of the thoracic aorta
- **Diagnostics**
    - *ECG*
        - Electrical alternans
            - Heart is "swinging" in the chest and each beat looks different due to changing in electrical vectors
    - On CXR can look like cardiomegaly
    - Echocardiogram - normal heart with large amount of fluid surround it
    - Clinical intervention:
        - r/o tamponade

CARDIAC TAMPONADE

- Result of effusion (usually that accumulates rapidly)
- *Beck's Triad:*
    - Muffled heart sounds
    - Jugular venous distention
    - Hypotension (low SBP)
- Requires pericardiocentesis

Shock

- Common denominator = decreased tissue perfusion

CARDIOGENIC SHOCK

- **Etiology**
    - Acute MI with persistent SBP < 90 mm HG
- **H & P**
    - Precordium would be quiet (heart is not pumping well)
    - Pallor, cool clammy extremities
- **Labs/Diagnostics**
    - Echocardiogram
    - US of chest would show decreased contractility
- **Clinical intervention**
    - Emergent CV consult (cath lab, surgery)
    - Dopamine
    - LVAD (LV assist device)

HYPOVOLEMIC SHOCK

- **Etiology**
    - Hemorrhage, dehydration
- **H & P**
    - Pallor
    - Orthostatic abnormalities in vital signs (tachycardia occurs before hypotension)
    - Hyperdynamic precordium and PMI (heart is pumping hard and fast)
- **Labs/Diagnostics**
    - CBC (looking for anemia)
    - CMP (looking at CO2, creatinine for dehydration)
- **Clinical intervention**
    - Mainstay is fluid resuscitation (blood/pRBC's)

SEPTIC SHOCK

- **Etiology**

- Infection
- Typically gram negative bacteria, but can be any bacterial infection

- **H & P**
  - T>101 or < 96
  - HR>90
  - RR>24
  - SBP<90 mm Hg
  - Skin erythema first, rash next, then pallor
  - Altered mental status
- **Labs/Diagnostics**
  - CBC with differential
  - leukocytosis with left shift
  - lactic acid >4
  - CMP to check for multiorgan failure
- **Clinical intervention**
  - Antibiotics – within 1-3 hours is the key!!!
  - Fluid
  - Supportive care

ANAPHYLACTIC SHOCK

- **Etiology**
  - Systemic inflammatory response system
- **H & P**
  - Flushing
  - Urticaria
  - Angioedema
  - Hypotension
- **Labs/Diagnostics - none**
- **Clinical intervention**
  - IV access
  - Fluids
- **Therapeutics**
  - Epinephrine
  - Steroids
  - H1 blocker (Diphenhydramine, aka Benadryl)
  - H2 blocker (cimetidine, ranitidine)

ORTHOSTASIS/POSTURAL HYPOTENSION

- **Etiology**
  - Hypovolemia can cause orthostasis
    - Dehydration, hemorrhage, volume depletion for any reason
  - Medications commonly cause orthostasis
    - Diuretics, antihypertensives, smooth muscle relaxants, etc.
  - Diabetes mellitus
    - Autonomic dysfunction

- Parkinson's Disease
  - Autonomic dysfunction

- **H & P**
  - Orthostatic vital sign changes
  - Tachycardia +/- hypotension
  - Remember that in a young person, the HR will go up long before the BP starts to fall; but in the elderly with little reserve they may occur concomitantly.
- **Labs/Diagnostics**
  - Tilt-table testing
  - Check CBC for anemia; check urine for concentration (increased specific gravity)
- **Clinical intervention**
  - Depends on cause
  - Fluids if volume depleted
  - Pressors (midodrine) can be given to drive BP up if autonomic
  - Fludricortisone can be used to increased sodium retention, if needed.

CHAPTER 12

Pulmonary Medicine – 12%

Pulmonary Embolism/DVT

It's difficult to talk about PE without talking about DVT, as the most common etiology for a PE is from the deep vein system of the lower extremities (secondarily from the upper extremities), so both are discussed here as a single topic.

- **Epidemiology**
    - 300k-600k incidence per year (poorly reported)
    - 1/3 recur within 10 years
    - 1/3 die within 1 month
- **Etiology --- **Know These Risk Factors****
    - Prolonged immobilization (> 3 day)
    - Surgery > 30 min. anesthesia (especially pelvic, LE surgeries)
    - Trauma to pelvis and/or lower extremities (even a bad hematoma)
    - Estrogen
        - Birth control pills, pregnancy and postpartum state
    - Cancer
        - Especially visceral (lung, pancreas, GI, GU)
    - History of DVT
    - Hematologic abnormalities
        - Antithrombin III deficiency, Protein C & S deficiency, etc)
    - Congestive heart failure
    - Recent travel
    - Age (>60)
    - Obesity
    - Smoking
    - Central venous catheter
- **H & P**
    - Tachycardia
    - Tachypnea
    - Hypoxia (mainly when up and ambulating)
    - Calf pain/LE edema/duskiness
- **Labs & Diagnostics**
    - *CXR*
        - Used primarily to rule out other causes of the presentation
        - Almost always is normal

        - Atelectasis is next most common finding (very nonspecific)
        - Very rare, but often in standard exam Q's:
            - Fleischner's sign – prominent pulmonary artery
            - Westermark's sign – oligemia distal to embolism
            - Hampton's hump – pleural based, wedge-shaped consolidation
    - *D-Dimer*
        - If low risk – negative D-Dimer will rule out PE/DVT
        - Nonspecific test so many false positives
            - Unfortunately, the same RF for DVT/PE cause elevation of Dimer
            - So it's utility is mainly in low risk patients
    - *Ultrasound lower extremities*
        - If suspected DVT – get lower extremity ultrasound venous dopplers
    - *Helical/high resolution CT of chest*
        - If moderate to high risk – may want to go to helical CT with contrast (contrast fills the pulmonary arteries and the clot causes a darker "defect" in the white contrast)
        - If creatinine is elevated – do not use contrast
        - If pregnant – avoid CT – might start with lower extremity ultrasound venous dopplers,
            - If positive, then presumptive PE
    - *V/Q scan*
        - If no DVT and still suspicious in patient who cannot have contrast
    - *Pulmonary Angiography*
        - If you must know if a PE exists– and cannot do above, pulmonary angiogram is "gold standard"
        - But it is contrast dye, so once again, not in pregnancy or renal insufficiency
        - Rarely performed in the emergency room
- **Clinical Intervention**
    - Heparin is given at time of diagnosis; low molecular weight if possible
    - Warfarin is begun and both are given for several days until INR is therapeutic
        - LMW heparin can then be stopped
        - Warfarin is continued for at least six months
        - Does not dissolve clot - just stops propagation
    - If saddle embolism – and need clot dissolved – will need t-PA
- **Therapeutics**
    - LMW heparin ok in pregnancy
    - warfarin Category D in pregnancy –should be avoided
    - patient will have to stay on LMWH through entire pg and postpartum period
- **Contraindications to T-PA, eg., Anything that would cause brain bleed**
    - Recent stroke/hemorrhage/known AVM
    - Brain cancer
    - Closed head injury of significance
    - Very recent surgery
- **Health Maintenance**
    - LMW heparin is used prophylactically on admission for patients who will have long surgeries; who will be immobilized; post-operatively to prevent DVT
    - Consider warfarin in patients with cancer, end stage renal failure and congestive heart failure as prophylaxis

- Refer to heme-onc if you suspect a thrombophilia:
  - *Pro C/S deficiency, AT III deficiency, Factor V Leiden*
- If repeated DVT:
- Greenfield filter to "catch" clots in inferior vena cava

- **Scientific concepts**
  - Virchow's Triad:
    - Venous stasis (sedentary)
    - Endothelial damage (trauma, surgery)
    - Hypercoagulable state (estrogen, thrombophilias, cancer, CHF)
  - PESI score *(see PEARL below)* to identify low risk
  - Well's Criteria *(see PEARL below)* to identify high risk

PEARL: *PERC rule* can "rule out" PE if all criteria are met (<2% chance):

- < 50 year old
- HR > 100 bpm
- Pulse ox > 95%Cancer history
- No unilateral leg edema
- No estrogen use
- No prior history of:
  - DVT/PE
- No recent lower extremity surgery/trauma

If Well's Score: > 6 (see below) = heparin is recommended even before testing; or if delay of 4 hours or more for testing.

- Symptom of DVT in LE (3 points)
- No other diagnosis to explain symptoms (3 points)
- HR > 100 bpm (1.5 points)
- Immobilization or surgery in past 4 weeks (1.5 points)
- Prior h/o DVT/PE (1.5 points)
- Presence of hemoptysis (1 point)
- Presence of cancer (1 point)

Obstructive Pulmonary Disease

COPD/EMPHYSEMA

- **Epidemiology**
  - 32 million persons in US
  - 4th leading cause of death
  - Major cause of disability
- **includes three types:**
  - Chronic bronchitis/COPD
  - Emphysema

  - Asthma (usually also included in obstructive pulmonary disorders, but covered separately)
- **Etiology**
  - ***Smoking***
  - Occupational exposure
  - Air pollution
- **H & P**
  - Chronic shortness of breath, cough
  - Barrel chest, distant breath sounds
  - Wheezing, rales, rhonchi
- **Labs & Diagnostics**
  - PFT's are the only way to diagnose COPD (see Chapter 6)
- **Clinical Intervention**
  - The only intervention that improves prognosis is oxygen
  - Peak flows during exacerbation – not used to make diagnosis
  - Duoneb therapy (albuterol plus ipratropium) nebulized therapy
  - Steroids PO/inhaled
    - Now longterm steroids PO are avoided, short-course therapies only
- **Therapeutics**
  - *Oxygen – only intervention that prolongs life
  - Albuterol – beta agonist = bronchodilator
  - Ipratropium – anticholinergic = dries mucous & bronchodilates
  - Corticosteroids – antiinflammatory
  - Theophylline – bronchodilator
  - Roflumilast - PDE-4 inhibitor – reduce inflammation
    - New
    - Only used if FEV1 < 50% predicted or frequent exacerbations of chronic bronchitis
    - Must be used with bronchodilator (no bronchodilating effect)
- **Health Maintenance**
  - Smoking cessation
  - Occupational smoke/inhalant avoidance (mask)
  - VACCINATE – influenza, pneumococcal, Tdap
- **Scientific concepts**
  - Infiltration of immune cells secreting substances which cause inflammation
  - Inflammatory mucous exudates in lumens of airways

COPD VS EMPHYSEMA (VERY GENERAL, OFTEN MENTIONED)

- **COPD (blue bloater)** = irreversible airflow limitation during expiration
  - Obese
  - Cough with expectoration
  - Rhonchi and wheezing
- **Emphysema (pink puffer)** = destruction of alveolar septa and destruction of terminal bronchioles
  - Thin; barrel chested
  - Little to no cough; no expectoration
  - Hyper-resonant breath sounds; occasional wheezing

CHRONIC BRONCHITIS

- **Definition:**
    - Defined clinically as cough with sputum expectoration
    - For at least 3 months a year
    - During a period of 2 consecutive years
- **Epidemiology**
    - Smokers!
    - Comorbidities increase risk, i.e. DM
    - Viruses & bacteria can exacerbate chronic bronchitis, i.e. AECB (acute exacerbation of chronic bronchitis); at this time antibiotics become indicated
- **H & P**
    - Chronic cough; productive of clear sputum
- **Labs & Diagnostics**
    - None needed; clinical diagnosis
- **Clinical Intervention**
    - Smoking cessation!
- **Therapeutics**
    - Usually just albuterol or albuterol/ipratropium inhaler for bronchospasm
    - If increase in sputum and yellow/green color, treat for bacterial cause
    - No difference in effects between respiratory FQ (levofloxacin, moxifloxacin); macrolides (azithromycin, clarithromycin) and Augmentin
- **Health Maintenance**
    - Smoking cessation!
- **Scientific concepts**
    - This is more an inflammatory chronic type problem with opportunistic bacterias/or viruses.
    - Treating the inflammation is key in reducing risk of secondary pneumonias and improving ventilation

BRONCHIECTASIS

- **Definition**
    - Irreversible airway inflammatory destruction
- **Etiology**
    - Mechanical obstruction (malignancy; mucous)
    - Infectious (Tuberculosis (TB), pneumonia, Mycobaterium avian complex (MAC)
    - Autoimmune (Cystic fibrosis, hypogammaglobulinemia)
- **H & P**
    - Chronic copiously productive cough
    - Hemoptysis
    - Digital clubbing
    - Wheezing
- **Labs & Diagnostics**
    - PFT's –obstructive pattern
    - CXR – "honeycomb" pattern
    - Helical CT – thickened bronchial walls
- **Therapeutics**

- Inhaled corticosteroids
- Beta agonist inhaled therapy
- Macrolides (if pseudomonas suspected give Cipro)
- Vaccination for influenza

ASTHMA

- **Epidemiology**
  - 25 million with increasing prevalence among African-Americans; urban dwellers and children
- **Pathophysiology**
  - Inflammatory response of airways
  - Mast cells release inflammatory mediators
  - Airway bronchoconstriction
  - Mucous production
  - Edema of bronchioles
- **Etiology**
  - Smoke and pollution exposure
  - Genetically predisposed reactive airway disease
  - Exercise-induced
  - Viral-induced
  - GERD (irritation/inflammation from acid)
- ***Medications to Avoid in Asthma***
  - Aspirin and NSAID's
    - In atopic patients (with eczema), especially with nasal polyps
    - "Allergic triad"
  - Beta-blockers
  - ACE inhibitors
- **H & P**
  - Episodic or chronic SOB, cough, wheezing, chest tightness
  - Prolongation of expiratory phase
  - Wheezing diffusely (if focal, think foreign body or pneumonia)
- **Labs & Diagnostics**
  - *Acute*
    - Peak flows (NOT PFT's!) – normal is >80% of vital capacity in 1 second
    - FEV1:FVC ratio < 0.8
    - +/- CXR; *not usually indicated*
  - *Chronic*
    - Spirometry could be performed before and after bronchodilator
      - Complete or partial reversibility makes diagnosis
    - Histamine or methacholine challenge
      - Proves bronchoconstriction with "trigger"
- **Clinical Intervention** *(all drugs are covered in detail; Therapeutics, Chapter 4)*
  - *Acute* intervention
    - Rescue therapy
      - Beta agonists (relieve bronchoconstriction) = albuterol
      - Anticholinergics (reduce mucous) =atrovent
    - Steroids – high dose, short course oral; IM; IV

        - Epinephrine
            - Can be given SQ; racemic inhaled
    - *Chronic*
        - Inhaled steroids (**first line**)
        - Long acting bronchodilators
            - Inhaled beta agonists
                - Salmeterol (serevent)
            - Combined steroid/beta agonist
                - Advair
        - Inhaled mast cell stabilizers (prevent mast cell degranulation)
            - Cromolyn sodium
                - Nedocromil
        - Leukotriene modifiers
            - Montelukast
            - Safirlukast
                - Inhibit smooth muscle contraction
                - Inhibits mucous secretion
                - Inhibits inflammatory cell activation
        - Theophylline
            - Bronchodilator
            - Narrow therapeutic window
            - Problems with toxicity
                - Tachycardias/tachyarrhythmas
- **Health Maintenance**
    - Reduce allergen contact
    - Influenza and pneumovax vaccines
- **Scientific Concepts**
    - * Most important concept is that asthma by definition is reversible airway obstruction
    - * All asthmatics need a "rescue" inhaler
    - * Steroids are not for acute "rescue"

ASTHMA TABLE – NHLBI Guidelines (*condensed*) to highlight when changes need to occur.

Step 1	Step 2	Step 3	Step 4	Step 5	Step 6
Intermittent	Persistent (mild)	Persistent (moderate)	Persistent (mod, not well controlled)	Persistent (severe)	Persistent (severe) with poor control
Symptoms < 2 days/wk	Symptoms >2 days/wk	Daily		Several times daily	
No nighttime symptoms	1-2/month	1-2/weekly	< 7/week	nightly	
SABA use < 2 days/wk	SABA use > 2 days/wk	SABA use daily		SABA use several times daily	
Normal FEV1 between events	FEV1 >80%	FEV1 60-80%		FEV1 < 60%	
SABA prn	Low Dose inhaled corticosteroids (ICS)	Medium-dose ICS	Med-dose ICS + LABA or montelukast	High-dose ICS + LABA or montelukast	High-dose ICS + LABA or montelukast +oral steroids

**SABA as needed for symptoms*

- With viral URI, SABA every 4-6 hours up to 24 hours
- Consider short course of oral steroids if exacerbation from URI is severe or h/o severe exacerbations
- Frequent or increased use of SABA indicates need to Step Up
- Before stepping up, review compliance to regimen, inhaler technique, comorbid conditions (smoking)
- Refer to pulmonary or asthma specialist if Step 3 or greater

---

Restrictive Pulmonary Disease

Restrictive diseases generally have to do with infiltration of a substance into an organ – there are examples of this in the heart, lungs, liver, pancreas, adrenal, pituitary, etc. Any of these substances which are produced by the body infiltrate any and all organs; those that are inhaled (pneumoconiosis) involve only the lung, obviously.

Pay attention in the stem as to whether the item writer is telling you that this is occupational (acquired and probably inhaled); whether the patient has other autoimmune diseases (likely "idiopathic); or whether the patient has another infiltrative disease in his history (sarcoidosis, amyloid, etc). This will help you identify the likely diagnosis.

The bottom line is a restrictive disease causes a decrease in the total lung volume and vital capacity (the lungs have problem expanding when taking a deep breath --- opposite of what happens in asthma and COPD where the lungs expand but the patient has trouble getting air out)

IDIOPATHIC Pulmonary Disease

Idiopathic Pulmonary Fibrosis

- Causes stiff and noncompliant lungs
- Will reduce total lung capacity
- This is *not* an obstructive problem
- It is a "filling of the lungs" problem

INHALED Pulmonary Disease

THE PNEUMOCONIOSES (OCCUPATIONAL LUNG DISEASES)

- The common denominator in occupational lung diseases is inhalation of foreign bodies that in the short run cause little problem, but will cause chronic inflammatory responses that are very destructive when chronically activated. Diagnosis is made on biopsy during bronchoscopy.
- Pulmonary function tests would show a restrictive pattern of pulmonary disease.

Silicosis

- Inhaled silica (sand)
- Ingested by alveolar macrophages
- Causes chronic inflammatory process
- CXR shows coarse nodularity
    - *Hilar adenopathy*

Asbestosis

- Inhaled from insulation
- Very fine particles, so travel all the way to the periphery of the lungs
- Causing pleural plaques on CXR
- RF for mesothelioma

Berylliosis

- Manufacturing fluorescent light bulbs
- Same course of granulomatous changes of the lungs

Coal miner's lung *(not in blueprint)*

- Similar to silicosis
- Same findings on CXR although more significant
- Hx of being a coal miner would help, yes?

INFILTRATIVE Pulmonary Disease

These diseases are caused by chronic infiltration of the lungs with proteins (amyloid), or formation of nonspecific noncaseating granulomas (sarcoid); all are idiopathic and cause a multitude of sympto-

Sarcoidosis

- **Epidemiology**
  - Young to middle-aged
  - Scandinavian
  - African-American
  - Japanese
- **Etiology**
  - Every system is affected:
    - Rheumatologic symptoms, neurologic symptoms, dermatologic symptoms
    - Cardiac issues from infiltration of conduction system (arrhythmias)
    - Noninfectious non-caseating granulomatous disease in lungs
    - Differential includes: TB, Hodgkin's, metastatic lung cancer, etc)
- **H & P**
  - Cough/dyspnea
  - Fever
  - Arthralgia
  - Malaise
  - May be normal exam
  - Uveitis
  - Erythema nodosum
  - Lymphadenopathy/mediastinal nodes
- **Labs & Diagnostics**
  - Angiotensin converting enzymes **(ACE) is elevated in 60% of patients**
  - CBC = leukopenia; eosinophilia
  - Hypercalcemia/hypercalceuria
  - Increased ESR/CRP
  - Hypergammaglobulinemia
  - CXR – hilar lymphadenopathy and nodular lesions
  - Transbronchial biopsy = granulomas
- **Clinical Intervention**
  - Symptomatic treatment only
- **Therapeutics**
  - Steroids (if symptoms)
- **Scientific concepts**
  - most self-limited
  - no good treatment
  - 10% mortality from progressive fibrosis

Amyloidosis

- Typically thought of as a renal disease; this causes protein deposition in tissues (causing renal failure, but also deposits in skin, lungs, liver, heart, etc)

Acute Infectious Disorders

Tuberculosis – see I.D. Chapter 22 for detailed TB information
HIV-related pneumonias – see I.D Chapter 22 for HIV-related pneumonias

Acute Bronchitis

- **Epidemiology**
  - Common
- **Etiology**
  - 80% viral
  - 20% bacterial
    - Increased incidence in smokers
    - The usual suspects, (i.e, S. pneumo, H. flu, M. Cat)
- **H & P**
  - URI symptoms
  - Cough, nonproductive or clear to white sputum
  - +/- Bronchospasm
- **Labs & Diagnostics**
  - Not necessary; CXR would be normal (clinical diagnosis)
- **Clinical Intervention**
  - Albuterol if bronchospasm component
  - Reassurance
- **Therapeutics**
  - Cough suppressant
  - If you suspect pathogen in smoker/diabetic, Amoxicillin is still first line (although some might choose a respiratory quinolone, those should be reserved for pneumonias)
- **Health Maintenance**
  - Careful hand washing
  - Smoking cessation

PEARL: Please note that nothing about acute bronchitis is similar to chronic bronchitis; as is typical in medicine; presentation is different; epidemiology is different; pathogens are different; management is different. Remember to read the stem of a pulmonary question looking for clues about the problem's acute or chronic nature; this alone may help you answer the question!

Influenza

- **Epidemiology**
  - Epidemics every winter (influenza A & B)
- **Etiology**
  - Viral
- **H & P**
  - Sudden onset fevers, rigors
  - Myalgias, headache, arthralgias
  - Sore throat (scratchy), rhinorrhea

  - Followed in 3-4 days with cough, bronchospasm
- **Labs & Diagnostics**
  - Nasopharyngeal swab for type A/B
- **Clinical Intervention**
  - Supportive
  - Watch for secondary bacterial pneumonia
- **Therapeutics**
  - Only shorten symptoms slightly, doesn't prevent secondary infections
  - MOA – neuraminidase inhibitors:
    - oseltamivir (Tamiflu)– Influenza A & B – nasal spray or oral
    - zanamivir (Relenza) – powder to inhale
  - Former drugs – amantadine and rimantadine have significant resistance now and are no longer used
- **Health Maintenance**
  - Vaccination! all children, elderly, pregnant, asthmatics, chronic other diseases
  - Avoidance of sick contacts
- **Scientific concepts**
  - Vaccination is key pearl here!
  - Treatment may also be symptomatic and not require medication.
  - If using medication, must be given within 48 hours of onset – if longer onset, not indicated (waste of money, and potential side effects)

Pertussis

- **Epidemiology**
  - Thought eradicated through vaccination, but apparently it doesn't last
- **Etiology**
  - Bordetella *pertussis*
- **H & P**
  - Starts as URI
  - Paroxysmal cough with post-tussive emesis and "whoop"
  - Convalescent stage may last months
- **Labs & Diagnostics**
  - Nasopharyngeal swab
- **Clinical Intervention**
  - If respiratory distress (infants, small children), hospitalize for observation
- **Therapeutics**
  - Use a macrolide (clarithromycin; azithromycin)
- **Health Maintenance**
  - Very contagious – occurs in epidemics
  - Tdap every ten years to age 65 instead of tetanus booster
- **Scientific Concept**
  - *NEW - On October 27, 2010, the ACIP voted to recommend:*
  - Use of Tdap regardless of interval since the last tetanus or diphtheria containing vaccine
  - Use of Tdap in certain adults ages 65 and older, (*but very recently no age limit*)
  - Use of Tdap in under-vaccinated children ages 7 through 10 years

Acute Epiglottitis

- **Epidemiology**
  - Was common occurrence due to H. influenza in children
    - Now extremely uncommon among vaccinated children
  - More common now in adults, though still rare
- **Etiology**
  - H. influenza cellulitis of epiglottis causing airway obstruction
- **H & P**
  - Fever
  - Drooling; unable to control secretions
  - Cherry red epiglottis
  - Dysphonia/dysphagia
  - Tachycardia/tachypnea
  - No cough typically (unlike croup)
- **Labs & Diagnostics**
  - Blood cultures
  - CBC
  - May need CXR to r/o pneumonia (25%)
  - Lateral soft tissue neck plain films
- **Clinical Intervention**
  - Maintain airway
  - Early placement of endotrach tube in child; adults usually manage better
- **Therapeutics**
  - Ceftriaxone, 1-2 gm. IV
- **Health Maintenance**
  - *HIB vaccine
- **Scientific concepts**
  - Vaccination has virtually wiped this out as a cause in kids

---

Pneumonia

Basic Tenets About Pneumonia:

- 8th leading cause of death in U.S.
- Mortality has improved since influenza and pneumococcal vaccine (health maintenance question!)
- Most pneumonias are viral (influenza)
- Most common bacterial cause of pneumonia is strep pneumonia
- Joint Commission and CDC, Medicare Services, and American Thoracic society have measures for management:
  - **Blood cultures performed BEFORE administration of antibiotics**
  - **Antibiotics must be begun within 6 hours of patient arrival**
  - **Smoking cessation counseling must be done**
- Presentation for viral and bacterial are different – pay careful attention below
- Antibiotic therapy is empirical; sputum culture takes 48 hours, AFB even longer – so treatment against most likely pathogen is everything here – make sure you memorize treatments for the appropriate pathogen

MICROBIOLOGIC DIFFERENTIAL DIAGNOSIS OF PNEUMONIA

History	Associated Organisms
Chronic obstructive lung disease (COPD)	S. pneumoniae, **Haemophilus influenzae**, Moraxella catarrhalis, **Legionella** spp.
Postinfluenza	S. pneumoniae, **S. aureus**, Streptococcus pyogenes, H. Influenzae
Aspiration	Mixed aerobic, **Klebsiella**
Alcoholism	Streptococcus pneumoniae, **Klebsiella**, M. tuberculosis
Anatomic abnormality of lung parenchyma (bronchiectasis, cystic fibrosis	**Pseudomonas aeruginosa**, S. aureus
Obstruction of large airway	Anaerobes, S. pneumoniae, H. influenzae, S. aureus
HIV infection	**Pneumocystis jiroveci,** cytomegalovirus, Cryptococcus spp., Histoplasma spp., Coccidioides spp.
Injection drug use	**S. aureus**, **MRSA**, anaerobes, M. tuberculosis, S. pneumoniae
Incarceration	M. tuberculosis
Marijuana smoking	Aspergillus spp.
Neutropenia	Aspergillus spp.
Asplenia	S. pneumoniae, H. influenzae
Desert travel, southwest United States	Coccidioides spp., Hantavirus (Sin Nombre virus)
Farm Exposure	Aspergillus spp.(barns, hay)
Exposure to bat or bird droppings, construction sites, caves	Histoplasma capsulatum
Exposure to birds	Chlamydia psittaci

Those in bold are most important to know. (MRSA = methicillin resistant staph aureus)

OVERVIEW OF THE MANY CAUSES OF PNEUMONIA

Viral Etiologies

- Acute bronchitis
- Influenza
- Viral pneumonia
- HIV-related

Bacterial Etiologies

- *Typicals*
    - Strep Pneumoniae
    - Hemophilus Influenza
    - Moraxella Catarrhalis
- *Atypicals*
    - Mycoplasma pneumoniae
    - Chlamydia

Mycobacterial Etiologies

- M. Tuberculosis

Fungal Etiologies *(look for something about immunocompromised status in the PMH of the patient)*

- Pneumocystis jerovicii (PCP)
- Aspergillus spp.
- Candida spp.
- Mucor spp.
- Cryptococcus neoformans
- Coccidioides spp.

BACTERIAL PNEUMONIA (CAP, healthcare-acquired, aspiration)

Community Acquired Pneumonia (CAP)= bacterial pneumonias acquired as an outpatient

- **Epidemiology**
    - Still 8th or 9th leading cause of death overall and 6th due to infectious disease
- **Etiology**
    - Typical = S. pneumonia, H. influenza, M. catarrhalis
    - Atypical = Legionella, Chlamydia, Mycoplasma
    - Tuberculosis covered separately in Infectious Disease Chapter XXX
- **H & P**
    - Fever T>100.4 (or hypothermia T<96.8 in critically ill) with rigors
    - Tachypnea, dyspnea, hypoxia
    - Cough (usually productive)
    - Change in color of sputum in COPD patient
    - Egophany
    - Increased tactile and vocal fremitus

- **Labs & Diagnostics**
    - *CXR*
        - Air Bronchograms
    - *Sputum analysis – gram stain, culture & sensitivity*
        - 40-50% sensitivity if correct collection:
        - "Ok" for analysis = pmn's and no epithelial cells
        - Vs. "spit" = few pmn's and epithelial cells
        - Blood cultures x 2 in adult, x 1 in child
            - (10-25% have bacteremia)
    - *Urinary antigen assay*
        - As high as 50-80% sensitivity for pneumococcus
    - *Bronchioalveolar lavage (BAL)*
        - Invasive, not done in ED, for specific therapy – but do not delay antibiotics in order to obtain
- **Clinical Intervention – who warrants admission?**
    - *CURB-65*
        - Confusion = 1 pt
        - Urea (renal failure) = 1 pt
        - RR > 24 = 1 pt
        - SBP<90 or DBP < 60 = 1 pt
        - Age > 65 = 1 pt
    - *Risk of death:*
        - 1-2 pt = 3% (OP may be considered)
        - 3 = 17% (IP best)
        - 4 = 42% (ICU consideration)
        - 5 = 57% (ICU)
- **Therapeutics**
    - See Clinical Therapeutics (Chapter 4) for drug indications – Bugs & Drugs
- **Health Maintenance**
    - Pneumovax
        - Asthmatics
        - Eldery
        - Splenectomy (or functionally asplenic, i.e. sickle cell, spherocytosis)
        - Immunocompromised (by disease, or medication)
    - Influenza vaccine for patients at risk for pneumonia (see ID)

HEALTHCARE AQUIRED PNEUMONIA (Nosocomial)

- Any patient with pneumonia who has been hospitalized within 90 days of onset
- Any patient with pneumonia from nursing home
- Any patient at increased risk of *pseudomonas* infection

ASPIRATION PNEUMONIA

- Alcoholics
- Neurologic disorders (abnormal gag/swallow)
- Increased risk of *gram negative aspiration* from stomach

PEARL: *Legionella and Chlamydia are intracellular (will not show up on gram stain)*

- Legionella can cause a "relative" bradycardia (heart rate not as high as temperature would suggest it should be)
    - Legionella causes abdominal pain, diarrhea
- In younger individuals who are markedly ill (18 year olds without comorbidities) think GAS (group A strep), very lethal form of pneumonia – associated with toxic shock syndrome; mortality as high as 38%
    - (This is what Jim Henson the Muppet maker died from)
- Similar symptoms in young people that lead rapidly to death from pneumonia are from MRSA (methicillin resistant staph aureus)
- Varicella virus causes pneumonia primarily in adults. This pneumonia is an indication of dissemination of the virus. All adults with varicella pneumonia must be hospitalized. Illness from varicella in pregnancy causes very high morbidity and mortality.

Neoplastic Disorders

PULMONARY NODULES – single lesion < 3 cm in size

- **Epidemiology**
    - 30% malignant
    - 70% benign
- **Etiology**
    - Infectious granuloma – most common
    - Infection
    - Vascular lesion
    - Cancer
- **H & P**
    - Typically asymptomatic
    - Possible cough/hemoptysis
- **Labs & Diagnostics**
    - CXR (compare to previous)
    - Serial CXR q 3 mos to observe
    - CT if high risk (suspicious lesion)
    - Biopsy if suspicious on CT
- **Clinical Intervention**
    - Referral for biopsy if indicated (suspicious CT)
- **Health Maintenance**
    - Stop smoking!
- **Scientific concepts**
    - *Benign* = Round, smooth, central calcium "popcorn" pattern
        - Growth; double < 1 mos or > 2 years (either very quick or very slow)
    - *Malignant* = Irregular, speculated
        - Growth; Double > 1 month < 2years

LUNG CANCER (Bronchogenic Carcinoma)

- **Epidemiology**
    - Increases with smoking duration and age
    - Most common cause of cancer *death* US and worldwide
    - *Not* most common cancer! lower incidence than breast, prostate, colon
        - but higher death rate
- **Etiology**
    - Small cell carcinoma (central tumor)
    - Non-small cell carcinoma
    - Adenocarcinoma (peripheral tumor)
    - Squamous cell carcinoma (central tumor)
    - Large cell carcinoma (peripheral tumor)
- **Risk Factors**
    - SMOKING!
    - Age
    - Radiation
    - Asbestos (combined with smoking)
    - HIV
- **H & P**
    - Chronic cough
    - Hemoptysis
    - Dyspnea
    - Weight loss
    - Anemia
    - Hoarseness
    - Superior Vena Cava Syndrome
        - From lymph node enlargement impeding flow of lymph
        - Swelling of neck and face; may compromise airway
- **Labs & Diagnostics**
    - CXR
    - CT chest
    - Sputum Cytology
    - Biopsy
- **Health Maintenance**
    - STOP SMOKING!!!
- **Scientific Concepts**
    - Paraneoplastic syndromes associated with lung cancer
        - Small cell **(most common)**
        - SIADH (syndrome of increased ADH)
        - Dermatomyositis
        - Cushing syndrome
        - Eaton-Lambert syndrome (Myasthenia Gravis like syndrome)
        - Acanthosis nigricans
        - Hypercalcemia
        - hypoglycemia
- **How to remember histology:**
    - "S" = squamous and small cell = "Sentral"; Others are peripheral

CARCINOID TUMORS – (this probably belongs in GI, but the NCCPA puts it here for some reason (?)

- **Etiology**
  - Neoplasm arising from neuroendocrine cells
    - Appendix #1
    - Small bowel #2
    - Rectum #3
    - Bronchus #4
- **H & P**
  - Vasomotor flushing – *almost 90% have facial flushing episodes that spread to trunk*
  - Dizziness, tachycardia, hypotension – paroxysmal
  - Diarrhea with abdominal bloating
  - Bronchospasm, intermittently (maybe that is why it is in pulmonary?)
  - Facial telangiectasia
- **Labs & Diagnostics**
  - Marker = 5-HIAA (serotonin metabolite)
  - Imaging: CT of abdomen; octreotide scan; CXR
- **Clinical Intervention**
  - Surgical resection of tumor can be a cure
  - If metastasis, palliative surgery
- **Therapeutics**
  - Chemotherapy
  - Management of symptoms (H2 blockers like ranitidine, famotidine)
  - Albuterol for bronchospasm
- **Scientific concepts**
  - Paroxysmal symptoms (like pheo) but OPPOSITE – *this one causes **HYPO**tension, pheo causes HYPERtension*
  - Flushing is major clue
  - Diarrhea is second clue
  - Should remind you of serotinergic syndrome, yes? *(but patient not on SSRI's!)*

Pleural Diseases

MESOTHELIOMA

- **Epidemiology**
  - Due to asbestos exposure (plumbers, remodelers, Navy prior to OSHA regulations)
  - Increased risk of mesothelioma in asbestosis exposure in a smoker
- **Clinical presentation**
  - Cough
- **Labs & Diagnostics**
  - CXR shows pleural plaques
- **Clinical Intervention**
  - Referral to oncology/pulmonary medicine
- **Treatment**
  - Surgery, chemotherapy, external beam radiation

PLEURITIS/PLEURISY

- **Epidemiology**
  - Common; usually follows an upper respiratory infection or bronchitis
- **Clinical presentation**
  - Sharp pleuritic-type chest pain with deep breathing
  - No pain to palpation of ribs/costochondral margins (this would be costochrondritis and has similar presentation)
  - Friction rub (not rales, crackles, rhonchi) – *sounds like velcro with each breath*
- **Labs & Diagnostics**
  - CXR – almost always normal, but a very tiny pleural effusion could be present
- **Clinical Intervention**
  - Pain relief
  - If splinting and not deep breathing, give patient an incentive spirometer to prevent pneumonia
- **Health Maintenance**
  - Incentive spirometer
  - Used to prevent atelectasis/pneumonia from splinting behavior

How can you tell the difference between a pleural and a pericardial friction rub?

Answer: Have the patient hold their breath; pleural rub will go away; pericardial rub will persist

PLEURAL EFFUSION

- **Epidemiology**
  - Result of other disease process (exudative)
  - Increased pulmonary pressures (transudative)
- **Etiology**
  - *Transudative (like water)*
    - Renal failure (third spacing of fluid from hypoalbuminemia)
    - Congestive heart failure
    - Liver failure (cirrhosis, third spacing due to hypoalbuminemia)
    - Hypothyroidism
  - *Exudative (purulent or proteinaceous)*
    - Malignancy
    - Pneumonia
    - TB
    - Autoimmune inflammatory (lupus, RA)
    - Pancreatitis
- **H & P**
  - Decreased breath sounds in area of effusion
  - Dullness to percussion
  - Egophany
  - Hypoxia varies with size of effusion and patient's pulmonary reserve

- **History**
    - Dyspnea, cough, pleuritic chest pain
- **PE**
    - Decreased breath sounds
    - Dullness to percussion
    - Egophany
- **Labs & Diagnostics**
    - CXR - blunting of the costophrenic angles
- **Clinical Intervention**
    - Observe
    - Thoracentesis – therapeutic/diagnostic
- **Scientific concepts**
    - *Light's criteria*
        - Pleural/serum protein < 0.5 (transudative) ; >0.5 (exudative)
        - Pleural/serum LDH < 0.6 (transudative) ; >0.6 (exudative)

PEARL: *Pleural Effusions:*

- Effusions are a consequence of fluid accumulating in the interstitium
- Due to gravity, there is "layering" out in the most dependent parts (when the patient is upright) which are the costophrenic sulci.
- It is important to note that the deepest sulcus is the posterior sulcus (you will find "blunting" of that sulcus on the lateral view of the CXR)
- See Chapter 10 on how to distinguish transudative from exudative effusions (and therefore, establish a shorter differential for "the most likely diagnosis")

Pneumothorax

PRIMARY PNEUMOTHORAX

- **Epidemiology**
    - Tall thin young male smokers
    - Marfan's syndrome
- **Etiology**
    - Spontaneous rupture of visceral pleura causing air to flow between the visceral and parietal pleura filling that virtual space
- **H & P**
    - Hyperresonance on auscultation/ hypertympanic on percussion
    - Rule out tension
        - ** Deviated trachea = tension pneumothorax (see below)*
- **Labs & Diagnostics**
    - CXR
- **Clinical Intervention**
    - Chest tube
- **Scientific Concepts**
    - Occurs "spontaneously"
    - Most typically in tall thin young men (Marfanoid), usually but not always a smoker –
    - the clue is *sudden onset* of pleuritic chest pain and dyspnea

SECONDARY PNEUMOTHORAX

- **Etiology**
    - Trauma
    - Central line placement
    - Emphysema (bleb rupture)
- **H & P** –same as primary
- **Labs & Diagnostics** -same
- **Clinical Intervention** –same
- **Formulating the Most Likely Diagnosis**
    - <u>Sudden onset</u> of pleuritic chest pain and dyspnea
- **Health Maintenance**
    - Post op CXR following all line placements
- **Scientific Concept**
    - Occurs most often in emphysemic patients (older epidemiology) from rupture of a bleb

TRAUMATIC PNEUMOTHORAX

- Occurs with trauma (duh) –
- Most often secondary to a rib fracture, could be a knife, ice pick, etc..

TENSION PNEUMOTHORAX

When a complete collapse of the lung is causing "tension" in the pleural space, and the empty lung is being "pushed" over

- **H & P**
    - The trachea gets shifted
    - Tracheal "tugging"

  *Life threatening emergency requiring immediate needle decompression
- **Scientific Concept**
    - The underlying pathology is decreased venous return to the heart due to the wildly increased pressures in the chest ---

PEARL: Chest tube placement depends primarily on the status of the patient; but in general also on the size of the pneumothorax

- For vital signs, the following would warrant tube placement: RR> 24, HR <60 or >120, Pulse Ox < 90%)
- For size of pneumothorax, >25% is the typically accepted number

Acute Respiratory Distress Syndrome

This is kind of like congestive heart failure without the heart involvement. There is damage to the alveolar air spaces which results in the patient becoming hypoxemic, with alveolar edema (but not due to increased LV or LA pressures). The heart size on CXR would be normal.

- **Etiologies**
  - Sepsis
  - Drowning
  - Opiate overdose
  - Trauma
  - Severe burns
  - Pancreatitis
  - S/p resuscitation
- **H & P**
  - Dyspnea
  - Chest pain
  - Cough
- **Labs & diagnostics**
  - BNP would be normal (see congestive heart failure section)
  - CXR would show diffuse alveolar infiltrates **but without cardiomegaly**
- **Clinical Intervention**
  - O2 does not work (hallmark of this process)
  - Mechanical ventilation or tracheotomy are needed

PEARL: *Pulmonary Hypertension (also covered in more depth in Chapter 10)*

- **Elevation of pulmonary vascular pressure causes:**
  - Primary pulmonary hypertension
  - Idiopathic or due to weight loss (and other) drugs
- **Secondary pulmonary hypertension**
  - *Left heart failure (CHF)*
    - causes pressure due to poor forward flow of blood
    - pressure back up into the left atrium
    - and eventually into the pulmonary vascular bed
  - COPD
  - Cystic Fibrosis
  - Pneumoconioses
  - Pulmonary embolism (acutely, obviously)
  - Near drowning

PEARL: *Cor Pulmonale (covered in Physiology, Chapter 10)*

Let the Latin help you – This is heart failure *(cor)* due to the lungs *(pulmonale).* The clue here is that the patient with cor pulmonale will have a pulmonary cause for pulmonary edema (heart size is normal, no evidence of heart failure, no cardiac history).

"Go confidently in the direction of your dreams. Live the life you have imagined."

–Henry David Thoreau

CHAPTER 13

Gastroenterology/Nutritional Deficiencies – 10%

Introduction to Gastroenterology Chapter

General Principles: The entire GI section is different from the rest. In this section, I will cover all the NCCPA topics and will cover several topics not in the Blueprint, but felt significant enough to include.

The first section will cover all the GI topics in terms of their anatomy on physical exam, and the organs that cause those disease states. The next section will be covered in terms of their presenting symptoms instead of a laundry list in alphabetical order of all the topics. This is meant to highlight the fact that symptoms that may appear to be GI in origin may, in fact, be cardiac, or pulmonary, or autoimmune, etc.

The last section covers nutritional deficiencies, a specific topic in the Blueprint.

If you are not up to speed on hepatology labs, please review the section on LFT's in Chapter 6.

Diagnosis by Anatomy

Differential Diagnosis by Location

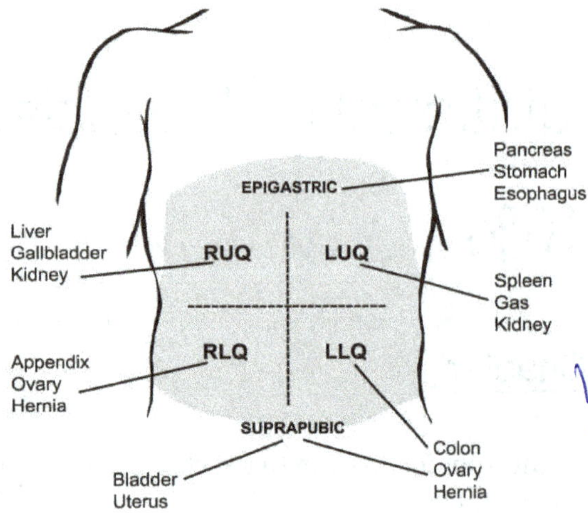

RIGHT UPPER QUADRANT

The Liver

PEARL: *Liver*

The liver functions to produce or synthesize:

- Albumin
- Coagulation factors
- Conjugation of bilirubin

The liver enzymes increase in the serum if damage to hepatocytes (which may not affect the liver's function for a very long time):

- AST
- ALT
- Alk p'tase
- GGTP/5'nucleotidase

Hepatitic Liver Enzyme Pattern (liver disease)	Cholestatic Enzyme Pattern (biliary disease)
Very high ALT > AST (100 x's normal)	Mild elevation ALT>AST (2-3 x's normal)
Mild elevation alk p'tase	Very high alk p'tase
Mild (if any) elevation of GGTP	Elevation of GGTP

Acute Viral Hepatitis

- **Etiologies**
  - *CMV*
    - Infants, immunocompromised
    - Infectious mononucleosis
    - Typically young adults (self-limited hepatitis)
  - *HSV*
    - Often subclinical (asymptomatic, just feels "lousy")
  - *Hepatitis A, B, C, D*
    - All are covered below
- **H & P**
  - All patients with acute hepatitis have these symptoms (except Hep. C, which is asymptomatic!)
    - Malaise, anorexia, nausea
    - Dark urine
    - **Icterus/jaundice**
- **Labs & Diagnostics**
  - ALT>AST (20+ times elevated)
  - Bilirubin variably elevated
  - S. albumin, protime, coags all normal

Hepatitis A

- **Epidemiology/Etiology**
  - 65% of causes of Hepatitis in US
  - Fecal-oral (think foreign travel/flooded areas of US)
  - Mild disease (rarely fulminant)
  - No chronic carrier (infection) state
- **H & P**
  - As above
- **Labs & Diagnostics**
  - Positive IgM to HAV = acute infection
  - Immunity is suggested by IgG to HAV
- **Clinical Intervention**
  - No treatment is necessary, avoid ETOH and liver metabolized meds
- **Health Maintenance**
  - If not immune and traveling to area at risk, vaccinate

PEARL: *To remember that IgM goes up first:* M = miserable
When you are *acutely ill*, you are miserable. When your body makes antibodies to the antigen, you get better as Ig**G** is made and you feel **g**ood again. It works!

Hepatitis B *(See Chapter 6 for detailed Hep B Serology information)*

- **Epidemiology**
  - Clinical outcome depends on host defense
  - Chronic carrier (US) 5-10%
  - Major risk factor for cirrhosis and hepatocellular Ca if a chronic carrier (80% of all causes)
  - 90% of patients recover completely
  - Risk of chronicity related to age (90% infants) & immune status
- **Etiology**
  - IVDA (35%)
  - Sex (19%)
  - Transfusion (5%)
  - Needle stick (1%)
- **Clinical Intervention**
  - Monitor liver function
  - Avoid liver metabolized drugs; alcohol
- **Health Maintenance**
  - Vaccinate US children at 2, 4, 6 mos of age
  - Vaccinate health care workers
- **Scientific Concept**
  - Of patients with fulminant hepatitis - 50% are caused by Hep B

Hepatitis C

- **Epidemiology**
  - Most common blood-borne infection
  - Leading cause of chronic liver failure
  - Most common indication for transplant
  - 80% of infected patients develop chronic Hep C infection
  - 20% of these patients develop cirrhosis
  - 1-5% of chronic carriers develop hepatocellular carcinoma
- **Etiologies**
  - IV drug abuse – 40%
  - Transfusion – 5-10%
  - health care workers – 5%
  - Sexual activity – debatable – 10% by CDC estimates
  - Tattoos (?) – particular in prison systems
- **Labs & Diagnostics**
  - Screen with EIA – 97% sensitivity
  - If EIA positive – RIBA to confirm (checks for specific antigens)
  - Viral load testing
  - HCV RNA establishes chronicity as well as following therapeutic management

- Ongoing LFT's
- **Therapeutics**
  - *Pegylated interferon plus ribavirin*
    - Also follow early viral response (EVR)
    - And sustained viral response (SVR)
    - Which helps to direct the length of treatment
- **Health Maintenance**
  - No vaccine available
  - Screen patients with high risk for exposure
  - This is an asymptomatic disease until too late
- **Scientific Concept**
  - *Interferon treatment considerations:*
    - Patients with Depression
      - Interferon causes severe and profound depression with high risk of suicide
      - It used to be contraindicated in patients with depression – but now if under active management of psychiatry, may have interferon
    - Patients with Autoimmune Disease
      - Consider risk/benefit when determining "whether or not to start therapy
  - *Many new drugs being tested*
  - *FDA approval of two new drugs in 2011 to be added to standard therapies (above)*
    - Treats genotype 1 (majority of HCV patients)
    - Protease inhibitors
      - Bocepravir
      - Telaprevir
    - Best for patients who have responded to interferon and ribavirin but are not cured
    - Also used for those who did not respond at all

Hepatitis D

- **Epidemiology**
  - The virus can only replicate if HepB-sAg is present
  - <5% of chronic HBV carriers
- **Etiology**
  - IVDA/sexual contact?
- **Treatment** - none

Chronic Liver Failure

Hemachromatosis

- **Epidemiology**
  - Autosomal recessive
  - Onset ~ 50 yrs. in women
  - Males manifest disease earlier
    - Women "phlebotomize" every month until menopause!
    - Women have increased requirements for Fe during pregnancy & lactation

- **Etiology**
  - Increased intestinal absorption of iron causing "iron overload"
- **H & P**
  - Arthralgias
  - Hepatomegaly
  - Gray skin
  - Cardiomegaly/conduction disorders
  - DM
  - ED in men
- **Labs**
  - Elevated S. Ferritin
- **Clinical Intervention**
  - Weekly phlebotomy

Wilson's Disease

- **Epidemiology**
  - Autosomal recessive
  - Rare
- **Etiology**
  - Copper is deposited in tissues (liver, brain primarily)
- **H & P**
  - Usually presents with liver failure as few early signs
  - Kayser-Fleischer ring in iris
  - Conduction abnormalities of the heart
  - Always consider Wilson's in patient < 40 yr with parkinsonian symptoms (a little factoid I never knew before – learn something from doing PanceMaster Q's!)
- **Labs**
  - Low serum ceruloplasmin
- **Clinical Intervention**
  - Penicillamine
- **Scientific Concept**
  - Gene mutation identified – called the Wilson gene mutation (finally, something easy to remember!)

NASH (Nonalcoholic Steatohepatitis)/NAFL (Nonalcoholic Fatty Liver)

- **Etiology**
  - Obesity
- **H & P**
  - Asymptomatic
  - No h/o alcoholism, liver metabolized meds, illness, or other reason
  - Normal exam except for obesity/possibly hepatomegaly
- **Labs & Diagnostics**
  - Elevated LFT's – without other explanation
    - ALT > AST (distinguishes it from alcohol pattern of AST > ALT)
  - US shows "fatty liver"
  - Can be incidentally found on CT showing fatty infiltration of the liver

    - *Liver biopsy is the only way to confirm the diagnosis*
- **Clinical intervention/health maintenance**
    - **Weight loss**
    - Avoid alcohol

PEARL: *NAFLD (non-alcoholic fatty liver disease)* is present in 20% of the U.S. population. Of this 20%, 2-5% develop liver disease and possible cirrhosis from this NASH. No therapies exist; mainstay of treatment is to help the patient lose weight.

In alcoholic fatty liver, the patient may have *tender* hepatomegaly.

Alcoholic Cirrhosis

- **Epidemiology**
    - Common cause of chronic illness worldwide
- **Etiology**
    - 4 beers/day for 10 years is enough to kill the liver
- **Labs & Diagnostics**
    - Vitamin and calorie deficiency
    - Megaloblastic anemia (folate/B vitamin deficiencies)
    - AST > ALT (rarely above 300)
    - Increased bilirubin - 60-90% of patients
    - Prolonged PT/INR = poor prognosis
    - Hypoalbuminemia = poor prognosis
- **Clinical Intervention**
    - Abstinence
    - Thiamine replacement
    - Folic acid replacement
- **Scientific Concept --- complications of cirrhosis:**
    - Portal hypertension with splenomegaly
        - Caput medusae
    - Variceal bleeding (from above)
    - Ascites (osmotic secondary to hypoalbuminemia)
    - Spontaneous bacterial peritonitis (SBP)
        - Peritoneal infection from normal gut flora due to immunocompromised status
    - Encephalopathy (Wernicke's)

PEARL: *Alcoholic cirrhosis:*

- The classic picture of alcohol abuse on lab evaluation is the combination of any or all of the following:
    - *Macrocytic anemia*
        - Low H & H
        - MCV > 100
        - Due to chronic folic acid deficiency
    - *AST > ALT in a pattern of 2:1*

        - Recall that in liver disease from other reasons, the ALT > AST
            - i.e. AST = 300, ALT = 150
        - Usually not very high (all the liver cells are dead, so no enzyme left to leak!)
    - *Direct bilirubinemia (elevated direct fraction of bilirubin)*
    - *GGTP is 2 x elevated*
    - *Physical findings of cirrhosis*
        - Ascites, gynecomastia, plethoric facies, telangiectasias, splenomegaly with caput medusae

Hepatocellular Carcinoma

- **Etiology**
    - Anything that causes chronic inflammation
    - Chronic active Hep B, Hep C, alcohol
- **H & P**
    - Jaundice (increased direct fraction)
    - RUQ discomfort (usually no symptoms, like all cancers, so caught late)
- **Labs & diagnostics**
    - AFP is the marker
    - Usually abnormal transaminases
    - Direct bilirubinemia

- **Formulating Most Likely Diagnosis**:
    - Look for the risk factors *(above in etiology)*
- **Clinical Intervention**
    - Treatment of choice = partial hepatectomy (if no features of metastasis)
    - Radiofrequency ablation
    - Chemoembolization
    - No transplant for liver cancer
- **Health Maintenance:**
    - Hep B vaccination!
    - Alcohol is a risk factor; so decrease alcohol intake
        - Ask and intervene in alcohol abuse

PEARL: While uncommon in the US, liver cancer is very common in the rest of the world due to the endemic nature of Hepatitis B

The Gall Bladder

Cholelithiasis - *Stones in the GB (not in cystic duct)*

- **Epidemiology**
    - Female, fat, forty, fertile (how rude!)
    - Men get gallstones! Just saying...
- **H & P**
    - No fever
    - Post-prandial biliary colic – (occurs 1-2 hours after fatty meal)
    - Resolves on own
    - No Murphy's sign

    - Should be asymptomatic in between "attacks"
- **Labs & Diagnostics**
    - *Labs*
        - Alkaline phosphatase, bilirubin, AST, ALT all normal
    - *RUQ ultrasound will show stones without common bile duct (CBD)dilatation*
    - *HIDA scan if no stones found and high index that there is insufficient GB motility*
        - This is scheduled as an elective imaging study
        - Nuclear medicine (not in pregnancy or nursing)
    - *And/or cystic duct patency evaluation*
- **Clinical Intervention**
    - Elective surgical referral for cholecystectomy
        - Most often done laparoscopically now
    - If poor surgical risk give low fat diet
- **Scientific Concept:**
    - 80% cholesterol
    - Female, fat, fertile, forty
    - 20% "pigment" or bilirubin stones
    - Hemolytic anemias (rapid turnover of bilirubin) (see hemolytic anemia section)

Acute Cholecystitis

- **Etiology**
    - Stone in cystic duct
- **H & P**
    - Positive Murphy's sign
    - Jaundice
    - Low grade temp
- **Labs & Diagnostics**
    - Should have normal ALT/AST
    - Check lipase – should be normal if only cystic duct involved
    - RUQ US shows cystic duct dilatation *without* dilatation of CBD
- **Clinical Intervention**
    - Needs surgical referral
    - Laparoscopic cholecystectomy

Choledocholithiasis

- **Etiology**
    - Gallstone in CBD (common bile duct)
- **Labs & Diagnostics**
    - Elevated bilirubin (direct fraction)
    - Elevated alkaline phosphatase
    - Elevation of ALT/AST
    - Check lipase/amylase
        - Gallstones and alcohol are two most common RF for acute pancreatitis!
- **Clinical Intervention**
    - *Needs surgical referral*
        - Laparoscopic cholecystectomy
        - ERCP (endoscopic retrograde cholangiopancreatography)
        - Endoscopic means to retrieve gallstone in CBD

    - *If pancreatitis, prognosis is worse*

Ascending Cholangitis

- **Etiology**
    - Stone has caused inflammation/infection of bile ducts
    - Think of this as an abscess/cellulitis in the biliary tree
        - Transmigration of bacteria from the portal circulation
- **Labs & Diagnostics**
    - Leukocytosis with left shift
    - Increased transaminases (ALT/AST)
    - Increased total and direct bilirubin
- **Clinical Intervention**
    - RUQ US to look for CBD dilatation
    - ERCP for biliary decompression
        - Both diagnostic and therapeutic
    - Acute surgical intervention
    - This is a toxic patient, needs admission to ICU
        - IV fluids
        - Broad spectrum antibiotics
- **Scientific Concept**
    - Charcot's triad:
        - RUQ pain
        - High fever (>40C)
        - Jaundice
    - Reynolds's pentad:
        - RUQ pain
        - High fever (>40C)
        - Jaundice
        - AMS (altered mental status)
        - Hypotension

Cholangiocarcinoma

- **Epidemiology**
    - Uncommon
    - Adenocarcinoma more often than squamous cell cancer
    - Major risk factor is chronic disease of the biliary tract:
        - Ulcerative colitis
        - Primary sclerosing cholangitis (PSC) – increased risk in UC
        - Having both UC + PSC = increased risk of cholangiocarcinoma
        - Choledochal cysts
    - Tumor marker = CEA

PEARL: as a reminder, if you suspect this patient may be going to the O.R., you will want to order him to be NPO (no per oral intake); this may be your immediate intervention! It would be bad to have a family member giving him fluids just prior to his going to the O.R.

A 56 year old female patient presents with acute onset of RUQ pain for the past 6 hours which was colicky but has become constant.

VS : T 40C; HR 120; RR 22; BP 120/64

Patient appears ill and has epigastric and RUQ pain with positive Murphy's sign
Labs show leukocytosis with left shift. AST, ALT, Alk-ptase, lipase are all 5-10 x elevated.

What is the most likely diagnosis?

A. cholelithiasis
B. acute cholecystitis
C. choledocholithiasis
D. ascending cholangitis
E. acute pancreatitis

Answer: E.

***Discussion*:** This question is one of those mildly tricky ones where it looks like a gall bladder problem (and, in fact, is a GB problem) but it is causing a bigger issue, i.e what was choledocholithiasis is now a gallstone pancreatitis. This is, in fact the answer C. but the best answer has to do with the fact that the pancreas is now inflamed, and the surgeon would sure like to know this!

If the patient had, instead, acute cholecystitis, which of the following would you expect to find?

A. 10 times elevation of transaminases
B. 4-5 times elevation of lipase/amylase
C. RUQ US demonstrating gall stones without dilatation of the CBD (common bile duct)
D. high fever, hypotension, altered mental status
E. resolution of symptoms and normal PE

Answer: C.

***Discussion*:** A represents possible choledocholithiasis; B represents a gallstone pancreatitis; D represents ascending cholangitis; E. represents cholelithiasis.

Be very careful to read the words carefully when you are tired and answering these questions!

EPIGASTRIUM

Esophagus

Esophagitis *(this is the topic in the blueprint, there are many causes; will cover all briefly here, and most important in greater detail)*

- Reflux esophagitis
    - See GERD below
- Alcohol esophagitis (much the same as erosive gastritis)
    - Stop drinking!
- Infectious esophagitis (see odynophagia above)
    - Think immunocompromised, or patients who inhale or swallow steroids
        - Causes: Candida, CMV, HSV
    - Clinical Intervention
        - Upper endoscopy for diagnosis
        - Treat appropriately for yeast infection or viral infection

GERD

- Epidemiology
    - 10-20% of adults have sxs 1-7/wk
    - 50% develop reflux esophagitis
- H & P
    - Heartburn exacerbated by meals, bending over, recumbency
    - Increased incidence with increased abdominal girth
        - pregnancy
            - pregnancy also causes decrease lower esophageal sphincter tone due to smooth muscle relaxation
        - obesity
    - History of NSAID use
    - Regurgitation of sour tasting refluxate
    - Some relief with antacids
- Labs & Diagnostics
    - CBC, CMP, DRE (to r/o bleeding)
- Clinical Intervention
    - Treat empirically for 4 weeks – H2RA, PPI
        - Uncomplicated patient – typical sxs
        - No red flags (see ulcer above)
        - No dysphagia or odynophagia
        - Must have normal labs and normal PE
    - Endoscopy
        - Failure of empirical treatment
        - Any of above red flags

Barrett's Esophagus

- Definiton:
    - metaplasia of esophageal squamous epithelium
    - can progress to dysplasia and then to adenocarcinoma
- Epidemiology
    - Typically a white male with longstanding issues with reflux
- Etiology
    - Complication of GERD (10% with chronic reflux disease will develop BE)

    - Increased risk for adenocarcinoma of esophagus (0.8% annual incidence – 40 fold increased risk compared to patients without BE)
- Labs & Diagnostics
    - As for GERD/PUD
- Clinical Intervention
    - Upper endoscopy
        - "salmon colored change to the esophageal mucosa"
- Therapeutics
    - Long-term PPI therapy
    - endoscopic ablation
    - esophagectomy if high grade dysplasia is present of the Barrett's segment
- Health Maintenance
    - Regular surveillance with upper endoscopy by GI
    - No cure
- Scientific Concept
    - Squamous cells replaced with abnormal glandular-type epithelium
    - Thirty years ago, this was almost unheard of, most esophageal cancers were squamous cell (from smoking and alcohol, now from reflux disease) ---- see below

Esophageal carcinoma

- Epidemiology
    - 3:1 , men to women
    - 50-70 year old patients typically
        - Squamous cell
            - SE Asians, Blacks
            - Risk factor = Smoking, ETOH
        - Adenocarcinoma
            - Barrett's esophagus (White males)
            - Risk factor = GERD
            - See Barrett's esophagus above in GERD
- H & P
    - Significant weight loss is common
    - Dysphagia for SOLIDS only (90% present with this symptom)
- Labs & Diagnostics
    - Barium swallow
- Clinical Intervention
    - Endoscopy for biopsy and dx
    - Poor prognosis
    - Treatment options:
        - surgery
        - with preoperative chemotherapy and radiation

Achalasia & esophageal spasm (also discussed below in "dysphagia" section)

- Epidemiology
    - Much less common than GERD or other dysphagia etiologies
- H & P

- Dysphagia for SOLIDS AND LIQUIDS
- Diagnostics
  - Manometry
    - Assesses peristalsis (achalasia)
  - Endoscopy
    - Cancer suspicion, Schatzki's web

The Stomach

Peptic Ulcer Disease (PUD)

- Epidemiology
  - Most common risk factors:
    - H. Pylori
    - NSAID's
      - other risk factors include alcohol and smoking
  - Lifetime prevalence 10%
  - Slight male propensity (1.3 : 1)
  - Duodenal 5 X more than gastric
    - Duodenal 30-55 y.o.
    - Gastric 55-70 y.o.
- H & P
  - Benign abdominal exam if not perforated; mild epigastric discomfort
    - No masses should be palpable
  - DRE is done on ALL GI complaints – should be negative for blood
  - If perforated, peritoneal signs are present
    - Rigidity, guarding, decreased bowel sounds
- Labs & Diagnostics
  - CBC
  - H. Pylori testing (stool antigen is best, unless being scoped)
    - Stool antigen ->90% PPV
      - More sensitive than serum EIA
      - Cheaper than all the rest
    - Serology - EIA
      - still positive after treatment, so cannot be used for "test of cure"
    - Urea breath test
      - active infection - 90%PPV
    - Endoscopic biopsy
      - If upper endoscopy, H. Pylori will be done during endoscopy
  - DRE (as above in PE)
- Red Flags
  - Anemia (microcytic, anemia of Fe deficiency)
  - Positive hemoccult/hematemesis/melena
  - Weight loss (unintentional)
  - Persistent vomiting (suggests gastric outlet obstruction from scar from ulcer)
  - Progressive symptoms
- Clinical Intervention
  - May be empiric if <50, and no red flags

- EGD all patients with red flags
- EGD all patient with past h/o PUD
- EGD all patients >50 (per most authors)
- EGD all patients who fail empiric therapy

- Therapeutics
    - If empiric therapy, proton pump inhibitor (PPI), reassess in 4 weeks
        - Omeprazole, lansoprazole, etc.
        - H2RA (cimetidine, ranitidine) do not work as well, but are cheaper
    - Treat H. Pylori if positive (*know this triple therapy treatment*!)
        - Amoxicillin 1 gm. BID and
        - Clarithromycin 500 mg. BID and
        - PPI BID
            - all for 14 days
        - PCN allergic - substitute
            - Metronidazole 500 mg. BID
    - Follow up for eradication of H. Pylori
        - Patient completes two week therapy regimen
        - One month after treatment is completed; perform stool antigen test
            - Patient should remain off PPI until stool antigen is completed

Gastritis (this is the blueprint topic, many causes, see below):

Alcoholic gastritis
- Common with both acute alcohol "bingeing" or with chronic alcohol use
- Can result in erosive esophagitis with occult bleeding, Fe deficiency anemia, and ulcer formation

Atrophic gastritis
- Elderly, due to loss of mucosal barrier (this is why they are so prone to bleeding with NSAIDs (below) and steroids)
- No treatment, just be careful with giving the elderly meds that promote bleeding, atrophy

NSAID gastropathy
- RR in general population - 4.2
- Both a topical effect and non-topical effect (prostaglandin inhibition can cause gastritis and mask sxs)
- RF's
    - ***age
    - PUD/bleed
    - NSAID overuse
    - concomitant corticosteroids
- Clinical intervention
    - d/c NSAID and/or give with food and/or add PPI

Gastric Carcinoma
- Epidemiology
    - Most common cancer worldwide
    - #2 cause of cancer death *worldwide*
    - Uncommon in US

    - H. Pylori is strong risk factor
- H & P
    - Asymptomatic until late
    - Vague dyspepsia sxs with weight loss
- Labs & Diagnostics
    - CBC for Fe deficiency anemia
    - DRE
- Clinical Intervention
    - EGD all dyspepsia over age 50 if new, persistent or fails empiric treatment

The Pancreas

Acute Pancreatitis

- Etiology
    - gall stones and alcohol are equal in occurrence:
        - Alcohol – 50%
        - Gall stone (acute biliary pancreatitis) – 50%
    - ERCP can cause acute pancreatitis (would obviously occur after ERCP)
- H & P
    - Epigastric pain radiates into the back
    - Worse after eating, therefore, anorexia
    - Fever (75%)
    - Tachycardia (65%)
    - Epigastric pain with guarding & distention
    - Diminished bowel sounds (suggesting ileus)
    - Dehydration
    - AMS (altered mental status) is a very bad sign
    - Cullen sign – periumbilical bluish discoloration (due to leaking of pancreatic fluids)
    - Grey-Turner sign – flank bluish discoloration (two words like two flanks!) same cause – bleeding and leaking of pancreatic fluids – in flank, likely tail of pancreas
- Labs & Diagnostics
    - Lipase – 3X increase
        - Most specific for pancreas
        - May remain elevated for 10 days or more
    - Amylase
        - In saliva
        - May be elevated in:
            - Parotitis
            - Small bowel obstruction
            - Mesenteric ischemia
            - Renal failure
- Clinical Intervention
    - NPO
    - IV fluids
    - Pain control
    - If gallstone, cholecystectomy and/or ERCP may be needed
    - If alcohol, treat withdrawal

- Complications
    - Pseudocyst
        - "pseudo" because not lined with epithelial cells like a cyst
        - Formed due to "walling off" of the caustic enzymes by the body
        - Will cause distention, easy to see on US; or on CT
        - Management
        - most remit on their own with time and abstinence
            - if not, or if enlarging due to continued alcohol intake:
                - percutaneous drainage (IR)
                - or endoscopic drainage (GI)
    - Necrotizing pancreatitis
        - Ranson's criteria (identifies those at greatest risk of death)
            - WBC > 16,000
            - Age > 55 y.o.
            - Glucose > 200 (means pancreas no longer making insulin)
            - Low S. Calcium (calcium is being bound to fat and enzyme called "saponification", i.e. "soap formation"
            - LDH > 350 (recall, this means "cell lysis")
            - AST > 250 (damage to skeletal muscle)
    - Chronic Pancreatitis (see below)

Chronic Pancreatitis

- Etiology
    - alcohol
    - smoking
- H & P
    - chronic epigastric pain
    - steatorrhea (fat in stool due to malabsorption)
    - benign exam
- Clinical intervention
    - stop alcohol
    - may treat with pancreatic enzymes plus a PPI (very expensive),
    - low fat diet with vitamin supplementation
- Scientific Concept
    - As a diagnosis, this is completely different from acute pancreatitis.
    - This patient is chronically ill
        - has trouble with pain management
        - main medical issue is malabsorption of fat soluble vitamins and fat itself

Pancreatic Cancer

- Etiology
    - alcohol & smoking
- H & P
- Typical presentation
    - vague epigastric discomfort or
    - "knife-like" through to back or

- painless jaundice or
- occasionally a mass – recall that tumors may occur in the head of the pancreas (in the abdomen) or in the tail (retroperitoneal space) so could even give back discomfort ---- the symptoms are so vague it is usually caught late ----

- Labs & Diagnostics
  - CT with contrast
  - Tumor marker is Ca 19-9
- Clinical intervention
  - Whipple procedure (if patient surgical candidate)
  - chemotherapy
- poor prognosis no matter what

LEFT UPPER QUADRANT

There are no topics in the blueprint in the LUQ, but I would feel remiss if I did not discuss the most common cause of LUQ pain (gas) and a less common but lethal cause (splenic rupture, or splenic infarct)

Gas

- gas trapped in the splenic flexure is a very common cause of severe *atraumatic* LUQ sudden stabbing abdominal pain in an otherwise health patient with normal vital signs and labs

The Spleen

- after trauma, patient with LUQ pain should be considered to have a splenic rupture
- during infectious mononucleosis infection, spontaneous rupture is possible, and even minor trauma may cause splenic rupture
- splenic infarcts are possible in patients with coagulopathies (this is very uncommon)
- splenomegaly is a cause of LUQ pain in patients with leukemias, lymphomas, and would result in a palpable spleen tip on abdominal exam

LEFT LOWER QUADRANT

Large Bowel

Constipation (these topics are repeated below in "diagnosis by symptoms" section)

- Epidemiology
  - Iatrogenic (narcotics, calcium channel blockers, diuretics)
    - this is actually the MOST common cause of constipation
  - Irritable bowel syndrome – see below in chronic abdominal pain
  - Colorectal Cancer – keep this in the back of your mind in the patient who is older and may be at risk for colorectal cancer
  - Non-GI cause
    - Hypothyroidism – most common in young women, but has a second peak in older adulthood
    - CNS chronic diseases (multiple sclerosis, ALS, etc)

Fecal Impaction

- Epidemiology
  - Common in elderly
  - Hypothyroidism
  - Hypercalcemia
  - Medications
    - Calcium channel blockers (Verapamil, diltiazem)
    - Diuretics
    - Opiates
- H & P
  - Anorexia
  - Vomiting if obstruction
  - Severe (usually LUQ gas pains)
  - Palpable stool in LLQ/sigmoid
  - Can have leaking liquid stool around fecal impaction
  - DRE must be done
- Labs & diagnosis
  - Abdominal series (upright and KUB)
  - Look for air-fluid levels to suggest SBO
  - Patient is seen to be F. O. S. (full of poop)
  - If concern for metabolic cause obtain TSH, Ca+
- Clinical Intervention
  - Enema
  - If unable to pass tube due to rectal impaction, then digital disimpaction
- Health Maintenance is the key!
  - Do not give opiates without remembering to have patient increase fluids, raw veggies or give Miralax prophylactically

Diverticular disease

Diverticulosis

- Epidemiology
  - Increases with age (50% in age >80)
  - Asymptomatic if uncomplicated (2/3)
  - Complications occur in 1/3
    - GI bleed (diverticular hemorrhage)
      - **most common cause of LGI bleed in patients > 50 yrs.*
    - Diverticulitis
  - Believed due to chronic low-fiber diets
- H & P
  - Asymptomatic if not infected or bleeding
  - Abdominal exam should be normal
- Labs & Diagnostics
  - Usually an incidental finding on colonoscopy
  - May be discovered when patient presents with a complication

Diverticulitis

- Epidemiology/Etiology
    - 15-20% of pts with diverticulosis
    - Perforation of a diverticulum resulting in acute infection in bowel wall
- H & P
    - LLQ pain
    - Fever
    - Leukocytosis
    - Mainly a clinical dx
- Labs & Diagnostics
    - CBC showing leukocytosis (only 50% early)
    - If classic sxs, no imaging necessary
    - Plain films to look for abd free air or obstruction (would not show the diverticulitis --- only used to r/o bowel perforation)
    - *CT if sxs don't resolve in 2-4 days, or sooner if unable to tolerate PO medications*
    - **no Ba Enema or scoping acutely (may perforate inflamed bowel)
- Clinical Intervention
    - If discharged home:
        - treat empirically if strong clinical suspicion
        - close followup with return if not significantly improved in 48 hours for CT to r/o abscess
            - NPO day one, then advance diet as tolerated
            - low residue with eventual advancement to high fiber
    - Many require hospitalization (especially elderly)
        - IV antibiotics; then to PO
        - Rehydration
        - Pain control
- Therapeutics
    - **broad spectrum antibiotic+ anaerobic coverage (Cipro + Metronidazole)
        - PO if patient is stable and tolerating PO
        - Oral antibiotics for 7-10 days
    - admission and IV antibiotics if patient is not tolerating PO
        - still cipro and metronidazole

Diverticular hemorrhage

- Epidemiology
    - 5-15% of patient with diverticulosis
    - 50% of all lower GI bleeds **most common
    - 80-90% of episodes will be self-limiting
    - Elderly patient
- H & P
    - *acute, painless, large volume maroon or BRB in patient > 50 y.o. (usually much older, i.e. 70's or more)
    - Otherwise normal exam
    - Be sure to pay attention to any orthostatic vital signs you are given meant to tell you that the patient is/or is not hemodynamically stable!!!

- Labs & Diagnostics
    - CBC
    - remember HCT may not reflect amt of bleeding if volume depleted
    - Type and screen/cross
- Clinical Intervention
    - Colonoscopy is usually performed to stop bleeding (if not self-limited)
    - Surgical resection may be necessary if recurrent bleeds/admissions
    - GI consult is always recommended

Colorectal cancer

- Epidemiology/Etiology
    - 2nd most common cause of cancer DEATH (1st is lung)
    - Highest rate in N. America & Europe
    - Increased risk in pts migrating into "high-risk" countries
    - 90% of colorectal cancers occur in pts >50 y.o.
    - Family Hx exists in 25% of new cancers
    - Adenomas precede most cancers
    - Early cancer is asymptomatic
    - High fat/low fiber diets implicated
    - Greatly increased risk in pts with IBD (Ulcerative colitis)
- Risk Factors
    - Age
    - Adenomatous polyps
    - Family History
    - Familial adenomatous polyposis
    - HNPCC (hereditary nonpolyposis colorectal carcinoma
    - Peutz-Jeghers syndrome
    - Ulcerative Colitis history
- Health Maintenance
    - Screening detects early cancers
    - Microcytic anemia + >50 = colon cancer until proven otherwise
    - Weight loss and obstruction occur too late
- Screening Options for general population – beginning at age 50
    - Colonoscopy q. 10 years is most effective
    - Annual FOBT >50 y.o.
        - No red meat, NSAID's, Aspirin for three days prior to collection
        - Three consecutive stools
        - PPV 22-58% (found earlier though)
- Better than nothing for patients without insurance (still improves outcomes)
    - Flexible Sigmoidoscopy
        - Q. 5 yrs >50 y.o., plus yrly FOBT
    - Barium enema q. 5-10 years
        - Rarely used; misses small polyps; unable to biopsy
- Screening Special Populations
    - First degree relative with cancer >60
        - Screen at age 40 – colonoscopy preferred
    - First degree relative with cancer <60

        - Screen 10 years younger than age at dx
    - African-American ethnicity
        - screening begins at age 40-45
    - IBD patients
        - Colonoscopy 8 years after diagnosis
            - Risk exceeds the general population risk at 8 years
        - then every 1-2 years for life
    - FAP (familial adenomatous polyposis)
        - Autosomal dominant (so strong family history)
        - 100% colon cancer risk by age 50
        - Genetic screening after age 10
        - Refer to GI/surgery for total colectomy
    - HNPCC (hereditary nonpolyposis colorectal cancer)
        - Genetic testing is available
        - Clue is genetic pedigree that includes ovarian, uterine/endometrial and colon cancer
- Scientific Concept
    - **Tumor marker for colon cancer is CEA*

Toxic megacolon

- Etiology
    - severe ulcerative colitis
    - treatment with bile acid sequestrants (cholestyramine)
- H & P
    - massive distention of the belly
    - hypertympanic (lots of air in the bowel)
- Labs & diagnostics
    - KUB (flat plate of abdomen) will show
    - By definition, > 6 cm of dilatation of colon
- Clinical Intervention
    - GI/surg referral
    - Mortality rate if perforation occurs, is 50%!

Irritable bowel syndrome (see above in chronic abdominal pain)

- Etiology
    - unknown (most common in young women with h/o depression)
    - "functional" disorder (meaning, no organic disease is identified on workup)
- H & P:
    - normal (if anything is abnormal don't pick IBS!)
- Labs & diagnostics:
    - normal
- Formulating Most Likely Diagnosis:
    - months of GI issues with no known cause
- Clinical Intervention:
    - fiber, reassurance

IBS, particular diarrhea predominant, is often the diagnosis made in a patient who actually has celiac disease. Make sure you evaluate the patient for malabsorption (if Fe deficient, then celiac is in the differential)

SUPRAPUBIC/LOWER ABDOMEN

HERNIAS

Hiatal hernia

- GI diagnosis, actually
- occurs as a "defect" in the diaphragm allowing the lower portion of esophagus and stomach to "herniate" into the lower chest
- may be asymptomatic
- may increase GERD symptoms
- usually does not need any surgical intervention

Ventral hernia

- These hernias occur in the belly, usually midline (in that virtual space between the two abdominal rectus muscles
- do a sit up and look, you can see that line
- in obesity with increased abdominal pressure, the gut can protrude through this space and create a "hernia"
- Be on the lookout for words in the stem that suggest incarceration or strangulation
    - if not, then weight loss, and elective surgery if needed (remember, only if the patient is a good surgical candidate – this is pretty big surgery)

Incarceration

- Bowel is trapped in the hernia opening, it is "incarcerated" if it is unable to be reduced (pushed back into the abdomen)
- Surgical intervention
    - time frame has to do with concern for ischemia (see strangulation below)

Strangulation of a hernia

- Bowel is trapped and is "twisted" becomes ischemic
- Emergent surgical intervention

Incisional hernia

- Truly a surgical diagnosis
    - a result of abdominal surgery
    - the wound which was closed (usually many years ago), is now open in the deeper layers (skin is closed)
    - abdominal contents are palpable through this "hernia"
    - treatment would be surgical referral

- Clinical Intervention
  - check for incarceration (should be able to push contents back into abdomen)
  - complication would be strangulation
  - more likely in a small hernia, ironically, than in a very large one (as loop of bowel could get trapped and blood supply cut off)
  - CT should be ordered, if incarcerated, then a surgical emergency to prevent ischemia and necrosis

Inguinal hernia (more common in men than women)

- Indirect hernias are a result of the lack of closure of the inguinal ring after testes have descended into the scrotum at 28 weeks gestation – the opening left there can allow bowel to come down the ring and enter the scrotum (just like the testicles did when the man was a fetus).

- Direct hernias occur through a defect in the fascia of the abdominal wall with its sac noted to be medial to the inferior epigastric vessels. Direct inguinal hernias may occur in males or females, but males are ten times more likely to get a direct inguinal hernia

- See above for incarceration and strangulation complications
  - if not incarcerated or strangulated the clinical intervention would be elective repair of either type of hernia

Femoral hernia (not in blueprint)

- Femoral hernias occur just below the inguinal ligament, when abdominal contents pass through a naturally occurring weakness called the femoral canal.
- Femoral hernias are a relatively uncommon type, accounting for only 3% of all hernias.
- While femoral hernias can occur in both males and females, almost all of them develop in women because of the wider bone structure of the female pelvis

Fournier's Gangrene (not in blueprint, but should be!)

- Epidemiology/Etiology
  - rare, but life-threatening infection posing as inguinal hernia
  - men, 40-50 y.o.
  - increased risk in DM/ alcoholism; cancer
- H & P - diagnosis made on physical exam
  - presents with pain in groin, like a "groin strain" or inguinal hernia
  - swelling, suggestive of hydrocele or varicocele
  - after few days, fever, malaise, anorexia, severe pain
  - PE – signs of illness – tachycardia, severe pain
  - induration /bronzing of skin along symphysis, left groin, mass like area in inguinal ring; scrotum
  - edema and tenderness of skin of penis and scrotum
  - gangrene of tissues of rectum, scrotum, penis
- Labs & Diagnostics
  - leukocytosis with left shift
  - cultures have multiple gram negative and anaerobic pathogens

  - CT
- Clinical intervention
  - ICU admission for sepsis
  - immediate surgical intervention for I & D
  - broad spectrum antibiotics with anaerobic coverage
    - cipro & clindamycin or Flagyl (metronidazole)
  - hyperbaric oxygen
- Scientific Concept
  - rapidly progressing necrotizing fasciitis
  - involves perineum; perianal region, penis and scrotum
  - may be due to incarcerated hernia, but not necessarily associated at all, but presents as though it is a tender hernia initially

RIGHT LOWER QUADRANT

Appendicitis

- The appendix is at the end of the cecum, typically in the right lower quadrant
  - Retrocecal appendices can present with lower back pain.
- Epidemiology
  - patient is usually young (but can be any age)
- H & P
  - pain is at the umbilicus generalized at first
  - then focuses at McBurney's point
  - 1/3 the distance from the imbilicus and R ischial spine
  - patient may have low grade fever (not necessarily, though)
- Labs & Diagnostics
  - elevated or normal WBC count
  - either US or CT of abdomen (may be a clinical diagnosis of acute abdomen as well)
- Differential
  - Mesenteric Adenitis
  - Hernia (see above)
  - Ovary
    - Always consider an OB-GYN issue in a female with lower abdominal pain
    - Pelvic exam is indicated in any lower abdominal complaint
    - Pregnancy test is always indicated (unless hysterectomy or menopause)
    - Potentially serious diagnosis if missed in a female patient includes:
      - ovarian torsion
      - ectopic pregnancy/fallopian tube rupture

Inflammatory Bowel Diseases

Crohn's disease

- Often presents as more chronic type RLQ symptoms with other associated symptoms (see discussion in this chapter)

- Epidemiology
    - Idiopathic, autoimmune
- H & P
    - Rectal bleeding
    - Fever
    - Weight loss, anorexia
    - Nausea, vomiting
    - Malabsorption, vitamin deficiencies
    - May be manifestations in all organ systems (just like all autoimmune diseases):
        - Genitourinary: May include presence of skin tags, fistulae, ulcers, abscesses, and scarring in perianal region; nephrolithiasis, hydronephrosis
        - Musculoskeletal: Possible arthritis and arthralgia, particularly in large joints[
        - Dermatologic: May show pallor or jaundice, mucocutaneous or aphthous ulcers, erythema nodosum, and pyoderma gangrenosum
        - Ophthalmologic: May reveal episcleritis; uveitis/iritis
        - ENT: mouth ulcers (canker sores)
        - Growth delay: failure to thrive, pubertal delay
        - Hematologic: Hypercoagulable state
- Labs & Diagnostics
    - CBC ; CMP (electrolytes)
    - Inflammatory markers (C-reactive protein, ESR)
    - Stool studies
        - Rule out dysentery as a cause of symptoms
- Imaging
    - Plain abdominal radiography
    - Barium contrast studies (eg, small bowel follow-through, barium enema, enter-oclysis)
    - CT scanning of the abdomen
    - CT enterography or magnetic resonance enterography: Replacing small bowel follow-through studies
- Clinical Intervention
    - GI referral
    - Colonoscopy (ileocolonoscopy)
    - Interventional radiology for percutaneous drainage of abscesses
- Therapeutics
    - 5-aminosalicylates
        - mesalamine
    - Corticosteroids
        - Prednisone
        - For acute flares only – not longterm
    - Budesonide (Enterocort)
        - Oral or rectal
        - *less systemic absorption of steroid, so now approved for maintenance*
    - TNF-a inhibitors (monoclonal antibiodies)
        - Infliximab (Remicade)
        - Adalimumab (Humira)
        - certolizumab (Cimzia)
        - Any "imab" or "umab"

- For infection/abscess
  - Ciprofloxacin & Metronidazole
- Scientific Concept
  - *No NSAID's for patients with IBD
  - brand name Asacol has been taken off the market

Ulcerative Colitis ! strong correlation to primary sclerosing cholangitis

- Also idiopathic, and likely autoimmune
- Also extraintestinal manifestations
  - Anemia, arthritis, skin issues
- H & P
  - **Hallmark = bloody diarrhea*
  - Cramping abdominal pain
  - Tenesmus (urgent feeling of needing to defecate)
  - Fever, weight loss (less than in Crohn's)
  - Hemoccult positive during active disease
  - LLQ pain (recall that Crohn's is more often RLQ)
  - Anoscopy
    - ulcerations will be seen as this always involves the rectum
    - it spreads continuously proximally
    - anoscopy is not enough; need to examine the proximal colon to quantify the extent of disease (colonoscopy)
- Labs & Diagnostics
  - CBC – mild anemia of chronic disease (normocytic)
  - ESR elevated
  - C-reactive protein increased in active flare
  - Stool studies (r/o dysentery)
  - CT imaging often done to r/o abscess or other infectious process
- Clinical Intervention
  - Colonoscopy
  - Double contrast barium enema (not often done)
    - "lead pipe" colon
  - Total colectomy provides cure and removes risk of colorectal cancer
- Therapeutics
  - Same as Crohn's disease above
- Complications
  - Colorectal cancer
    - Dysplastic tissue in colon (not polyps)
    - Adenocarcinoma
    - Up to 34% risk 30 years from onset of disease
  - Toxic megacolon
    - Rare, but up to 50% mortality if perforation

Inflammatory Bowel Disease (IBD)	
Crohn's Disease	Ulcerative Colitis
Spares rectum	Rectum ALWAYS involved
Mouth-to-anus disease	Involvement only of colon
Skip lesions	Continuous lesion
Full thickness ulcers	Superficial friable ulcerated mucosa
Strictures/fistulae	
No cure	Cure = total colectomy
Medical management	Medical management
Significant malabsorption of B-12, Calcium, Vit. D	

Inflammatory Bowel Disease (IBD):

- Chronic diarrhea should always prompt thought about IBD
- UC is entirely curable with colectomy
- Crohn's is managed medically but not cured

OTHER SMALL BOWEL PROBLEMS

Small Bowel Obstruction

- Epidemiology
    - Common
    - Due to adhesions (prior abdominal surgery or infection, i.e. PID)
- H & P
    - Sudden onset of vomiting (no diarrhea)
    - No fevers, no other symptoms to suggest viral etiology
    - Either borborygmi (increased high-pitched bowel sounds) or no bowel sounds
- Labs & Diagnostics
    - Usual labs
    - Upright plain film of abdomen (not a KUB, should order abdominal series to look for air/fluid levels)
- Clinical Intervention
    - NG tube to suction
    - Patient is obviously NPO

  - Admission to surgery (may or may not need surgical intervention, but surgery should be consulted)

Celiac disease

- Etiology:
  - Autoimmune
  - Abnormal response to gluten intake causing destruction of the duodenal villi
    - decreased absorptive surface in the small bowel; causing malabsorption
    - first iron (absorbed in duodenum); if extensive can cause malabsorption of B-12 and Ca/Vit. D. in terminal ileum too
- Epidemiology
  - patients of Celtic, Northern European descent
- H & P:
  - history of intermittent diarrhea, bloating, abdominal cramping
  - PE is normal
- Labs & diagnostics:
  - malabsorption is the key; Fe, B12, Ca, Vit. D
  - anemia
  - antibody tests
    - tTG & endomysial antibody
  - mucosal biopsy of the small bowel is diagnostic
    - *shows "flat duodenal surface with absence of villi and villus atrophy"*
- Formulating Most Likely Diagnosis:
  - think "diarrhea predominant" irritable bowel syndrome
    - but celiac disease has malabsorption issues
- Clinical Intervention:
  - gluten free diet
  - what to avoid? (BROW – bananas, rye, oats (if not pure), wheat)
  - what can they eat?(CRAP – corn, rice, arrowroot, potatoes)
- Therapeutics/Health Maintenance
  - treatment is diet
  - periodic EGD
  - risk for small bowel lymphoma if left untreated

Ischemic bowel disease (mesenteric ischemia)

- Etiology:
  - usually embolism from the heart (a fib?), causing occlusion of the SMA (superior mesenteric artery)
  - typically a "vasculopathic" patient, i.e., prior stents, caths, shunts, clot history
- H & P:
  - Hx - sudden onset; typically post-prandial
  - PE- severe mid abdominal pain (out of proportion to temp, abdominal exam, etc)
- Labs & diagnostics:
  - CT angiography
- Formulating Most Likely Diagnosis:
  - Atrial fibrillation is the key, with sudden onset severe abdominal pain

    - differential includes bowel perforation, aortic dissection
- Clinical Intervention
    - usually observation with potential surgery or interventional radiology
    - remember that ischemic bowel (if not perfused) becomes necrotic bowel which becomes peritonitis which becomes death!

The Rectum – Pain in the butt!

- Anal fissure
    - painful "papercut" of anus, usually due to large hard stool (think IBS with bright red, painful rectal bleeding
    - most common occurrence is at the posterior midline of the anus
- Abscess/Fistula
    - consider Crohn's disease in young person (look for clues in stem about weight loss, malabsorption)
- Fecal Impaction
    - due to constipation, a large bowel obstruction, covered in constipation section, stool is often lodged in the rectal vault, may leak liquid stool around slightly open rectum
- Hemorrhoids
    - internal hemorrhoids usually do not hurt, but external ones throb, both types can bleed; both can thrombose
    - thrombosed hemorrhoids can be "lanced" but usually supportive therapy
        - sitz bath; Epson salts; Anusol cream; stool softeners to prevent straining
- Pilonidal disease (not in blueprint) – and not actually in the butt (but in gluteal cleft)
    - result of a congenital defect in the skin at the top of the gluteal cleft (not in the anal
    - sometimes there is a little dimple, hole, or tuft of hair
    - for obvious reasons, bacteria can infect the area causing an abscess
    - the abscess needs to be incised, drained, and treated with antibiotics
        - staph/ MRSA coverage
            - cephalexin plus TMP/SMZ (Bactrim)
            - but remember, the "cyst" and its likely tract is still there.
    - Health Maintenance
        - if recurrent pilonidal abscesses; patient needs referral to the surgeon for this most uncomfortable (and surprisingly extensive) surgery.
    - Scientific Concept
    - This is not a meningomyelocele
        - the cord is not exposed; there is no defect in the vertebral bodies themselves.

Diagnosis by Symptoms

DYSPHAGIA (difficulty swallowing)

- *Solids only*
    - cancer (squamous cell/adenocarcinoma)
    - stricture (Schatzki's webs)
- *Solids and liquids*
    - Motility disorder (achalasia, scleroderma, eosinophilic esophagitis)
- *Labs & Diagnostics*
    - R/O cancer with EGD (esophogastroduodenoscopy)
    - R/O motility disorders with barium swallow or manometry (pressure swallow test)

PEARL: Eosinophilic esophagitis is not in the blueprint; more recognized now as a common cause of inflammatory (allergic?) thickening of the esophagus; most common in young white men; treatment with inhaled (swallowed) steroids

PEARL: EGD (esophagogastroduodenoscopy) – no wonder we call it EGD, should always be done for dysphagia; it is both diagnostic and therapeutic (resection of rings and strictures; biopsy if needed)

ODYNOPHAGIA (painful swallowing)

- Candida, CMV, Herpes
- Immunocompromised (HIV)
- Inhaled corticosteroids (or even nasal if the patient doesn't rinse his mouth)
- Pill induced
- Tetracyclines, oral potassium, Alendronate or other bisphosphonates

PEARL: Odynophagia should always be scoped (EGD) – especially in immunocompromised, or if a pill is stuck.

HEMATEMESIS

<u>Esophageal Varices</u>

- *Etiology*
    - Chronic alcoholic with portal hypertension (plethoric facies, palmar erythema, gynecomastia, telangiectasias, abnormal transaminases, hypoalbuminemia)
- *H & P*
    - Painless hematemesis
    - Abnormal orthostatic vital signs
    - Increase in HR > 20 bpm when going from supine to standing
    - Decrease in SBP (falls 20 mm Hg) when supine to standing
    - Large amount of blood in emesis
    - May have hematochezia if brisk bleeding; rapid transit
- *Labs & diagnostics*
    - Loss of blood is usually severe – patient is orthostatic (hypotension/tachycardia)
- *Formulating Most Likely Diagnosis*
    - Painless hematemesis with abnormal vital signs

- *Clinical Intervention*
  - Life-threatening emergency
  - Upper endoscopy (EGD)
  - Banding or sclerotherapy
- *Therapeutics*
  - Type and cross for packed RBC's
  - Octreotide IV
    - Increases splanchnic vascular resistance by inhibiting the release of splanchnic vasodilator hormones (eg, glucagon, vasoactive intestinal peptide (therefore, reducing bleeding)
- *Health Maintenance*
  - Stop alcohol intake!
  - Reduce BP (usually beta-blockers)
  - 20-30% mortality with each bleed; if patient survives, 50-70% chance of recurrence

PEARL: Remember to check INR as this patient may have decrease in synthesis of all coagulation factors, (except Factor VIII) compounding the bleeding problem!

Mallory-Weiss Tear

- *Etiology*
  - No evidence of portal hypertension
  - More typically going to be a "normal" patient with excessive vomiting
  - Due to a small tear at the gastroesophageal junction or bleeding from a vessel irritated from retching
    - (Flu, acute alcohol intoxication, etc), but not due to varicose veins as varices
- *H & P*
  - Painless hematemesis (small amount of blood)
- *Labs & diagnostics*
  - Normal (no significant orthostasis)
- *Formulating Most Likely Diagnosis*
  - Painless hematemesis with normal vital signs
- *Clinical Intervention:*
  - Self-limited
    - Often upper endoscopy is done, but usually no intervention necessary
  - Always make sure vital signs and orthostatic BP and HR (if given) are normal before choosing this answer

Boerhaave's Syndrome

- *Etiology*
  - Effort rupture during retching/vomiting
- *H & P*
  - Severe sudden tearing sensation retrosternally
  - Orthostatic hypotension/tachycardia
- *Labs & diagnostics:*
  - CXR showing mediastinal air is a major clue!
  - CT scan to better image the mediastinum

- *Formulating Most Likely Diagnosis*
    - Severe sudden pain with vomiting or instrumentation
- *Clinical Intervention*
    - Type and screen/cross
    - Make sure you have IV access
    - Life-threatening emergency (bleeding into the anterior mediastinum)
    - Immediate surgical referral
- *Scientific Concept*
    - Iatrogenic perforation (while uncommon) causes 80-90% of all esophageal ruptures
    - Inadvertent occurrence during upper endoscopy
    - This is not called a Boerhaave's syndrome though

MELENA (UGI bleeding)

Definition: dark/coffee ground/black stool (not bright red) and/or hemoccult positive

- #1 Cause - Peptic Ulcer Disease (PUD)
- *Gastritis*
    - Due to NSAID's, prednisone, aging, alcohol
- *Cancer*
    - UGI cancers, i.e. gastric, esophageal
    - Colorectal cancer
        - If right sided may be melena; may also be occult and not visible at all!

HEMATOCHEZIA (Bright red bleeding from the rectum)

- *Hemorrhoids*
    - Bright red blood
    - Internal hemorrhoids may not hurt at all
    - External hemorrhoids may ache & throb, be palpable
- *Rectal fissure*
    - Bright red, painful passage of blood when passing stool
- *Diverticular hemorrhage*
    - Bright red; painless passage of dark blood
- *Colorectal cancer*
    - Usually not bright red; usually occult or black stools (melena)

PERSISTENT VOMITING

Most common GI causes:

- *Small Bowel Obstruction*
    - Adhesions
- *Large Bowel Obstruction*
    - Volvulus
    - Fecal impaction
    - Colorectal cancer
- *Gastric outlet obstruction*

    - Scarring across ulcer
    - Pyloric stenosis (in peds)
- *Gastroparesis (gastro= stomach, paresis = paralysis)*
    - Diabetes is #1 (causes hypomotility, i.e. peripheral neuropathy of the gut)
    - CNS reasons for hypomotility
        - Multiple sclerosis, ALS (amyotrophic lateral sclerosis), other chronic progressive CNS diseases
    - Treat with promotility agents
        - Metoclopramide
        - Domperidone
    - Gastric pacemaker

Non- GI causes of persistent vomiting:

- Uremia/Chronic renal failure
- Increased CSF pressures (masses, meningitis)
- Reye's syndrome (covered in peds)

HYPERBILIRUBINEMIA (If total bilirubin is > 3 = jaundice)

PEARL: When given an elevated T. Bili, check whether the elevated fraction is the direct or the indirect (you have to do simple math subtracting the direct from the total to get the indirect fraction). If the indirect fraction is elevated there is a short list of three possible etiologies, so memorize this list. If you find an elevated direct bilirubinemia it is potentially anything but these three!

<u>Indirect Bilirubinemia –</u>

- *Hemolytic Anemias*
    - Sickle cell, spherocytosis, G6PD, autoimmune hemolytic anemia
    - Physiologic jaundice of the newborn
- *Gilbert's syndrome*
    - Benign inherited absence of an enzyme not essential for much of anything
    - Clinical intervention is reassurance
    - Once diagnosed, it has no ramifications for the patient
- *Passive hepatic congestion (i.e., CHF, portosystemic shunting)*

<u>Direct Bilirubinemia</u>

- *Liver metabolized drugs (hundreds and hundreds)*
- *Alcohol*
- *Obstruction to flow of bilirubin (cholelithiasis)*
    - Gallstones
    - Pancreatic tumor (head of pancreas)
- *Primary biliary cirrhosis*
- *Primary sclerosing cholangitis*

DYSPEPSIA (these topics are covered elsewhere in this chapter in more detail)

Causes

- Peptic Ulcer Disease (PUD) – gastric or duodenal ulcers
- Gastritis
- Gastric Cancer – rare in the United States; most common in patients with untreated H. Pylori
- GERD
- Pancreatitis (acute or chronic)
- Pancreatic cancer

HICCUPS

- ***Definition***
    - < 48 hours is typical
    - 48 hours is protracted
    - 1 month is intractable

Causes of protracted/intractable hiccups

- *GI*
    - Liver dome tumors
    - Subphrenic abscesses
    - Peritoneal infections
- *CV*
    - Acute MI (inferior wall)
    - Thoracic aneurysm
- *Mediastinal*
    - Recurrent laryngeal nerve irritation
    - Phrenic nerve irritation
- *Renal*
    - Uremia
- *CNS lesions*
- *Multiple drugs*
- *Treatment*
    - Thorazine (chlorpromazine)

PRURITIS

Causes

- Cholestasis/choledocholithiasis
- Primary biliary cirrhosis
- Primary sclerosing cholangitis
- Renal failure, i.e. uremia
- Hematologic cancers (leukemias & lymphomas)

Acute Diarrhea

PEARL: Acute Infectious and Inflammatory Diarrhea:

- Most causes of acute diarrhea are self-limited
- In a healthy host no treatment necessary
- In non-healthy host (dehydrated infant, other comorbidities):
- The bacterial can be treated with various antibiotics
- The best way to hydrate a human is orally; give oral rehydration solutions
- The way to prevent infection is to wash your hands, cooking utensils

Viral vs. Bacterial usually noted by a few differences:

- **Viral**
    - No PMN's in viral stool
    - Large volume, watery stools; not bloody
    - Often associated with short episode of vomiting
    - Fever is common
- **Bacterial/Inflammatory**
    - Increased fecal leukocytes
    - Frequent, small volume, bloody stools
    - Fever is common

Non-Inflammatory Diarrhea

- **H & P**
    - Large volume
    - Watery
    - No blood
    - No leukocytes
    - Flu-like symptoms
- **Etiologies**
    - Chemical/osmotic/electrolyte
    - Magnesium citrate (bowel prep)
    - "Turista" – drinking the water in Mexico
        - High mineral content causes osmotic diarrhea
    - May need culture to distinguish it from enterotoxigenic E. coli infection

VIRAL ETIOLOGIES

Rotavirus

- *Epidemiology*
  - Pediatric
- *Clinical intervention*
  - Oral rehydration (no antibiotics)
- *Health maintenance*
  - Vaccine available

Norovirus

- *Epidemiology* – most common cause of gastroenteritis
  - "Vomiting disease"
  - *Cruise ships ----- fecal/oral*
- *Clinical intervention*
  - Oral rehydration

PARASITIC ETIOLOGIES

Giardia

- *Epidemiology*
  - Most common parasitic diarrhea
  - Drinking from fresh water stream (beavers)
- *Labs & Diagnostics*
  - EIA/serology of stool
- *Clinical Intervention/Therapeutics*
  - Metronidazole

Cryptosporidium

- *Epidemiology*
  - Self-limited if normal immune system
  - Severe symptoms in immunocompromised (i.e., HIV/AIDs)
- *Labs & Diagnostics*
  - EIA /serology of stool (like giardia)
- *Clinical Intervention*
  - Oral rehydration/supportive/ no Rx

Inflammatory/Infectious Diarrhea

- **H & P**
  - Small volume stools
  - Frequent
  - Bloody
  - Many leukocytes
  - Fever and chills

- Cramping abdominal pain
- **Etiologies**
    - Staph enterotoxin
- **Epidemiology**
    - "Food poisoning" – improper storage of food
- **Labs**
    - Check electrolytes
- **Clinical Intervention**
    - Supportive (no Rx)
        - *Do not use anti-diarrheal meds – can cause dissemination and bacteremia*

Bacillus Cereus

- *Epidemiology*
    - From cooked rice not stored properly
- *Labs* – None
- *Clinical intervention* – Supportive

Vibrio Cholera

- *Epidemiology*
    - Inadequate sanitation (after floods/hurricanes)
- *H&P*
    - Rice water stools
- *Labs & Diagnostics*
    - Order specific culture on stool sample
- *Clinical Intervention*
    - Oral rehydration
    - Azithromycin
        - Not a cure, but shortens length of symptoms

PARASITIC/PROTOZOAL INFECTIONS

Entamoeba Histolytica

- *Etiology* – Entamoeba *histolytica*
- *Epidemiology*
    - Fresh water; rivers;
    - Fecal-oral; poor sanitation
- *H & P*
    - Diarrhea and abdominal cramping
    - Liver abscess is most common complication
- *Labs & Diagnostics*
    - Stool ova & parasites (not found on culture), must order separately
    - Antigen PCR from serum is better
    - Abdominal CT to r/o liver abscess
- *Therapeutics*
    - metronidazole
    - drainage of abscess

BACTERIAL

E Coli 0157-H7 – "Shigatoxin"

- *Epidemiology*
    - Undercooked hamburger meat
- *Treatment is supportive (no specific tx)*

Antibiotic Associated Diarrhea

PEARL: Antibiotic-associated diarrhea (AAD) has become a huge problem most recently in hospitalized patients. Risk factors include age (the elderly), length of hospital stay, and treatment with broad spectrum cephalosporins, penicillins, and clindamycin. Be on the lookout for the words in the stem that clue you to one of the top three listed below:

Clostridium dificile
Clostridium perfringens
Staph aureus

- *Epidemiology*
    - 33% - C. dificile
    - 15% - C. perfringens
    - 10% - Staph aureus
- *Etiologies*
    - Antibiotic therapy
        - Broad spectrum cephalosporins and penicillins
        - Clindamycin
        - Newer fluoroquinolones
        - PPI therapy
    - Hospitalization
        - Transferred from healthcare workers to patients
        - Incidence increases with length of stay
    - immunocompromised host
- *Therapeutics*
    - Metronidazole is first-line
    - Vancomycin is next (oral is best)

Others

Campylobacter jejuni

- *Epidemiology*
    - One of the most common causes of infectious diarrhea
    - Undercooked poultry; unpasteurized milk
- *H & P*

  - Diarrhea, cramping, abdominal pain, and fever within two to five days after exposure to the organism.
  - The diarrhea may be bloody and can be accompanied by nausea and vomiting.
  - The illness typically lasts one week.
- *Treatment*
  - Usually not needed/ self-limited
  - Azithromycin/erythromycin if early in illness or immunocompromised status

Shigella
- *Epidemiology*
  - Fairly common
  - Gram negative rod
- *Cause*
  - Fecal-oral route
  - Unwashed veggies; drinking pool water, changing diapers
- *H&P*
  - Dysentery (bloody frequent stools)
- *Labs & Diagnostics*
  - Stool culture
- *Clinical Intervention*
  - None, self-limited
  - If severe, amoxicillin, Bactrim
- *Health Maintenance*
  - Hand washing
- *Scientific Concept*
  - <u>Do not use motility agent</u>

Salmonella
- *Causes*
  - Handling turtles, undercooked chicken
- *H&P*
  - Dysentery (fever, bloody stools)
- *Labs & Diagnostics*
  - Stool culture
- *Clinical Intervention* – none, self-limited
  - In high risk (sickle cell, cancer, infants, elderly) can be treated with multiple meds

---

Chronic Diarrhea

BLOODY

- Inflammatory Bowel Disease (covered above and below in detail)
- Crohn's disease
- Ulcerative colitis

NON-BLOODY

- **Malabsorption Syndromes**
  - Celiac sprue
  - Chronic pancreatitis (steatorrhea)
- **Irritable bowel syndrome**
- **Laxative Abuse**

Carcinoid tumor

- *Description*
  - Slow-growing type of neuroendocrine tumor
  - 10% of carcinoid tumors of the midgut (jejunum, ileum, appendix, and cecum) are associated with carcinoid syndrome
- *H & P*
  - Due to secretion of serotonin 5-HT causing
    - Flushing
    - Diarrhea
    - Abdominal cramping
    - Peripheral edema
  - Depletion of tryptophan leading to niacin deficiency (pellagra)

ACUTE ABDOMINAL PAIN

Ischemic Bowel Disease (mesenteric ischemia)

- *Description/Etiology*
  - Really more of a "cardiac" disease
  - Usually an embolism from atrial fib with clot to the superior mesenteric artery
- *H & P*
  - Causes severe abdominal pain, out of proportion to exam
  - Causes "ischemia of the small bowel, and if not "fixed" in time, will cause necrosis and eventual peritonitis
- *Imaging:* CT with contrast
- *Clinical Intervention*
  - Needs acute surgical intervention if bowel does not become perfused

Appendicitis

- *Anatomy*
  - The appendix is at the end of the cecum, typically in the right lower quadrant
    - (Although retrocecal appendices can present with lower back pain)
- *Epidemiology*
  - Patient is usually younger (but can be any age)
- *H & P*
  - Pain is at the umbilicus, then focuses at McBurney's point.
    - 1/3 the distance between imbilicus and R ischial spine

  - Patient may have low grade fever
  - Elevated or normal WBC count
- *Clinical Intervention*
  - NPO
  - Order either US or CT of abdomen (may be a clinical diagnosis of acute abdomen as well)
  - Emergent surgical referral for appendectomy

CHRONIC ABDOMINAL PAIN

Irritable Bowel Syndrome

- *Diagnosis of exclusion*
- *H & P*
  - The patient has a history of chronic abdominal pain,
  - Both diarrhea and constipation (mucous in stool may be ok)
  - Normal abdominal exam
- *Labs & Diagnostics*
  - Normal labs; therefore:
  - No malabsorption
  - No anemia, folate or B12 deficiency
  - Negative hemoccult
  - No abdominal PE abnormalities
  - No weight loss
  - No blood in stool (unless hemorrhoid or fissure)
- *Imaging* – none
- *ROME criteria (for diagnosing)*
  - 3 months of continuous or recurring symptoms of abdominal pain or irritation that:
    - May be relieved with a bowel movement,
    - May be coupled with a change in frequency, or
    - May be related to a change in the consistency of stools.
  - Two or more of the following are present at least 25 percent (one quarter) of the time:
    - A change in stool frequency (more than 3 bowel movement per day or fewer than 3 bowel movements per week)
    - Noticeable difference in stool form (hard, loose and watery stools or poorly formed stools)
    - Passage of mucous in stools
    - Bloating or feeling of abdominal distention
    - Altered stool passage (e.g. sensations of incomplete evacuation, straining, or urgency)

Inflammatory Bowel Disease *(covered in more detail earlier in this chapter)*

Crohn's disease & Ulcerative Colitis

- *Most important is to distinguish IBS from IBD (Crohn's and UC)*
- *H & P*

    - Blood in stool
    - Weight loss
- *Malabsorption is a clue*
- *Family history*
    - Clues in the "stem" that tell you this is not a benign functional disorder

Colorectal Cancer *(covered in detail earlier in this chapter)*

- *H & P*
    - Mostly asymptomatic
    - Can have change in patterns of stooling, i.e. diarrhea/constipation
    - Positive hemoccult
- *Scientific concept*
    - Fe deficiency anemia is a clue!

Constipation

- *Etiologies*
    - Iatrogenic (narcotics, calcium channel blockers, diuretics)
        - this is actually the *most* common cause of constipation
    - Irritable bowel syndrome – see above in chronic abdominal pain
    - Colorectal cancer – keep this in the back of your mind in the patient who is older and may be at risk for colorectal cancer
- *Non-GI cause*
    - Hypothyroidism – most common in young women, but has a second peak in older adulthood
    - CNS chronic diseases (multiple sclerosis, ALS, etc)

Fecal Impaction

- *Etiologies*
    - Common in elderly
    - Hypothyroidism
    - Hypercalcemia
    - Medications
        - *Calcium channel blockers (Verapamil, diltiazem)*
        - *Diuretics*
        - *Opiates*
- *H & P*
    - Anorexia
    - Vomiting if obstruction
    - Severe (usually LUQ gas pains)
    - Palpable stool in LLQ/sigmoid
        - *Can have leaking liquid stool around fecal impaction*
    - DRE must be done
- *Labs & diagnosis*
    - Abdominal series (upright and KUB)
    - Look for air-fluid levels to suggest SBO
    - Patient is seen to be F. O. S. (full of poop)
    - If concern for metabolic cause, TSH, Ca+

- *Clinical Intervention*
  - Enema
  - If unable to pass tube due to rectal impaction, then digital disimpaction
- *Health Maintenance is the key!*
  - Do not give opiates without remembering to have patient increase fluids, raw veggies or give polyethylene glycol (Miralax) prophylactically

---

Nutritional Deficiencies

Vitamin B deficiency overall causes the same vague complaints. (Any specific to the vitamin will be listed below.) All Vitamin B deficiencies cause mouth sores; cheilitis (cracks at the corners of the mouth), and glossitis.

Thiamine Deficiency (Vit. B1)

- *Etiology*
  - Alcoholism
- *H & P*
  - Altered mental status (Wernicke's encephalopathy)
  - Congestive heart failure (wet Beri-Beri)
- *Clinical intervention*
  - Give thiamine either 100 mg. PO (if asymptomatic) or IV (if altered mental status)

Riboflavin Deficiency (Vit. B2)

- *Scientific Concept*
  - Found in milk/B vitamin fortified breads/grains – rarely deficient in isolation – almost always occurs as a total Vit. B deficiency
- *H & P*
  - Same as all B vitamins; no special findings
- *Clinical Intervention*
  - Dairy products/supplementation with B vitamins

Niacin Deficiency (Vit. B3)

- *Etiology*
  - Found in protein; so deficient in patients who do not, or cannot take in proteins
- *H & P*
  - Causes Pellagra
    - *Dermatitis* (dark dry scaly spots in sun exposed areas)
    - *Diarrhea* – can be severe
    - *Dementia* (memory loss, psychosis
- *Clinical intervention*
  - oral niacin (usually with other B vitamins as well)

B5 Pantothenic Acid
↳ hypoglycemia

Pyridoxine (Vit. B6) Deficiency

- *Etiology*
    - Isoniazid (INH therapy for TB prophylaxis)
- *H & P*
    - *Peripheral neuropathy (plus usual Vit. B skin changes)*
- *Clinical Intervention*
    - Always give pyridoxine daily with INH treatment

Vitamin B12 (Cobalamin) Deficien and Folate Deficiency

Please see Chapter 23 (Hematology) for detailed discussion of both B-12 and Folic acid deficiency anemias

Vitamin C (ascorbic acid) Deficiency

- *Etiology*
    - Poor diet in citrus products
    - The elderly (lose taste buds for sour)
    - Alcoholics (as in all nutritional deficiencies)
    - Urban poor (due to prohibitive cost of fresh produce)
- *H & P*
    - Scurvy
        - *Gingival bleeding; gingivitis*
        - *Perifollicular hemorrhages*
        - *Petechia, purpura*
        - *Poor wound healing*
- *Treatment*
    - Oral replacement, tolerated well, water soluble so little concern for toxicity

Vitamins A, D, E, K are fat soluble vitamins; can be stored for extended length of time, so can cause toxicity problems; deficiencies almost always due to fat malabsorption by the gut or due to pancreatic insufficiency

Vitamin A deficiency

- *Etiology*
    - Fat malabsorption
    - Chronic pancreatitis
- *H & P*
    - Night blindness
    - *Poor wound healing*
- *Clinical intervention*
    - Supplementation

Vitamin D Deficiency

- *Etiologies*
    - Lack of sun exposure
    - Renal failure (unable to metabolize to active Vit. D3)

- Malabsorption of fat soluble vitamins in terminal ileum
- There is a current epidemic of vitamin D deficiency

- *H & P*
  - Rickets in kids, osteopenia (osteomalacia) in adults
- *Clinical intervention*
  - Supplement both Calcium and Vitamin D3

Vitamin E Deficiency

- *Etiology*
  - Fat malabsorption
  - Chronic pancreatitis
- *H & P*
  - Multiple somatic issues
  - Mainly poor wound healing
- *Clinical intervention*
  - Supplementation is easy, but malabsorption poses problem anyway

Vitamin K Deficiency

- *Etiology*
  - Deficiency of dark green leafy vegetables needed weekly (easy to be deficient)
  - Also produced in colon (15%), so decreased in chronic antibiotic use (think acne treatment)
  - Reverses the effects of warfarin (so if deficient, you will have easy bruising)
  - Common in alcoholics
- *H & P*
  - Easy bruising, gum and skin bleeding (epistaxis, gingival bleeding)
  - Increased INR
- *Clinical intervention*
  - Dietary replacement is best
  - Vitamin K – either orally or IM

Good to know:

Anything that causes chronic inflammation anywhere along the GI system causes cancer:

- Alcohol = mouth cancer, esophageal (squamous cell) cancer, stomach cancer, pancreatic cancer, liver cancer – alcohol is the inflammatory carcinogen
- Smoke =mouth cancer, esophageal (squamous cell) cancer, stomach cancer, pancreatic cancer
- HCl acid = esophageal cancer (adenocarcinoma)
- H. Pylori = gastric cancer
- Hep B sAg, Hep C = liver cancer
- In general all alcoholics will be deficient of all B vitamins
- In general, the most malnourished are the very old (they can't chew as well, have lost taste buds for sour, and have malabsorption due to atrophic guts, etc.

CHAPTER 14

Orthopedics & Rheumatology – 10%

Introduction to Orthopedics

PEARLS:

- Fractures are almost always due to trauma or fall; if not, consider bone cyst or tumor (pathologic fracture)
- Tendonitis is due to overuse – usually no single traumatic injury – the clue to this answer is that the nature of the problem is chronic and insidious and worse with the action that caused it in the first place
- In each section of the chapter, overuse syndromes will appear first, followed by traumatic injuries.

- **Imaging in ortho:**
    - Plain film is indicated for almost all orthopedic complaints (acute, chronic, traumatic or atraumatic)
        - But will only show bony injuries (including an avulsion chip from ligament tear) but will not show ligamentous/tendon damage otherwise
    - CT will be used for bony injuries (occult fx of any bone)
    - MRI will be used to look at tendons/ligaments/soft tissue
    - Arthroscopic surgery can be both diagnostic and therapeutic

- **Management of ortho injuries:**
    - *RICE for all injuries:* rest, ice, compression (bracing), elevation
    - *MICE is newer acronym :* modified activity, ice, compression, elevation
    - *NSAID's for all injuries*: careful in renal failure or congestive heart failure
    - Steroid injections are common --- only one or two for most joints – exception might be low back

<u>The following orthopedic problems are commonly missed or cause complications if missed and *must be reviewed* for the test:</u>

- Cauda equina (covered in lumbar spine)
- Subcondylar humeral fracture/radial head fractures (covered in elbow, humerus fractures)
- Scaphoid/navicular fracture (covered in wrist)
- Compartment syndrome
    - Most typically in forearm and lower leg fractures, covered just below
- Femur fracture complications

  - Bleeding
  - Fat embolism
- Fracture with significant risk of bleeding
  - Pelvic fracture
  - Femur fracture
  - Humeral fracture

Orthopedic Trauma and Overuse Syndromes

Compartment Syndrome

- *Etiology/epidemiology*
  - Most common in tib/fib fractures/crush injuries and radial/ulnar fractures/crush injuries
- *H & P*
  - Early symptoms --- extreme pain with movement/palpation, coolness of extremity; decreased pulses
  - Late symptoms – absence of distal pulse; paralysis; numbness
- *Labs & Diagnostics*
  - Compartment testing (needle inserted into compartment to measure pressure)
- *Most Likely Diagnosis*
  - Consider in any anterior compartment tense-ness with pain on movement of distal structure (hand or foot, wrist or ankle)
- *Clinical Intervention*
  - Fasciotomy to relieve pressure
- *Health Maintenance*
  - Caution patient with crush injury of these compartments about warning symptoms
- *Scientific Concept*
  - Complications
    - Muscle and nerve ischemic necrosis
    - Limb contracture = Volkmann contracture
    - Renal failure

PEARL: The cycle of events leading to acute compartment syndrome begin when the tissue pressure exceeds the venous pressure and impairs blood outflow. Lack of oxygenated blood and accumulation of waste products results in pain and decreased peripheral sensation secondary to nerve irritation. Besides possible loss of the limb; renal failure and death may occur due to rhabdomyolysis.

THE SPINE

Cervical Spine (not in blueprint, but should be!)

Torticollis

- *Etiology*
    - Usually from "sleeping wrong" or simply unknown
- *H & P*
    - Unilateral spasm/contraction of sternocleidomastoid (SCM)
    - No radicular symptoms
- *Labs & Diagnostics* – none needed
- *Therapeutics*
    - NSAID's
    - Ice/Heat
    - Self-limited

Whiplash (Cervical Strain)

- *Etiology/Epidemiology*
    - Usually motor vehicle accident – acceleration/deceleration
    - Sports related is common as well
- *H & P*
    - No radicular symptoms; bilateral SCM and top of trapezius (top of shoulders)
    - Neuro exam is normal (no radicular symptoms)
- *Labs & Diagnostics*
    - If indicated, plain films of c-spine – *must be able to see C7!!!*
- *Therapeutics*
    - NSAID's
    - Ice/heat
    - Soft collar
    - ***Physical Therapy***
- *Health Maintenance*
    - Follow up for resolution

Cervical Radiculopathy

- *Etiology/Epidemiology*
    - Nerve root impingement
    - Usually due to osteoarthritis/degenerative disease
- *H & P*
    - C5 – Deltoid – abduction of arm
    - C6 – Biceps – flexion of arm
    - C7 – Triceps – extension of arm
    - C8 – Interossei's - include thumb
- *SPECIAL TESTS*
    - Spurling's test– axial load compression with lateral bend to neck – reproduces radicular symptoms
- *Labs & Diagnostics*

- MRI for cord visualization
- CT for bony visualization (spurs)

- *Most Likely Diagnosis*
    - Based on neurologic examination showing radicular symptoms
- *Clinical Intervention*
    - PT
    - Immobilization
    - NSAID's
    - Steroid injection?
- *Scientific Concept*
    - complete resolution in 6-12 weeks for most

Cervical Fractures

- C1 – Jefferson (seen on odontoid view) -- diving injury – hyperflexion injury
- C2 – Hangman – hyperextension injury
- C7 – Clay Shoveler's – snapping neck backward

PEARL: What is cervical radiculopathy?

Nerve root dysfunction, which is usually secondary to chronic pressure or invasion of the root, causes a radicular syndrome of pain and segmental neurologic deficit.

It causes pain, numbness, and eventually atrophy of the musculature of the upper extremity; pain radiating to the shoulders and into hand, caused by irritation and compression of the cervical nerve roots by a protruding intervertebral disk, tumor, osteophyte. Made worse with cough, sneeze.

Thoracic Spine

Thoracic Outlet Syndrome

- *Etiology/Epidemiology*
    - Compression of brachial plexus; women 20-50 y.o.
- *H & P*
    - Numbness
    - Weakness
    - Upper extremity "sense of swelling" without edema
- *SPECIAL TEST*
    - *Adson's* – extend arm and externally rotation

Thoracic Compression Fractures

- *Etiology/Epidemiology*
    - Osteoporosis (elderly female > elder male)
    - Prednisone therapy
    - Heparin therapy
- *H & P*

    - Pain, usually point specific
    - Loss of height in asymptomatic
- *Labs & Diagnostics*
    - PA and lateral plain film
- *Clinical Intervention*
    - NSAID's
    - Kyphoplasty
- *Therapeutics*
    - Consider bisphosphonates
- *Health Maintenance*
    - Calcium & vitamin D (found as effective as therapy with alendronate)
    - Dexa scanning of patients at risk for osteoporosis
- *Scientific Concept*
    - Most common in T10-L2 levels --- thoracic > lumbar in osteoporosis without trauma

Lumbar Spine

PEARL: Always look for clues that the question is describing cauda equine syndrome which would require emergent MRI and surgical intervention.

Symptoms include: saddle anesthesia, loss of bowel control (check rectal sphincter tone, check for "anal wink"), either urinary incontinence or urinary retention; abnormal neurologic exam

Back Strain/Sprain

- *Etiology/Epidemiology*
    - Precipitated by twisting and lifting
- *H & P*
    - Low back spasm worse with activity (rising from sitting/flexion); better with rest
    - Normal neuro exam
- *Labs & Diagnostics*
    - Not necessary to image unless concomitant other issues (steroid use; cancer history, etc)
    - Most Likely Diagnosis
    - R/O cauda equina
- *Clinical Intervention*
    - Physical Therapy
- *Therapeutics*
    - NSAID's
    - Epidural injection
- *Health Maintenance*
    - Abdominal muscle exercises
    - Back stretching exercises
    - Good body mechanics when lifting/bending/twisting

Low Back Pain

The NCCPA has put this in the blueprint separately from back sprain/strain, so I have tried to think of other reasons besides muscular spasm that cause low back pain. These are listed in order of importance to r/o first:

- **Cauda Equina (see above)** – Decreased sphincter tone (urethral and rectal) & saddle anesthesia
- **Abdominal Aortic Aneurysm** – Abnormal peripheral pulses in patient with RF for atherosclerotic disease
- **Diskitis** – Fever with back pain (especially in IV drug users and immunocompromised patients)
- **Metastatic Bone Cancer** – H/o cancer
- **Ankylosing Spondylitis** – Young man with SI joint pain; low grade fevers/malaise
- **Compression Fracture (Osteoporosis)** – Loss of height; or sudden pain
- **Bladder infection**
- **Herniated disc (see below)**
- **Degenerative Joint Disease** – Older patients; overused joints
- **Spondylolisthesis** – Gymnasts (discussed below)
- **Scoliosis** – Adolescents

Herniated Nucleus Pulposis

- *Etiology/Epidemiology*
  - Poor abdominal musculature
  - Flexing forward with twisting motion is most common etiology
  - Can occur as "overuse" with repetitive lifting/twisting
- *H & P*
  - If radicular symptoms – sciatica; decreased DTR's
  - *DRE needed to check rectal sphincter tone (always is included on OSCE of "patient" with radicular sx)
- *SPECIAL TESTS*
  - Straight leg raise; cross leg raise
  - L4 – Quad – knee extension
  - L5 – anterior tibialis – heel walking
  - S1 – Gastrocnemius – toe walking
  - DTR's
    - L4 – patellar reflex
    - L5 -
    - S1 – achilles reflex
- *Labs & Diagnostics*
  - Plain films
  - MRI
    - Emergent if symptoms of cauda equina
    - Elective if chronic pain to look at discs and cords

  - EMG if indicated
- *Most Likely Diagnosis*
  - R/O cauda equina syndrome
- *Clinical Intervention*
  - Rest, ice/heat
  - NSAID's
  - Steroids
  - Antispasm drugs(cyclobenzaprine or diazepam)
- *Physical Therapy (PT)*
  - Orthopedic referral if not improving with PT
- *Health Maintenance*
  - Abdominal muscle strengthening
  - Maintain good weight/decrease abdominal girth
  - Good body mechanics (information to patient)

Spinal Stenosis

- *Etiology/Epidemiology*
  - Osteoarthritis causing bony spurs (osteophytes) which pinch when the spinal column is straightened (narrowing the lumen)
- *H & P*
  - Pain with standing/walking; relieved with sitting
  - (Very similar to symptoms of claudicating lower extremity pain of peripheral arterial disease (PAD)
- *Labs & Diagnostics*
  - Plain film, then MRI
- *Most Likely Diagnosis*
  - Normal ankle branchial indexes (ABI's) rule out PAD
- *Clinical Intervention*
  - Surgical referral

Spondylolisthesis/Spondylolysis

- *Etiology/Epidemiology*
  - Stress fracture
  - Typical in small gymnasts from hyperextension of spine
- *H & P*
  - Normal exam except for focal pain
- *Labs & Diagnostics*
  - Plain films – oblique and lateral
- *Clinical Intervention*
  - Rest (out of gymnastics)
  - Conservative --- most resolve without treatment
  - PT

The Shoulder

Rotator Cuff Tears

- *Mechanism of Injury*
  - Age >40
  - Overuse; overhead torque
- *H & P*
  - Shoulder pain for months!!
  - No AROM due to pain
  - PROM is normal
- *Labs & Diagnostics*
  - Plain film
  - MRI
- *Clinical Intervention*
  - Rest
  - NSAID's
  - PT
  - Steroid injection (only one in pt > 50 y.o.)
  - Surgical intervention if all else fails
- *Scientific Concept*
  - Supraspinatus
  - Infraspinatus
  - Teres minor
  - Subscapularis

Anterior Shoulder Dislocation

- *Mechanism of Injury*
  - Fall or direct hit from behind (most common in young men in sports and elderly women who fall)
- *H & P*
  - Obvious deformity – "squared off shoulder" – humeral head palpable in front of shoulder
  - Usually neurovascularly intact
- *Labs & Diagnostics*
  - Shoulder xrays - Y view
- *Clinical Intervention*
  - Procedural sedation
  - Closed reduction
  - Get pre- and then get post-reduction films after closed reduction
  - Immobilization in sling
- *Scientific Concept*
  - The shoulder is the most frequently dislocated joint
  - Fracture of posterohumeral head is a Hill Sachs deformity – and many times only visible on post-reduction films

AC Separation

- *Mechanism of Injury*
  - Direct fall on lateral shoulder
- *H & P*
  - Pain over AC joint
  - Lifting arm is possible but painful
- *Labs & Diagnostics*
  - X-ray with weights
- *Clinical Intervention*
  - Grade 1 & 2 – immobilize
  - Grade 3 – surgical repair?
- *Scientific Concept*
  - Grade 1 – ligament strained only
  - Grade 2 – tear of AC ligament and sprain of coracoclavicular ligament
  - Grade 3 – tear of both ligaments

Clavicular Fracture

- *Etiology/Epidemiology*
  - Most common of pediatric fractures due to fall or being struck
- *H & P*
  - Unable to lift arm; deformity visible and palpable
- *Labs & Diagnostics*
  - Plain films
- *Clinical Intervention*
  - Cradle sling or Figure of 8
- *Scientific Concept*
  - "If the bones are in the same room, they will heal!"

Humeral Fracture (Radial Nerve Threatening)

- *Etiology/Epidemiology*
  - Trauma
  - Rarely, pathologic due to cancer or cyst
- *H & P*
  - Severe pain in humerus; shoulder
  - Usually too painful to move
  - Holds arm against body
- *Most important*
  - Check radial pulse; perfusion to fingers
  - Check radial nerve function
  - Dorsiflexion at the wrist
- *Labs & Diagnostics*
  - Plain films
- *Clinical Intervention*
  - Sling

- Coaptation splint (a splint that is hard plastic and wraps shoulder to elbow and attaches arm to chest with velcro wrap
- ***Scientific Concept***
    - Most common cause of radial nerve injury

The Elbow

Elbow tendinitis is the blueprint topic; and the next topic in the list is epicondylitis (epicondylitis in the elbow is an elbow tendinitis, so here is elbow tendinitis/epicondylitis:

(I would be remiss if I didn't also discuss elbow pain after trauma, and olecranon fracture, so I will, even though it is not in the Blueprint)

Epicondylitis

- *Etiology/Epidemiology*
    - Lateral = "tennis elbow" – overuse syndrome – extension of the wrist
    - Medial = "golfer's elbow" –overuse syndrome – flexion of the wrist
- *H & P*
    - Pain to palpation over epicondyle with flexion (or extension) of wrist
- *Labs & Diagnostics*
    - If trauma, get xray
- *Clinical Intervention*
    - NSAID's/steroid injection
    - PT
    - Splint
    - Avoid the action that caused the problem in the first place

Olecranon Fracture

- *Etiology/Epidemiology*
    - Falling directly onto elbow
- *H & P*
    - Pain to palpation directly over olecranon process
    - Marked swelling and bruising
    - Often a concomitant olecranon bursa injury
- *Labs & Diagnostics*
    - Plain films
- *Clinical Intervention*
    - Nonoperative care for simple fractures is usually successful
        - "Skillful neglect" in those who are poor surgical candidates
        - Will lose some full extension, but even widely displaced fractures heal well
    - Fractures with significant displacement (>2 mm) or comminution in young healthy individual usually requires surgical intervention

Other fractures/injuries presenting as "elbow pain":

- Radial head fractures(below, in forearm)
- Supracondylar humeral fractures (in pediatrics)

- Olecranon bursitis (discussed in bursitis section)

The Forearm

Radial Head Fracture

- *Etiology/Epidemiology*
  - Fall on outstretched hand (FOOSH injury)
- *H & P*
  - Pain and edema of elbow
  - Unable to pronate or supinate
- *Labs & Diagnostics*
  - Plain films show fat pad sign
- *Clinical Intervention*
  - Splinting and follow up

Monteggia fracture (not on blueprint)

- *Mechanism of injury*
  - FOOSH
- *H & P*
  - Pain over proximal forearm; swelling/ecchymosis
- *Labs & Diagnostics*
  - Plain film
    - Proximal ulnar fracture (closer to elbow)
    - Dislocation of radial head
- *Clinical Intervention*
  - Do not send home with splint – requires surgical intervention

Galeazzi Fracture *(not on blueprint)*

- *Mechanism of injury*
  - FOOSH
- *H & P*
  - Pain over distal 1/3 of radius and wrist; swelling/ecchymosis
- *Labs & Diagnostics*
  - Plain film
    - Distal shaft radial fracture (closer to wrist)
    - *Radio-ulnar subluxation*
- *Clinical Intervention*
  - Surgical intervention

PEARL : The acronym, MUGR <"mugger"> (Monteggia = ulnar fx; Galeazzi = radial fx)

The Wrist

Carpal Tunnel Syndrome

- *Mechanism of Injury*
    - Overuse (typing, driving, flexed wrist) fluid retention (pregnancy)
- *H & P*
    - Sensory parethesia reproducible with testing
        - Thumb to 3rd, 4th digit
    - Motor
        - Thenar muscle atrophy
- ***SPECIAL TESTS*** = Tinel's sign and Phalen's sign
    - Tinel's = tapping (over the dorsal wrist to elicit tingling)
    - Phalen's = flexion (of wrist; to 90 degrees and causes tingling/numbness)
- *Labs & Diagnostics*
    - EMG (electromyography)/NCV (nerve conduction velocity)
- *Clinical Intervention*
    - Wrist splint/limit activity/surgery
    - No surgical intervention while patient pregnant – wait until postpartum to see if it resolves without intervention
- *Therapeutics*
    - NSAID's
- *Health Maintenance*
    - Occupational intervention/PT/OT
- *Scientific Concept*
    - There are two tight "tunnels" in the wrist where the nerve goes through; if fluid, inflammation, nerve gets pinched
    - Carpal tunnel is due to entrapment of median nerve at the wrist

de Quervain's Tenosynovitis

- *Etiology/Epidemiology*
    - Overuse
    - Stretching and swelling, usually occupational
- *H & P*
    - Tender in region of distal radius
- ***SPECIAL TEST*** = Finkelstein test is diagnostic
    - Finkelstein – make a fist with thumb inside; and laterally flex the wrist (putting tension on the ligament attaching thumb) – severe pain
- *Labs & Diagnostics*
    - Plain film (r/o bony pathology)
- *Clinical Intervention*
    - Thumb spica splint
    - NSAID's
    - Steroid injection

Ganglion Cyst

- *Etiology/Epidemiology*
    - Cyst on synovial sheath

- *H & P*
    - Mainly painless bump; moves with tendon
- *Labs & Diagnostics*
    - Plain film (should not be visible, do it to r/o bone pathology)
- *Clinical Intervention*
    - Observation
    - Reassurance
    - Surgical excision if painful
- *Scientific Concept*
    - "Bible cyst" in the past because if you smash it with a bible it bursts and goes away – we don't treat them this way anymore!

Scaphoid Fracture *(also called navicular fracture)*

- *Mechanism of Injury*
    - Fall on outstretched hand (FOOSH)
- *H & P*
    - Pain at anatomical "Snuff box" (base of thumb at wrist)
- *Labs & Diagnostics*
    - Plain film
- *Clinical Intervention*
    - If pain at snuff box, and xray negative – thumb spica splint
    - Repeat xray in 7-10 days or do CT or bone scan

PEARL: *Navicular/Scaphoid Fractures:*

- Most of scaphoid is covered in cartilage
    - Blood supply cannot penetrate cartilage
- Entrance of vessel to scaphoid is distally (which is weird, on the finger side) and most fractures occur in the proximal 1/3
    - Far away from the supply
- Avascular necrosis is very common, especially if not immobilized
    - Always err on the side of immobilization

Colle's Fracture

- *Mechanism of Injury*
    - Falling forward on outstreched hand (FOOSH)
    - The most common traumatic wrist injury
- *H & P*
    - Pain and deformity of wrist
    - Dorsal angulation of distal radial fracture
- *Labs & Diagnostics*
    - Plain film
- *Clinical Intervention*
    - Sugar tong splint (to prevent pronation/supination)
    - If displaced, will need ORIF (open reduction, internal fixation)
- *Scientific Concept*
    - Colle's is more common than Smith's just because of the way we usually fall

Smith's Fracture

- *Mechanism of Injury*
    - Falling backward, putting hand out behind
- *H & P*
    - Pain and deformity
    - Reverse of Colle's with volar angulation of distal radial fracture
- *Labs & Diagnostics*
    - Plain film
- *Clinical Intervention*
    - Sugar tong splint
    - ORIF if badly displaced

The Hand

Boxer's (5th MC fx)

- *Mechanism of Injury*
    - Striking something/someone with a closed fist
- *H & P*
    - Check for sensation and capillary refill
    - Make sure not "open" from abrasion/laceration over injury
    - Injury from striking a mouth with lac by a tooth is particular prone to infection
- *Diagnostic*
    - Plain film, check for displacement
- *Clinical Intervention*
    - Ulnar gutter splint, followup with ortho for casting/pinning if needed

DuPuytren's Contracture (Viking Disease)

- *Epidemiology*
    - Northern European/Nordic descent
- *H & P*
    - Permanent flexion of a finger (4th, 5th, typically) over the palm
- *Labs & Diagnostics*
    - None, clinical diagnosis
- *Clinical Intervention*
    - Observation if minimal dysfunction
    - Collagenase injections with manipulation to break up adhesions
    - Surgical release of adhesions
- *Scientific Concept*
    - The skin adheres to the fascia; which pulls on the flexor tendon

Gamekeeper's Thumb

- *Mechanism of Injury*
    - Trauma; thumb gets pulled backward(skiier's thumb) and ulnar collateral ligament gets torn

- *H & P*
    - Pain, swelling, ecchymosis on ulnar side of MP joint
    - Laxity with radial stress to MP of thumb
- *Labs & Diagnostics*
    - Plain film to r/o avulsion fracture
- *Clinical Intervention*
    - Thumb spica splint
    - Surgical intervention if complete tear
    - Refer to ortho, thumb is the most important digit we have= refer all thumbs!!!!

Phalangeal Complications of Disease/Injury

Phalangeal fractures

- PIP Joint dislocations/sprains
- Most common joint injured in fingers
- Usually "jammed"
- Splint

Mallet Finger

- Extensor tendon injury
- "Jammed finger"
- Distal phalax is pulled down and unable to straighten it
- Splint

Boutonniere Deformity

- Tear in extensor tendon at PIP
- Unable to extend PIP (boutonniere is a clip used to attach a flower – s-shaped)
- Associated with Rheumatoid Arthritis
- Surgical repair if warranted

Trigger Finger

- Associated with rheumatoid arthritis or DM
- Inflammatory tendonitis
- Steroid injection

Phalangeal Infections

Felon

- Infection of the entire pad of the finger
- Must be opened (vertically) and drained
- Antibiotic (cover staph)

Herpetic Whitlow

- Herpes simplex (usually patient has blisters elsewhere)
- Common in health care workers (wear gloves!)
- Subepidermal blister on pad of finger
- Tender but not swelling over entire pad as in felon
    - Never becomes felon
- Treat with antiviral (acyclovir)

Paronychia

- Infection around nail itself but pad of finger is fine
- I & D, +/- antibiotics (drainage is key followed by warm soaks)
- Can extend over time if not treated to become a felon

The Hip

Hip Fracture

- *Etiology/Epidemiology*
    - In elderly, common, and due to minimal trauma; typically a fall
    - In younger, typically due to significant trauma, falls (I have seen fall while sky diving, skateboarding, falling from a roof)
- *H & P*
    - Limb is shortened and externally rotated
    - Make sure to check for neurovascular viability in the distal extremity
- *Labs & Diagnostics*
    - Plain film
    - May need CT to evaluate further
    - ***Get pelvic films as well, commonly associated injury***
- *Clinical Intervention*
    - ORIF (open reduction internal fixation)
- *Health Maintenance*
    - LMWH (low molecular weight heparin) prophylactically after surgery – pulmonary embolism from DVT is COMMON!!
- *Scientific Concept*
    - Femoral head is uncommon
    - Femoral neck and intertrochanteric much more common, esp. in females

Posterior hip dislocations

- *Mechanism of Injury*
    - High impact trauma (motor vehicle accident)
- *H & P*
    - Limb is shortened and internally rotated
- *Labs & Diagnostics*
    - Plain film
    - +/- CT (high impact, so high likelihood of fracture)
- *Most Likely Diagnosis*
    - 90% are posterior
    - Anterior dislocation is quite rare (the cup is deep anteriorly and shallow posteriorly)
- *Clinical Intervention*
    - Procedural sedation +
    - Closed reduction +
    - Post reduction films
- *Scientific Concept*
    - 25% of time, there is a knee injury

The Knee

Patellofemoral Syndrome

- *Mechanism of Injury*
  - Insidious onset due to poor muscle tone
- *H & P*
  - Pain with climbing stairs; getting out of a chair
  - Crepitus with flexion of knee
  - Vastus medius weakness
- *Labs & Diagnostics*
  - *Plain film (include sunrise films)*
- *Most Likely Diagnosis*
  - Chondromalacia of patella is key
- *Clinical Intervention*
  - PT/ quad strengthening (short arc weight lifting)
  - RICE/MICE

Meniscal Tears

- *Mechanism of Injury*
  - Twisting while flexing (climbing up into bed of truck; steep stair)
- *H & P*
  - "Pop" heard or felt
  - Joint line pain (medial vs. lateral)
  - Locking is key to this one
  - Effusion develops slower than an ACL, but usually present by 24 hours
- ***SPECIAL TEST***
  - McMurray's – supine – flex knee, rotate it (both ways to see which hurts) extend in rotation - pain
  - Apley's - prone, knee at 90, axial load with rotation -- pain
- *Labs & Diagnostics*
  - Plain films (just because)
- *Most Likely Diagnosis*
  - "Locking" of knee is key
  - Pain with walking up stairs
- *Clinical Intervention*
  - NSAID's
  - Brace
  - If continuing problems of locking: arthroscopic surgery (diagnosis and remove fragments)

Tibial Plateau Fracture

- *Mechanism of Injury*
  - More than 50% of patients who sustain a tibial plateau fracture are aged 50 years or older.
  - The increased frequency of tibial plateau fractures in older females is due to the increased prevalence of osteoporosis in these individuals.
  - Tibial plateau fractures in younger patients are commonly the result of high-energy injuries

- *H & P*
  - Full clinical assessment is required, including evaluation of the soft tissues to determine whether a compartment syndrome is present and whether the patient has sustained a neurovascular injury
  - Check distal pulses (popliteal artery damage is possible)
- *Labs & Diagnostics*
  - Plain film
- *Clinical Intervention*
  - Many require surgical repair
  - Often concomitant injury to meniscus; and collateral ligaments
- *Scientific Concept*
  - Dislocation-relocation injuries are more common with medial plateau injuries and carry an increased risk of peroneal nerve damage.

Patellar Fracture

- *Etiology/Epidemiology*
  - 20-50 year olds; direct fall onto knee cap
- *H & P*
  - Severe pain; swelling; hemarthrosis
  - Check for ability to extend knee against gravity (extensor mechanism)
- *Labs & Diagnostics*
  - Plain film with *sunrise view*
- *Most Likely Diagnosis*
  - Distinguish from patellar bursitis (from kneeling); fracture is from direct trauma (severe trauma)
  - Distinguish from patellofemoral syndrome which is an "overuse" insidious syndrome
  - Distinguish from patellar dislocation
- *Clinical Intervention*
  - Early surgical intervention for early movement/keep integrity of joint if:
  - Disruption of the extensor mechanism or more than 3 mm of separation between primary fracture fragments

Patellar Dislocation

- *Etiology/Epidemiology*
  - Direct trauma or "cutting" movement
- *H & P*
  - Acute pain; on inspection patella may be laterally or medially displaced
- *Labs & Diagnostics*
  - Plain film
  - MRI if recurrent
- *Clinical Intervention*
  - Immobilization improves function later
  - MICE
  - PT

<u>Cruciate Ligament tears *(not in blueprint!)*</u>

ACL (Anterior Cruciate Ligament)

- *Mechanism of Injury*
    - Twisting of knee with foot planted ; tibia forced forward
- *H & P*
    - 75% have significant hemarthrosis (if none, likely not ACL, then look at meniscus or collateral ligament)
- ***SPECIAL TESTS***
    - *Anterior Drawer Sign* – flex knee to 90 degrees (while supine); sit on foot; hands on calf; pull lower leg forward (should be almost no movement, if it moves, ACL is likely torn)
    - *Lachmann's* – knee at 30 degrees (supine), hand holding femur, other hand on tibia, pull forward (should not move), if it moves, ACL likely torn
    - *Pivot Shift Test* – knee in full extension (supine), slowly flex while applying internal rotation and valgus stress (subluxation occurs at 20 degrees). Patient has to be relaxed, so rarely actually works!
        - Just so you know, most patients have such huge joint effusions and such severe pain, they will never let you do these tests during acute phase of injury!
- *Labs & Diagnostics*
    - Plain film (just because)
    - MRI if not improving
- *Clinical Intervention*
    - PT
    - Brace
    - Surgical repair if active/sports/ unstable

PCL (Posterior Cruciate Ligament)

- *Mechanism of Injury*
    - Twisting injury with foot planted
- *H & P*
- ***SPECIAL TESTS***
    - *Posterior Drawer Sign* – bring tibia to midline (will be sagging posteriorly), then move it – very lax posteriorly
    - *Sag Sign* – knees flexed at 45 degrees, the one with PCL tear will "sag" backwards, causing a dimple below patella
- *Labs & Diagnostics*
    - Plain film (just because)
    - MRI if not improving
- *Clinical Intervention*
    - PT
    - Brace

PEARL: Before doing either the anterior or posterior drawer sign; do the sag sign first. All you do is look --- to see if the tibia is sagging. If it is, you have a PCL tear, and if it is and you don't recognize it first, when you move the tibia forward it will move, and you may mistakenly believe this suggests an ACL.

Collateral Ligament Tears *(also not in blueprint!)*

- *Mechanism of injury*
  - Hit in side of knee or falling with "flexion" laterally (the knee isn't supposed to flex that way!)
- *H & P*
- ***SPECIAL TESTS***
  - Varus or valgus laxity with stress
- *Labs & diagnostics*
  - Plain film = avulsion fracture
  - MRI if unstable or persistent problems

Baker's Cyst *(not in blueprint!)*

- *Scientific concept*
  - Communication with joint space
  - Fluid moves posteriorly out of knee into a "cyst" area in the popliteal fossa
  - Due to osteoarthritis of the knee
- *H & P*
  - Pain in popliteal fossa
  - Fullness or bulge in popliteal fossa
  - Comes and goes with arthritic inflammation;
- *Clinical Intervention*
  - Not removed
  - RICE/MICE
- *Scientific concept*
  - DVT is often in the differential
  - Sometimes "ruptures" and can cause LE swelling- then need to r/o DVT

The Ankle

Ankle sprains

- *Mechanism of Injury*
  - Inversion injury (woman "falls off her high heeled shoe", athlete inverts ankle)
- *H & P*
  - Swelling laterally
  - Ecchymosis
  - If sprain, is able to bear weight after injury
- *Labs & Diagnostics*
  - Plain films
- *Clinical Intervention*
  - Splint
  - PT
  - RICE/MICE
- *Scientific Concept*
  - Sequence of injury in order of most common ligament injured:

        - ATF anterior talofibular ligament
        - Then CF calcaneofibular ligament
        - Then PTF posterior talofibular ligament
    - *don't miss proximal fibular fracture (Maisonneuve)*
    - *don't miss achilles rupture*
    - *don't miss proximal 5th MT fracture*
- *Ottawa Criteria*
    - Used for deciding who needs imaging (has likely fracture)
    - 97-99% sensitivity/specificity
    - Unable to bear weight for 4 steps
    - Bony tenderness posterior to either malleolus
    - Bony tenderness over 5th metatarsal
    - Bony tenderness over medial forefoot

Ankle fracture (uni-, bi-, trimalleolar)
- *Mechanism of Injury*
    - Trauma/fall or inversion injury
- *H & P*
    - Point tender over medial or lateral malleolus (or both)
    - Unable to bear weight after injury
- *Labs & Diagnostics*
    - Plain films
- *Clinical Intervention*
    - Splint/ then cast
- *Scientific Concept*
    - Unimalleolar (if fibula, just needs walking boot or crutches and followup)
    - Bimalleolar – splint/cast - stirrup
    - Trimalleolar – surgical repair – unstable – splint with stirrup + posterior short leg
        - if surgical repair; wound problems are common – esp. in diabetic patient

Achilles Tendon Rupture
- *Mechanism of Injury*
    - Push off from rest , i.e., basketball jump shot
- *H & P*
    - Tender to palpation of achilles tendon area
    - "Step off" if complete tear
- ***SPECIAL TEST***
    - Thompson test – prone, squeeze calf – no movement of foot (should cause dorsi-flexion of foot if intact)
- *Most Likely Diagnosis*
    - " I thought someone hit me in back of foot with baseball bat"
- *Clinical Intervention*
    - Splint initially with foot in partial plantar flexion
    - Surgical repair if complete tear
- *Scientific Concept*
    - Quinolones can cause spontaneous Achilles tendonitis and rupture!

The Foot

Stress Fractures

- *Etiology*
  - Overuse (runners); pain with walking
- *Diagnostics*
  - Initial X-ray may be negative; post-op shoe, stop running!
- *Clinical Intervention*
  - Repeat X-ray in 7-10 days to look for sclerosis fracture line if pain not improving

Plantar Fasciitis

- *Mechanism of Injury*
  - Overuse, walking on concrete with poor sole support (nurses especially)
- *H & P*
  - Severe pain with first steps in morning; improves with a couple steps
- *Labs & Diagnostics*
  - X-ray to r/o stress fracture of MT's
  - Heel spur usually seen
- *Clinical Intervention*
  - Heel cup
  - NSAID's
  - Steroid injection

Morton's Neuroma *(not in blueprint!)*

- *Etiology/Epidemiology*- unknown
- *H & P*
  - Burning pain between toes
  - "Marble" between 3rd and 4th MTP (base of toes)
- *Labs & Diagnostics*
  - Plain films (just because)
- *Clinical Intervention*
  - Rest, ice, injections
  - Excisional removal of neuroma

5th Metatarsal Fracture (& Jone's Fracture)

- *Mechanism of Injury*
  - Inversion injury (associated with ankle sprains)
- *H & P*
  - Pain at base of 5th MT
  - Swelling and bruising of lateral foot
- *Labs & Diagnostics*
  - Plain film to r/o Jones fracture
- *Clinical Intervention*
  - Non-weight-bearing
  - Referral to orthopedics for recheck
- *Scientific Concept*
  - If styloid avulsion; usually heals without problem

- Lisfranc fracture (not in blueprint!)
  - Hyperflexion of forefoot (forefoot ends up bent underneath foot; usually during a trip and fall)
  - Bruising of mid forefoot; swelling; focal tenderness
  - Tarsal and metatarsal dislocation with fractures

Calcaneal Fracture *(not in blueprint!)*

- *Mechanism of Injury*
  - Fall from a height, landing directly on heel – severe pain
- *Diagnostics*
  - Should image both feet
- *Clinical Intervention*
  - X-ray lumbar spine for compression fracture (10%)
  - Remember to look for other fractures in a traumatic event
    - Distracting pain in heel may make patient unaware of back pain

---

Orthopedic Infections

Septic Arthritis (Native Joint)

- *Etiology/Epidemiology*
  - Children – staph aureus/strep
  - Sexually active – chlamydia/GC
  - IVDU – staph, MRSA
  - >50 y.o. – staph aureus/strep
- *H & P*
  - Relatively sudden onset
  - Red, hot, swollen, PAINFUL with joint movement
  - Both AROM and PROM cause severe pain
  - Fever +/-
- *Labs & Diagnostics (see Chapter 10, and Rheumatology for synovial fluid analysis)*
  - Synovial fluid analysis
    - Gm stain
    - Cell count (>100,000)
    - Crystals (neg)
    - Glucose (low)
- *Most Likely Diagnosis*
  - Distinguish from bursitis (only pain with palpation of bursa, not movement of joint)
  - Distinguish from gout – gout has crystals on fluid analysis
- *Clinical Intervention*
  - Surgical opening and irrigation/debridement of joint
- *Therapeutics*
  - Coverage as indicated by empirically (above), gm stain, or cultures
  - Typically vancomycin and third generation cephalosporin

Septic Arthritis (in prosthetic joint)

- *Have high index of suspicion in any sudden joint pain without trauma in a replaced joint*

- +/- fever, chills
- AROM and PROM of joint is very painful
- Joint is usually warm, with effusion, and often "pink"

- *Labs & Diagnosis*
    - CBC, ESR, CRP
        - CRP has best sensitivity and specificity
    - Plain film looking for gas, bony involvement
    - Synovial fluid analysis
        - Do not need cell count of 100,000 in a prosthetic joint
        - Gram stain positive
    - Clinical Intervention
        - Antibiotics pending
            - Open debridement or
            - Surgical explantation of joint
        - Empiric, and then directed at culture results
        - ID should be involved

Acute/Chronic Osteomyelitis

- *Most important distinction in osteomyelitis is whether it is:*
    - Acute (sudden onset of fever and pain)
    - Chronic (developing in a chronic infection of skin/soft tissue)
- *AND, is it likely:*
    - Post-traumatic (47%)
    - Associated with DM (34%)
    - Hematogenous (19%)
        - Sickle cell anemia
            - Interesting ID note: in SS disease one of the most common infections is osteo due to salmonella
- *Most Likely Diagnosis*
    - Occurs in knee
        - IV drug use
            - Staph aureus; staph epidermidis; MRSA; pseudomonas
    - More commonly occurs in spine
        - Diabetes Mellitus
        - The elderly (thoracic and lumbar spine)
        - Secondary to other infection (usually chronic in onset/nature)
    - In kids - -staph more likely
- In adults – gram neg (?) and in immunocompromised, TB is a thought

---

Other Orthopedic Topics

Osteoporosis

- *Etiology/Epidemiology*
    - Most common metabolic bone disorder
- *H & P*
    - Compression fractures of thoracic spine
    - Hip fractures

- *Labs & Diagnostics*
  - Dexa Scan - Tscore
    - "Normal" bone density = 0 = bone density of 35 y.o. caucasian female
    - Normal range = −1.0 to +1.0
    - Osteopenia = −1.0 to – 2.5 (unless fracture, then = osteoporosis)
    - Osteoporosis = < −2.5 (this has confused some, i.e. −2.8 = osteoporosis)
- *Risk Factors*
  - Age
  - Caucasian
  - Small frame
  - Smoking
  - Heparin/steroids
  - Low calcium/Vitamin D
- *Clinical Intervention*
  - Calcium and Vitamin D supplement
  - Weight bearing exercise (not swimming)
- *Therapeutics*
  - Bisphosphonates (alendronate)
  - Stomach upset/GI bleed common
  - Take on empty stomach; remain upright for 30 minutes after
- *Scientific Concept*
  - Vitamin D deficiency is an epidemic!
  - Depo-provera causes bone loss

Osteoarthritis (Degenerative Joint Disease)

- *Etiology/Epidemiology*
  - Overuse
  - Obesity
  - Aging of joints
  - Past history of trauma/infection of joint
- *H & P*
  - Pain in morning; quickly relieved with activity
  - Returns if too much activity
  - No fevers, no redness
  - Bony swelling (Heberden's nodes –occurs in DIPs)
- *Labs & Diagnostics*
  - X-ray shows "osteophyte formation with narrowing of joint spaces" (due to loss of cartilage)
- *Most Likely Diagnosis*
  - *Not* red, hot, boggy like septic or rheumatic joint
- *Clinical Intervention*
  - Only "cure" is total joint replacement
  - Attempts with "Synvisc" (synovial fluid type material); didn't work
- *Therapeutics*
  - Pain relief
  - RICE/MICE
  - Chrondroitin (dietary supplement/complementary medicine)

- *Health Maintenance*
    - Weight loss

Aseptic Necrosis/Avascular Necrosis of Bone

- *Etiology/Epidemiology*
    - Lack of blood supply to bone; sometimes due to trauma; due to steroid use
- *H & P*
    - Pain in joint (usually hip and referred pain to the knee)
    - No fevers (aseptic)
    - Decreased ROM
- *Labs & Diagnostics*
    - MRI/CT/nuclear medicine (bone scan)
- *Clinical Intervention*
    - Depends on extent of bone loss
- *Scientific Concept*
    - Most commonly occurs in femoral heads
        - Have high index if patient on steroids
        - Other risk factors: alcohol, trauma, sickle cell anemia
        - Have high index in high risk fractures (scaphoid, hip)
    - Jaw osteonecrosis from bisphosphonates when used to treat multiple myeloma and cancers (does not seem to happen with osteoporosis dosages)

Bursitis

- *Etiology/Epidemiology*
    - Bursa sacks exist in multiple places in and around joints, tendons, ligaments and between bone and skin to protect structures
- *Most common types:*
    - Olecranon bursitis
    - Prepatellar bursitis
    - Trochanteric bursitis
- *H & P*
    - Swelling beneath skin over the olecranon, patella, lateral hip (less visible on the hip)
    - Point tenderness --- definitely not an effusion within the joint
- *Labs & Diagnostics*
    - Can drain for comfort
    - *If red, send for culture and gram stain*
- *Most Likely Diagnosis*
    - Differentiate a benign bursitis (inflamed)
    - Vs. an infected bursa (red, hot, warm, patient with fever, pain with palpation of bursa itself, but not joint pain)
    - Vs. septic joint (re, warm joint; pain with any movement of joint)
- *Clinical Intervention*
    - Drain, or just treat with compresses and NSAID's;
    - If infected get fluid for culture; drain for pain relief
- *Therapeutics*
    - NSAID
- *Health Maintenance*
    - Knee pads when kneeling
    - Avoid leaning on elbow

Bone Cysts/Tumors

Benign Tumors:

- Do not have "Sarcoma" in the name
- Still cause pathologic fractures
- Not malignant
- Identified on plain films
    - Osteoma
    - Osteochondroma
    - Aneurysmal bone cyst

Malignant Primary Orthopedic Tumors

Osteosarcoma

- *Etiology/Epidemiology*
    - Boys > girls; 10-25 y.o.
- *H & P*
    - Long bone pain
    - Pathologic fracture of long bone
- *Labs & Diagnostics*
    - Sunburst appearance on xray
- *Clinical Intervention*
    - Removal of limb
    - Oncology referral

Chondrosarcoma ***(not in blueprint!)***

- Malignant cartilage tumor (chondro = cartilage)
- 35-50 year old men & women

Introduction to Rheumatologic Diseases

PEARL: Rheumatologic/Autoimmune Diseases:

- All are systemic illnesses and involve all organ systems
- Patient will have positive review of systems (think autoimmune disorder, endocrine disorder, or psychiatric disorder when the patient has complaints in all systems)
- The only disorder that can be diagnosed on first visit to the clinic would probably be Giant Cell Arteritis (Temporal arteritis)
- All the rest are insidious in onset; with waxing and waning symptoms; diagnosed after months to years of repeated evaluations

- All patients have generalized malaise, anorexia, weight loss, fevers (low grade), and just feel poorly
- Labs are mainly nonspecific; and multiple criteria are needed to diagnose the disease
- RA and SLE are most common in women; "the seronegatives" are more common in men

Rheumatoid Arthritis

- *Etiology*
  - Autoimmune disorder of young women
  - 3:1, women:men (so occurs in men too)
  - Systemic illness as well as joint arthropathies
- *H & P*
  - Joint redness, swelling, bogginess
  - Particularly MCP's, PIP's, wrists, and feet --- *symmetrical
- *Labs & Diagnostics*
  - CCP (cyclic citrullinated peptide) – 96% pos
  - RF (rheumatoid factor) – 80% pos
  - Elevated ESR (erythrocyte sedimentation rate)
  - Elevated C-reactive protein (especially during acute flare)
- *Formulating the Most Likely Diagnosis*
  - Distinguish from SLE (lupus) with diagnostics
    - ANA negative
    - RF and CCP positive
    - Both cause small joint symmetrical arthritis
- *Therapeutics*
  - <u>NSAID's</u>
    - SE: GI upset, ulcers
  - <u>Methotrexate</u>
    - SE: folate inhibitor, ***contraindicated in pregnancy
  - <u>Tumor Necrosis Factor α inhibitor</u>
    - Expensive, reactivates latent TB
      - Apply PPD and treat with INH if positive
- *Health Maintenance*
  - Physical therapy; exercise; joint rest
  - Folic acid supplementation for all patients on methotrexate

Systemic Lupus Erythematosus

- *Etiology*
  - Autoimmune (F:M, 9:1)
  - Incidence: 1:1000 White women, 1:250 African-American women
  - 1:40 in daughter of mothers with SLE
- *H & P*
  - Symmetric small joint redness, swelling, bogginess (similar distribution as RA – difficult to distinguish)
  - Systemic symptoms
- *Labs & diagnostics*
  - ANA

- False positive VDRL/RPR
- Elevated ESR
- Elevated C-reactive protein in acute flare
- Proteinuria (if renal involvement)

- *Formulating Most Likely Diagnosis*
  - Must have four or more of the following criteria
    - Arthralgias
    - ANA
    - False positive VDRL
    - Serositis (pleuritis, pericarditis)
    - Proteinuria (nephropathy)
    - Canker sores
    - Anemia
- *Clinical Intervention*
  - Referral to rheumatology
  - Referral to nephron if proteinuria
  - Referral to cardiology if any cardiac complaints
- *Therapeutics*
  - Prednisone (mainstay of therapy)
  - Hydroxychloroquine (anti-malarial) – doesn't work very well, 25-50% response rate
  - Azothiaprine (potent immunosuppressant)
- *Health Maintenance*
  - Avoid sun exposure

Rheumatoid Arthritis	Systemic Lupus Erythematosis
Young women 3 : 1 men	Young women 9 : 1 men
Rheumatoid nodules	Rash in sun exposed areas
Small joint arthralgias	Small joint arthralgias
RF 80%, CCP 96%	ANA 100%, anti-DS DNA
Leukopenia	Anemia, leukopenia, low Plts
Pulmonary symptoms	Renal and CNS abnormalities
	Antiphospholipid syndrome

The Seronegative Spondyloarthropathies

PEARL: The seronegative spondyloarthropathies include reactive arthritis, ankylosing spondylitis, psoriatic and colitic arthritis. It is called "seronegative" because in the historical understanding of these diseases, the patient had arthritis syndromes and an elevated ESR suggesting a rheumatologic disease, but the ANA and RF (the only two tests available 50 years ago) were negative. As it turns out, 50 years later, a human leukocytic antigen was discovered to be the culprit: HLA-B27.

These are called spondyloarthropathies because they involve the central spine and large joints. Recall that RA and SLE involve the small joints of the hands and feet.

So, when you get a question about a patient who has large joint or back pain; high sed rate; systemic symptoms (like all rheumatologic diseases), but negative ANA and RF; select one of the seronegative spondyloarthropathies. Order a serum HLA-B27!

Reactive Arthritis (Formerly called Reiter's Syndrome)

- *Etiology*
  - Prior infection with chlamydia, Yersinia, campylobacter, shigella, salmonella
- *H & P*
  - Iritis/conjunctivitis
  - Urethritis
  - Arthritis (knees)
  - "Can't see, can't pee, can't climb a tree, can't sleep with me (chlamydia)"
- *Labs & Diagnostics*
  - HLA-B27 positive
  - Elevated ESR
  - Neg ANA/RF (seronegative disease)
- Formulating Most Likely Diagnosis
  - Above constellation of symptoms weeks to months after diarrhea or chlamydia urethritis
- Clinical Intervention
  - Immunosuppressive drugs
  - Rheumatology referral

Ankylosing Spondylitis

- *Etiology*
  - Autoimmune; HLA-B27
  - Young men, 20-40 years of age
- *H & P*
  - Low back pain with SI joint pain
- *Labs & Diagnostics*
- *(Called the "seronegative spondyloarthropathies" because the ANA and RF are negative)*
  - Neg ANA

- Neg RF
- Elevated ESR
- Positive HLA-B27
- L-S X-rays show fusion of the S-I joint, and eventually a "Bamboo" spine
    - Fusion of the spine from distal to proximal

- *Formulating Most Likely Diagnosis:*
    - Likely to get info about a prior chlamydia (or urethral discharge) or infectious diarrhea – remember, even if appropriately diagnosed and treated, some with HLA-B27 will still develop this autoimmune response, unfortunately
- *Clinical Intervention*
    - Immunosuppressive drugs
- *Therapeutics:*
    - Prednisone
    - Tumor necrosis factor inhibitor

Colitic Arthritis

- Associated with inflammatory bowel diseases (Crohn's and Ulcerative Colitis)
- Most common extra-intestinal complication of their bowel disorder
- Treat the bowel, and the joints improve

Psoriatic Arthritis

- Associated with psoriasis
- Nonderforming arthritis
- Textbooks say that the psoriasis precedes the arthritis; rheumatology PA's around the country tell me that the arthritis frequently precedes the psoriatic plaques
- Either way, for the exam, there would have to be some clue that the patient has psoriasis to be able to get this one correct, i.e. the patient has "purple plaques with a silvery scale on the extensor surfaces of the elbows and knees," with arthritic symptoms and positive HLA-B27!

Other "Non-Classified" Autoimmune Disorders

Scleroderma (Systemic Sclerosis)

- *Etiology*
    - Autoimmune disorder causing squamous cell destruction
- *H & P*
    - Thickening of skin of face and hands; esophagus; telangiectasias, Raynaud's phenomenon
- *Labs & diagnostics*
    - May have (usually either or both):
        - Positive ANA
        - Positive RF
- *Formulating Most Likely Diagnosis*
    - Dysphagia is biggest clue; as well as skin thickening of face and hands
- *Clinical Intervention*
    - Immunosuppressive drugs

- *Therapeutics*
    - Very difficult; directed at problem
    - No good treatment available: no cure
    - Esophagus – manage as GERD or achalasia
    - Raynaud's – manage as in PVD – CCB's, avoid cold, stop smoking
    - Overall – immunosuppressant (Methotrexate, cyclosporine, prednisone)

Sjogren's Syndrome

- *Etiology*
    - Autoimmune destruction of the nasolacrimal and salivary glands in a female with autoimmune disease
    - 50 y.o. woman with underlying autoimmune disease
- *H & P*
    - Corneal abrasions/keratitis sicca
    - Poor dentition, gingival dryness, irritation
- *Labs & diagnostics*
    - Positive ANA
- *Clinical Intervention*
    - Treat symptoms of dry eyes, dry mouth and dry skin/mucous membranes
- *Therapeutics*
    - <u>Direct at complaints</u> – no cure
    - <u>Mild symptoms</u>
        - Lubricant drops for eyes; lemon drops for mouth; emollient cream for skin
    - <u>Moderate symptoms</u>
        - Lubricant ointment for eyes; lemon drops – dental surveillance, fluoride treatments to prevent dental caries
    - <u>Severe symptoms</u>
        - Cyclosporine drops for eyes; humidifier, lemon drops, dental visits

Muscular Disorders/Dysfunction

Polymyositis

- *Etiology*
    - Autoimmune chronic inflammatory myopathy
- *H & P*
    - Symmetric proximal muscle weakness
- *Labs & diagnostics*
    - CPK
    - Muscle biopsy
    - Electromyography (EMG)
- *Formulating Most Likely Diagnosis*
    - Proximal muscle weakness is the key
- *Clinical Intervention*
    - Immunosuppressives
- Therapeutics
    - Prednisone, sun avoidance

- *Scientific Concept*
    - ***Dermatomyositis***
        - A polymyositis-like disorder with purple "heliotrope" rash over eyelids and in a "shawl-like" distribution of the upper chest
        - 25% risk for occult malignancy
            - Colorectal cancer/lung cancer is most common

Polymyalgia Rheumatica

- *Etiology*
    - Inflammatory myopathy
- *H & P*
    - Elderly patient
    - Pain in shoulder and pelvic girdle (with relatively normal exam, pain out of proportion)
    - Fevers; myalgias, anorexia, malaise
- *Labs & diagnostics*
    - Elevated ESR (normal muscle biopsy, if done)
- *Formulating Most Likely Diagnosis*
    - *Pain* in shoulder and pelvic girdle in elderly patient with fevers and elevated ESR
- *Therapeutics*
    - NSAID's
    - Prednisone

PEARL: Polymyalgia Rheumatica is associated with Giant Cell Arteritis – so look for it in the past medical history!

Fibromyalgia

- *Etiology*
    - Functional disorder of GABA receptors ("amplifies" pain)
- *H&P:* normal
- *Formulating the Most Likely Diagnosis*
    - Chronic, muscular pain, without systemic symptoms except fatigue (i.e. no fevers, swelling, etc)
- *Labs & Diagnostics*
    - All testing will be "negative" or normal
- *Clinical Intervation: (see below in treatment)*
- *Treatment*
    - Exercise
    - Pregabalin (Lyrica)
    - Duloxetine (Cymbalta)
    - Sleep aids

PEARL: Do not give opiates (adding another problem --- opiate addiction)

Crystal Synovitis

Gout

- *Etiology*
  - Deposition of uric acid crystals in joint space
  - Causes inflammation (*not* infection)
  - Kidney is responsible for excreting uric acid.
  - As kidney function decreases incidence of gout increases.
- *H & P:*
  - Red, hot swollen 1st MTP (base of great toe), occurs less commonly in ankle, wrist, etc. (but can occur in any joint)
- *Labs & diagnostics*
  - Synovial fluid analysis shows *needle shaped crystals with negative birefringence
- *Formulating Most Likely Diagnosis:*
  - Location (big toe)
  - In typical patient (middle aged obese man with poor diet, alcohol)
  - Crystals in synovial fluid
- *Clinical Intervention*
  - Manage diet and risk factors; treat pain; treat arthritis
- *Treat Arthritis*
  - NSAID's (Indomethacin) (SE: stomach upset)
  - Colchicine (SE: GI upset, 80% vomiting and diarrhea)
    - Now dosed differently:
      - Colcrys, 1.2 mg now, then 0.6mg x 1 more dose
- *Therapeutics (see Scientific Concept below)*
  - Allopurinol
  - Probenecid
- *Health Maintenance*
  - Gout dietary instruction – (reduce shellfish, organ meats, high fat foods)
  - Reduce obesity
  - Reduce alcohol intake
  - Stop meds that increase risk of gout: thiazides, low-dose aspirin, niacin (all drugs that most gout-prone middle aged men would take!)
- *Scientific Concept*
  - Most humans are under-excreters of uric acid, and would benefit from Probenecid
    - However, it requires > 2 liters of urine output a day
    - Therefore, more than 2 liters of fluid a day to prevent uric acid stones.
  - Most humans are, therefore, instead treated with allopurinol that reduces production of uric acid (which still helps the body get rid of the uric acid).

PEARL: Do *not* treat acute gout with allopurinol ---- may precipitate many joints with gout --- wait until patient is finished with gout flare, has tried diet, and stopped gout-precipitating drugs before starting allopurinol

Pseudogout

- *Etiology*
    - Calcium pyrophosphate deposition in joint spaces, especially in elderly with osteoarthritis
- *H & P*
    - Large joint arthritis
- *Labs & diagnostics*
    - Synovial fluid finding crystals with positive birefringence
- *Formulating most likely diagnosis:*
    - Distinguish from a septic joint with synovial fluid analysis
- *Therapeutics:* none

PEARL:

- *Birefringence* is the term given to the "bending" of polarized light under a polarized light microscope; one crystal bends it one way, the other crystal bends it another way
    - Gout
        - **N**eedle shaped crystals with **N**egative birefringence
    - **P**seudogout
        - **P**rism shaped crystals with **P**ositive birefringence
- Distinguish crystal synovitis from septic arthritis
    - Clinically may look the same
    - Synovial fluid analysis is necessary for definitive diagnosis
        - Cell count = ~ 30,000 for crystal synovitis; ~ 100,000 or more for septic joint
        - Most WBC's will be monocytes in crystal synovitis; pmn's in septic joint
        - Gram stain negative in crystal synovitis; positive in septic joint

Classification of Synovial Fluid Analysis

Synovial fluid may be classified into normal, noninflammatory, inflammatory, septic, and hemorrhagic:

	Normal	Osteoarthritis	Inflammatory	Septic
Volume (ml)	<3.5	>3.5	>3.5	>3.5
Viscosity	High	High	Low	Mixed
Clarity	Clear	Clear	Cloudy	Opaque
Color	Straw	Straw/yellow	Yellow	Mixed
WBC	<200	<2,000	5,000-75,000	>100,000
Polys (%)	<25	<25	50%	>80%
Gram stain	Neg	Neg	Neg	Often positive

*Crystal analysis would be performed; if positive, will identify gout and pseudogout

VASCULITIC SYNDROMES

- *Basic tenets of all vasculitic syndromes:*
    - Discovered after weeks/months of symptoms
        - No single clinical test (except for vascular biopsy)
    - All cause similar vague symptoms
        - malaise
        - fatigue
        - fevers (low grade, typically)
        - anorexia, weight loss
    - All vasculitic syndromes involve all the arterials of the body
        - Each individual syndrome has a propensity toward either the large (aorta), medium (kidney parenchyma), or small (pulmonary, glomerular) arteries of the body
    - All are diagnosed with a biopsy (pulmonary, renal, liver, vascular, temporal artery)

Giant Cell Arteritis/Temporal Arteritis

- *Etiology*
    - Autoimmune vasculitic syndrome involving large vessels (aorta, carotids, temporal artery)
- *H&P*
    - Unilateral HA/eye pain
    - Painful temporal artery on palpation
    - May have absent pulse
- *Labs/diagnostics*
    - ESR (>100)
    - Temporal artery biopsy
- *Clinical intervention*
    - Immediate administration of prednisone (60-120 mgm PO)
    - You have 40 hours after prednisone to get biopsy performed so do not delay therapy
- *Therapeutics*
    - Prednisone, high dose, short course

PEARL: ***Complication of temporal arteritis* = Monocular blindness if not treated

Polyarteritis Nodosa

- *Etiology*
    - Autoimmune vasculitis
- *H & P*
    - Weight loss
    - Livedo reticularis (a purplish lacey, i.e. "reticular" blotching that to me looks like mottling)
    - H/o Hepatitis B infection

- *Labs & diagnostics*
    - Elevated ESR/CRP,
    - Elevated BUN & Creatinine
    - HepB Ag positivity
    - Biopsy of affected area is definitive (ANA & RF are NEGATIVE)
- *Formulating Most Likely Diagnosis:* clinically very difficult---
    - Vague somatic symptoms suggest autoimmune disorder generally, but there is no single clue to PAN that they could give you on a Q
- *Clinical Intervention*
    - Rheumatology referral
- *Therapeutics*
    - Prednisone

CHAPTER 15

Women's Health - 8%

Gynecology

Gynecological Cancers

Cervical Dysplasia

(I have decided to put both the topics of cervical dysplasia and cervical cancer together; they are listed separately in the Blueprint, but are really a continuum of the same disorder, making difficult to separate)

- *Etiology*
  - HPV, primarily types 16, 18 ...etc.
- *H & P*
  - Asymptomatic until it is too late (like almost all cancers)
- *Labs & diagnostics*
  - Pap smear
  - HPV typing
- *Formulating Most Likely Diagnosis*
  - Suspect this if patient has not had pap in years, and has friable cervix
- *Clinical Intervention*
  - If pap abnormal, colposcopy with biopsy
  - If severe dysplasia LEEP (loop excision electrocautery procedure)
- *Health Maintenance*
  - Pap smear screening

Cervical Cancer
- *Etiology*
  - HPV types 16, 18, 31, 33, 35
- *Epidemiology*
  - Squamous cell carcinoma
  - Cancer of *young* women
- *Risk Factors (risk that acquiring the HPV will lead to cancer)*
  - Early age at first intercourse
  - Multiple sexual partners
  - Immunocompromised status
  - Prior history of severe dysplasia or carcinoma in situ

 - moking
- *H & P*
  - May be normal
  - May have cervical bleeding after intercourse (post-coital bleeding)
  - May have friable lesion on pap smear visibly
- *Labs & diagnostics*
  - <u>Screening</u>
    - PAP Smear (may be "thin prep", cells collected and suspended in a liquid solution improves visibility of cells on evaluation)
  - <u>Diagnosis</u>
    - Colposcopy with biopsy
- *Formulating Most Likely Diagnosis*:
  - Suspect in any young woman who has not had pap testing regularly and has any bleeding or cervical lesion
- *Therapeutics*
  - LEEP (loop excision electrocautery procedure) for abnormal cells
  - Cold cone if CIS (carcinoma in situ)
- *Health Maintenance:*
  - PAP smear screening guidelines

PEARL: ** Adenocarcinoma of the cervix is very uncommon, but particularly lethal; it is in the endocervix, probably not related to HPV, and difficult to evaluate and treat

Vulvar Cancer

- *Etiology*
  - Squamous cell cancer
  - Likely HPV infection related (HPV types 16, 18, etc)
  - Likely in an older woman; still relatively uncommon
  - But increasing in incidence
- *H & P*
  - Painless ulcer (may bleed)
- *Labs & diagnostics*
  - perform a biopsy
- *Formulating Most Likely Diagnosis*
  - any painless ulcer should be biopsied
- *Clinical Intervention*
  - After biopsy
  - Refer to gyn onc surgeon for excision of tumor or treatment
  - Surgical excision
  - Cryocautery
- *Therapeutics*
  - Imiquimod (aldara) – intradermal injection
  - 5-fluorouracil – topical cream
- *Health Maintenance*
  - HPV vaccine
  - Barrier contraception to avoid HPV acquisition in young women
  - Regular pelvic examination

Endometrial Cancer

- *Etiology*
  - Relatively common after menopause
- *H & P*
  - May be normal
  - Bleeding, even a spot is not ok after menopause (>1 year after last menses)
- *Labs & diagnostics*
  - Endometrial Biopsy
- *Formulating Most Likely Diagnosis*
  - <u>Any postmenopausal bleeding is endometrial cancer until proven benign by endometrial biopsy.</u>
- *Clinical Intervention*
  - Referral to Gyn Onc
  - Hysterectomy / Bilateral Salpingoophorectomy
- *Therapeutics*
  - Chemotherapy
  - Radiation therapy
- *Health Maintenance*
  - Advise patient to report any vaginal bleeding at all after menopause.

Ovarian Cancer

- *Etiology*
  - Epithelial, stromal and germ cell cancers
- *Epidemiology*
  - Relatively uncommon compared to others (breast & endometrial)
  - Unless
    - BRCA1 mutation = 45% lifetime risk
    - BRCA2 mutations = 25% lifetime risk
- *H & P*
  - Any ovary palpable in a woman > 60 yrs. is probably abnormal
  - Any ovary > 5 cm. is considered abnormal and should have transvaginal ultrasound
- *Labs & diagnostics*
  - CA-125 is a marker (elevated in 80% with epithelial cancer)
    - Not found in 50% with early disease
    - Elevated for many other "benign" reasons
  - Transvaginal Ultrasound for mixed echogenic mass on ovary; or ovarian enlargement
  - Excisional removal of ovaries and uterus
- *Clinical Intervention*
  - Referral to Gyn Onc
  - Hysterectomy/ Bilateral Salpingoopherectomy
- *Therapeutics*
  - Chemotherapy and radiation
- *Health Maintenance*
  - Regular pelvic examination

Disorders of Menstruation

PEARL: In order to understand abnormal bleeding patterns, you must truly understand what is happening during a normal menstrual cycle (as painful as learning this may be)

The menstrual cycle can be looked at as causing two different changes:

- Ovarian follicle development (not useful for this talk, more related to fertility)
- Endometrial development (all about DUB)

Day 1–14 = Estrogen Dominant

- Ovary begins developing follicles =follicular phase
- The endometrium thickens in response to estrogen = proliferative phase
- Release of LH due to "magic" (said by expert in the field responding to an audience question!) LH surge = ovulation

Day 14-32 = progesterone dominant

- Dominant follicle "shell" develops into the corpus luteum = luteal phase
- Endometrium changes and becomes more vascular = secretory phas
- If no pregnancy occurs, corpus luteum "degenerates", progesterone levels fall and
- Menstruation begins (shedding of endometrium); the cycle starts over at day 1

AMENORRHEA

When evaluating a patient for amenorrhea, consider that there are "four compartments":

- I - Outflow tract (hymen, endometrium)
- II - Ovaries (estrogen)
- III - Pituitary (FSH/LH)
- IV - Hypothalamus (not measurable with lab testing)

Primary Amenorrhea

- *Etiology*
    - #1 – pregnancy (recall, that pregnancy can occur even if she has not reached menarche yet, as ovulation occurs prior to the first menses)
    - imperforate hymen
    - Turner syndrome, or other congenital defect
    - Eating disorder
- *H & P*
    - Check for secondary sex characteristics (Tanner development)
    - If no development at age 14; consider Turner syndrome

  - Pelvic exam to r/o intact hymen; to palpate for uterus and ovaries
- *Labs & diagnostics*
  - SHCG
  - TSH, prolactin
  - FSH and estradiol
- *Clinical Intervention*
  - Depends on what is discovered:
    - If intact hymen = surgical referral
    - If no sex development and no estradiol = referral to endocrine
    - If eating disorder = psych referral
- *Formulating the most likely diagnosis*
  - Imperforate hymen (compartment I)
  - Turner syndrome, or other congenital defect (compartment II)
  - Eating disorder (compartment III & IV)

Secondary Amenorrhea

- *Etiology*
  - #1 PREGNANCY
  - #2 hypothyroidism
  - #3 hyperprolactinemia
  - #4 bulemia/anorexia
  - Premature ovarian failure
  - Endometrial atrophy (Asherman's syndrome)
- *H & P*
  - Pelvic exam
- *Labs & diagnostics*
  - HCG
  - TSH, prolactin
  - FSH/LH; estrogen
  - Ultrasound
- *Formulating Most Likely Diagnosis*
  - Asherman's syndrome (endometrial atrophy) – compartment I
  - Premature ovarian failure (FSH >40 in female <40 yrs) –compartment II
  - Hypothyroidism – compartment III
  - Hyperprolactinemia – compartment III
  - Bulemia/anorexia – compartments III & IV
- *Clinical Intervention depends on etiology*

DYSFUNCTIONAL UTERINE BLEEDING

- **Definition**
  - Abnormal vaginal bleeding in the absence of any pathology of the gyn organs
- *Etiology*
  - Diagnosis of exclusion, but 90% due to anovulation
- *H & P*
  - *Really should be normal; it is a diagnosis of exclusion*
- *Labs & diagnostics*

    - HCG
    - Pap smear
    - Endometrial biopsy (will be "proliferative")
    - Ultrasound
- *Formulating Most Likely Diagnosis*
    - Again, r/o other causes, like cancer
- *Clinical Intervention*
    - Hormonal
        - Supplement the luteal phase of the cycle with progesterone each month about the time the women should ovulate x 10 days, then let her "with-draw"
- *Therapeutics:* progesterone d 14-24

If estrogen causes thickening of the endometrium, and progesterone causes vascularity of the endometrium, and withdrawal of that progesterone causes shedding (bleeding), what do you think would happen if a woman would fail to ovulate for, say, 52 days?

Answer: DUB

***Discussion*:**

- Estrogen predominant endometrial thickening (with no secretory phase, no progesterone, and no withdrawal bleed, i.e. no ovulation) = hyperplasia of the endometrium
- Hyperplasia of the endometrium (thickening) and eventually leaking of that thick heavy endometrium = dysfunctional uterine bleeding
- Therefore, the most common cause of DUB is anovulation!
- Remember --- we "run out" of eggs before we "run out" of estrogen -- hence, perimenopausal bleeding due to anovulation is very common.

If a woman was 43 and having very irregular periods due to anovulation, and you did not want to put her on the pill, how could you manage her DUB?

***Discussion*:** By giving her (and her uterus) progesterone from day 14-25 --- and then stopping it -- mimicking for her what ovulation should have done for her -- this is called "cycled progesterone"-- much safer than birth control pills for older women (or smokers).

How do you tell the difference between DUB or hyperplasia and endometrial cancer?

Answer: You cannot -- not without an endometrial biopsy.

Endometrial biopsy is a commonly done procedure where the PA inserts a straw-like pipelle through the cervix and "samples" the endometrium of the uterus.

It is day 45 of a woman's cycle, and a PA has done an endometrial biopsy. The pathology report returns showing "proliferative" endometrium. What important piece of information does this tell you?

Answer: That she has not ovulated yet (on day 45 of her cycle) .

What is this called? Anovulation

How do you treat it? Cycled progesterone

It is day 45 of a woman's cycle, and a PA has done an endometrial biopsy. The pathology report returns showing "atypical hyperplasia" of her endometrium. What does this suggest?

Answer: It is much more suspicious for endometrial cancer than just plain hyperplasia and she should be referred to GYN for D & C to evaluate the endometrium more carefully

Do you recall the term "unopposed estrogen"?

Answer: Anovulation causes unopposed estrogen (because progesterone is not produced to "oppose" the estrogen activity in the uterus. Unopposed estrogen can occur within our bodies as well (next Q)

What else increases the body's own production of estrogen? (Which could increase the concentration of estrogen relative to progesterone and cause an amount of "unopposed" estrogen?

Answer: Morbid obesity. Estrone is produced in adipose tissue and is converted to estradiol.

What other patient population would have increased risk of endometrial cancer?

Answer: Infertility patients whose problem is anovulation.

PEARL: We run out of "eggs" before we run out of estrogen, making it very common to have DUB after age 38.

DYSMENORRHEA

Primary Dysmenorrhea

- *Etiology*
    - Prostaglandin mediated pain
- *H & P*
    - Normal
- *Labs & diagnostics*
    - None (if discharge is present, r/o PID)
- *Formulating Most Likely Diagnosis*
    - Young patient shortly after menarche, occurs every month with menses
- *Clinical Intervention*
    - NSAID's
    - Birth control pills

Secondary Dysmenorrhea

- *Etiology*
    - Endometriosis #1
- *H & P*
    - Normal
- *Labs & diagnostics*
    - Cultures
    - US
- *Formulating Most Likely Diagnosis*
    - Older patient who has had menses without problem for several years, now with dysmenorrhea and w/u negative
- *Clinical Intervention*
    - Laparoscopy

ENDOMETRIOSIS

- *Etiology*
    - Is implantation of tissue within the pelvis (and sometimes extra-pelvic) which respond to estrogen and cause pain
- *H & P*
    - Not palpable on pelvic exam
    - Not diagnosed with laboratories
    - And not visible on ultrasound
    - The only way to diagnose it is with laparoscopy
    - Both diagnostic and therapeutic as laser can be used to ablate as many visible implants as possible.
- *Labs & diagnostics*
    - Laparoscopy
- *Formulating Most Likely Diagnosis*
    - Months of dyspareunia, dysmenorrhea, pelvic pain and infertility
- *Clinical Intervention*

  - Lap with ablation of implants
  - Medication to suppress estrogen
- *Therapeutics*
  - Leuprolide (Lupron) is a GNRH agonist that competes with LH and FSH at the pituitary and lowers estrogen levels.
  - Lack of estrogen causes problems with hot flushes short-term, and with osteoporosis long-term.

PREMENSTRUAL SYNDROME

- *Epidemiology*
  - Women who are menstruating (obviously!)
  - Symptoms occur about a week or so before menses, and resolves after.
- *H & P*
  - Emotional symptoms:
    - Depression
    - Irritability
    - Anxiety
    - Insomnia
    - Angry outbursts
  - Physical symptoms:
    - Bloating
    - Food cravings
    - Breast tenderness
    - GI changes/constipation or diarrhea
- *Definition*
  - Must be present for 5 days prior to menses for at least three months
  - Ends within for days after menses finished
  - Must interfere with daily life
- *Clinical Intervention*
  - Treat individual symptoms, i.e. diuretics, antidepressants
  - Exercise
  - Calcium, Magnesium, B vitamin supplements

Disorders of the Uterus

Leiomyoma (Fibroids)

- *Etiology*
  - Benign, vascular tumors which can grow both inside and outside the uterus causing bulky tumors, or if inside, causing menorrhagia
- *H & P*
  - Bimanual exam can reveal an enlarged, or irregular nontender uterus
- *Labs & diagnostics*
  - Ultrasound
- *Formulating Most Likely Diagnosis*

- Ultrasound is diagnostic

- *Clinical Intervention*
  - Surgery
  - Removal of fibroid
  - Embolization of blood supply to fibroid
  - Medication to suppress estrogen
    - Leuprolide (Lupron)
- *Therapeutics*
  - Leuprolide (see endometriosis above)

Adenomyosis
- *Etiology*
  - Unknown
  - Endometrium (instead of being completely shed) invades the myometrium (like endometriosis of the uterus)
  - Women > 30 years old with children
  - C-section increases risk
- *H & P*
  - Menorrhagia (heavy periods)
  - Dysmenorrhea (painful periods)
  - Dyspareunia (painful intercourse)
  - Pelvic may be normal or mildly enlarged uterus without mass
- *Labs & diagnostics*
  - Transvaginal US
  - MRI (not typically done)
- *Formulating Most Likely Diagnosis*
  - Consider this in women with the above who have normal laparoscopy (or just do not think about it at all, it is not a Family Practice topic!)
- *Clinical Intervention*
  - Send to OB/GYN – most common treatment is Hysterectomy

Disorders of the Ovary

Ovarian Cysts
- *H & P*
  - Painless (may be incidental finding on ultrasound without pain)
  - Unilateral pain (more typically presents with either RLQ or LLQ pain)
- *Labs & diagnostics*
  - US (abdominal and transvaginal ultrasound with doppler)
- *Formulating Most Likely Diagnosis*
  - Clear fluid-filled cyst on ultrasound at mid-cycle or in luteal phase
- *Clinical Intervention*
  - Usually none needed except pain relief
  - Unless > 5 cm. or in a menopausal woman, then referral to r/o cancer

- *Therapeutics*
  - Birth control pills may inhibit ovulation and reduce risk
- *Health Maintenance*
  - if > 5 cm or in a menopausal woman, should be referred

Types of Ovarian Cysts

- **Functional Cysts**
  - Normal, occur each month
  - Usually not painful
  - Incidental finding
  - No intervention
- **Corpus Luteum Cysts**
  - Normal in second half of cycle (luteal phase)
  - Produce progesterone
  - If pregnant, persist through first trimester
  - Incidental finding
    - Occasionally bleed and cause pain
  - Diagnose with US; no intervention
- **Dermoids cysts**
  - Germ cell tumors
  - 15% malignant
  - Composed of teeth and hair
  - Painless, incidental finding
    - Most common cause of torsion (heavy and twist easily)
  - US shows "calcifications" and mixed echogenic mass on ovary
  - Elective referral to GYN surgery for removal
- **Endometriomas**
  - Palpable; nontender
  - US shows solid mass
  - Always associated with endometriosis

Polcystic Ovarian Syndrome

- *Epidemiology*
  - Most common endocrinopathy in women
  - 5-10% of women 23-45 y.o.
  - Genetic predisposition
- *H & P*
  - Oligomenorrhea/amenorrhea
  - Infertility
  - Hirsutism/acne
  - Insulin resistance
  - Obesity
  - Enlarged ovaries
- *Labs & Diagnostics*
  - LH/FSH
  - Increased ratio, 3:1
  - Testosterone and DHEA levels
  - Insulin resistance panels

- US shows "string of pearls" (multiple tiny follicles)

- *Clinical Intervention*
  - GYN/endocrine
- *Treatment*
  - Birth control pills
  - Spironolactone
    - Decreases conversion of androstenedione to testosterone in peripheral tissues
  - Metformin
- *Health Maintenance*
  - Diet and exercise

PELVIC FLOOR PROBLEMS (PUBOPCOCCYGEAL MUSCLE ATROPHY)

Pelvic floor relaxation can result in any of the following:

Cystocele – Prolapse of the bladder
Rectocele – Prolapse of the rectum
Uterine Prolapse – Prolapse of the uterus

- *Etiology*
  - Poor pubococcygeal muscle tone due to aging, pregnancy
- *H & P*
  - Pelvic exam reveals prolapsing bladder, rectum or uterus (see below and illustration)
- *Clinical Intervention*
  - Pessary
  - Surgery
- *Health Maintenance*
  - Kegel exercises to contract pubococcygeal muscles may help

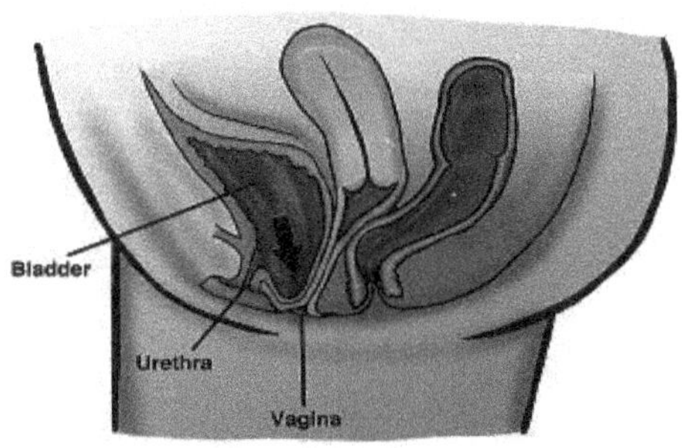

Infectious diseases

For specific information on the infectious diseases, see ID Chapter 22

Cervicitis

- *Etiology*
    - iInfection
    - Trauma
    - Inflammation (soaps, douches, etc)
- *H & P*
    - Friable cervix with or without discharge on speculum exam
- *Labs & diagnostics*
    - Wet prep - for WBC's, trichomonas
    - KOH – for candida yeast infection
    - Cultures
        - Culture specific for GC/Chlamydia
        - *Vaginal cultures for other pathogens (staph, strep B, etc)*
- *Formulating Most Likely Diagnosis*
    - WBC's on wet prep with friable cervicitis
- *Clinical Intervention*
    - If positive for bacterial infection = treat appropriately
    - If inflammatory, avoid irritants
    - If trauma, observation

Vaginitis

- *Etiology*
    - Candidiasis
    - Bacterial vaginosis (BV)
- *H & P*
    - Pelvic exam reveals vaginal discharge (look for itching (yeast) or odor (BV), itching (trichomoniasis/yeast)
- *Labs & diagnostics*
    - Wet prep – for trichomonas, WBC's
    - KOH – for candida yeast
- *Formulating Most Likely Diagnosis*
    - Use info in stem from H & P and results of wet prep/KOH
- *Therapeutics*
    - Directed at type of infection, i.e. bacterial vs. fungal
        - <u>Trich –</u> Treat with metronidazole 2 mg. PO
        - <u>BV –</u> Treat with oral or vaginal metronidazole (oral is 250 mg. TID for 7 days; vaginal is one applicatorful BID x 7 days)
        - <u>Candida –</u> Miconazole or terconazole cream (one app x 7 days, or short course 3 days) or diflucanazole 150 mg. PO x 1

Pelvic Inflammatory Disease

- ***Description***
  - An infection of the pelvis
  - Different from endometritis which is confined to the endometrium, PID is a peritoneal infection
- *Etiologies:*
  - #1 Gonorrhea
  - #2 Chlamydia
  - #3 anaerobes, Bacterial Vaginosis, E. Coli
- *Risk Factors*
  - Multiple sex partners
  - Recent instrumentation (endo biopsy, hysteroscopy, etc)
  - IUD
  - Previous PID
- *H & P*
  - Fever with pelvic pain
  - +/- discharge
  - Rebound tenderness
  - Cervical motion tenderness
  - +/- adnexal mass and tenderness
  - Dyspareunia (painful intercourse)
- *Therapeutics*
  - Rocephin 250 mg, IM plus Doxycycline 100 mg BID x 14 days
- *If severe infection, or failed OP therapy & nonpregnant:*
  - Cefotetan 2 gm. IV BID or Cefoxitin 2 gm IV QID PLUS Doxy 100 BID x 14 days
- *If pregnant*
  - Hospitalize, IV gentamycin & clindamycin

Metritis (Is this endometritis? I will assume so)

- *Etiology*
  - Infection, typically within the first week after delivering a baby
- *H & P*
  - Fever, pain on palpation of uterus
- *Labs & diagnostics*
  - CBC
  - Cultures of vaginal discharge, if present
- *Therapeutics*
  - Antibiotics to include gram negative coverage + metronidazole

INFERTILITY

- One year of unprotected intercourse with successful conception
- Order noninvasive testing first, i.e. semen analysis and basal body temperatures before any invasive testing, i.e. hysterosalpingogram.
- Patients with PCOS, other complicated infertility issues should be referred.

CONTRACEPTIVE METHODS

Natural Family Planning

- Regular menses is necessary
  - Failure rate with perfect use – 1-3%
  - Failure rate with typical use 20-40%

Barrier Methods

- Contraindications
  - Latex allergy, for cervical cap – history of dysplasia
- Male condom – 4-12%
- Diaphragm – 4-20%
- Cervical cap – 10-20%

IUD

- Paragard =0.6%
- Mirena (progesterone) = 1.5%
- Best users
  - Monogamous, have children
- *Contraindications*
  - Current infection
  - Pregnancy
  - Uterine anomaly

Oral Contraceptive Pills--Ortho-Evra--Nuvaring

- Failure rate – 3%
- *Contraindications*
  - DVT/PE, CVA, CAD, Afib
  - DM>20 yrs
  - Breast cancer
  - Pregnancy
  - Lactation <6 wks
  - Liver disease
  - Immobilization
  - Smoking >35
  - Uncontrolled htn

Progesterone Only Contraception (inj/oral/cream)

- Failure rate = 7%
- *Contraindications*
  - DVT
  - DUB
  - Liver disease
  - Breast cancer

Depo-Provera

- *Contraindications* – same as all progesterone only products
    - IM injection q. 3 months
- SE's
    - Weight gain
    - Irregular bleeding
    - Depression

Bilateral Tubal Ligation and Vasectomy

- Failure rate – 0.4-1.8%
- ***Not a reversible method***
- BTL
    - If pregnant – high incidence of ectopic pregnancies
    - Risk of anesthesia/bowel perforation with BTL

A 17-year-old patient requests birth control; she has a single sexual partner, this is her third in the past year. She is healthy with no chronic medical problems.

Which of the following is the most appropriate therapeutic intervention for this patient?

A. Oral contraceptive pills
B. Diaphragm
C. Condoms
D. Mirena IUD
E. Oral contraceptive pills plus condoms

Answer: E.

Discussion: OCP plus condom is the best idea for this 17 year old. Remember to review all five choices to make sure that there is not a better answer below. Having a 16-year-old use a condom to protect her is a better choice.

A 32-year-old patient requests birth control. She has three children; is divorced. She is a one ppd smoker. She does not think she wants more children, but is not ready for permanent sterilization.

Which of the following is the most appropriate therapeutic intervention for this patient?

A. Oral contraceptive pills
B. BTL/vasectomy
C. Condoms
D. Mirena IUD
E. Oral contraceptive pills plus condoms

Answer: D.

***Discussion*:** Mirena IUD is a good option for this patient; she is a smoker, so avoid estrogen. Condoms are good, but not as good as Mirena. Mirena is obviously reversible with removal.

A 42-year-old female presents for permanent sterilization. She is diabetic and a smoker. She has had one myocardial infarction. She has mild renal insufficiency.

What is the most appropriate clinical intervention for this patient?

A. Oral contraceptive pills
B. Bilateral tubal ligation
C. Vasectomy for her partner
D. Mirena IUD
E. Oral contraceptive pills plus condoms

Answer: C.

***Discussion*:** She is a surgical risk; she should certainly not take ocp's; Mirena is an option, but for permanent sterilization, the best option is vasectomy for her husband. Local anesthesia; no risk of bowel perforation.

PEARL: The only antibiotic felt to truly decrease the efficacy of the pill is rifampin. Good to know!

Menopause

Longterm sequelae of lack of estrogen

- Osteoporosis
- Vaginal atrophy/bladder sxs

Management

- Estrogen only – if no uterus
- Both estrogen *and* progesterone – if uterus

Benefits of HRT

- Osteoporosis prevention/reduction in hip fracture risk
- Lipid improvement
- Reduces risk of colon cancer

Osteoporosis

- *Epidemiology*
    - Most common metabolic bone disease in US
- *H & P*

  - Asymptomatic (may have pain with compression fracture of the vertebra column)
- *Labs & Diagnostics*
  - S. PTH, S. Ca, S. Ph, Alk p'tase are *normal*
  - Demineralization occurs in TRABECULAR bone:
    - Thoracic spine
    - Hip
    - Pelvis
    - Wrist
- *Risk Factors*
  - Age
  - Female gender
  - Caucasian
  - Small frame
  - Sedentary lifestyle
  - Low lifetime ca intake
  - Hyperthyroidism
  - Smoking
  - Caffeine intake
  - Heparin
  - Steroids
- *Diagnosis - Dexa (bone densitometry)*
  - T score of +1.0 to -1.0 normal
    - Density = 35 y.o. normal female
  - T score - 1.0 to -2.5
    - Osteopenia
    - If a fracture exists – moves to osteoporosis
  - T score < - 2.5
    - Osteoporosis
- *Therapeutics*
  - Calcium & Vitamin D
  - Weight-bearing exercise
  - Estrogen
  - Bisphosphonates
    - Alendronate (Fosamax) - GI SE's - weekly
    - Risedronate - lesser GI SE's - weekly
    - Ibandronate – once a month
  - SERMS (Evista)
    - Selective estrogen receptor modulators
    - Do not stimulate receptors of breast and uterus (safer)
    - Side effects usually preclude treatment

Breast Disorders

(in order of most common occurrence)

Fibrocystic Disease

- *Etiology*

-
    - Most common cause of lump #1
    - Estrogen dependent cyst formation
- *H & P*
    - Smooth, mobile, mass
- Labs & diagnostics:
    - US of breast
- Formulating Most Likely Diagnosis
    - Young patient with mobile, smooth slightly painful lump that recurs monthly
- Clinical Intervention
    - None or aspiration
- Health Maintenance
    - Reduce consumption of caffeine, teas, chocolate

Fibroadenoma

- *Etiology:* unknown
- *H & P*
    - palpable mass; mobile
- *Labs & diagnostics*
    - US shows solid; biopsy is definitive
- *Formulating Most Likely Diagnosis*
    - young patient painless mass; cancer unable to be ruled out without a biopsy
- *Clinical Intervention*
    - removal of fibroadenoma

Breast Cancer

- *Etiology*
    - adenocarcinoma (may be BRCA 1,2 positive or not)
- *H & P*
    - palpable mass, "fixed", nontender
- *Labs & diagnostics*
    - mammogram
    - US
    - biopsy (is definitive)
- *Formulating Most Likely Diagnosis*
    - mammography showing "spiculated lesion"
    - BIOPSY is definitive
- *Clinical Intervention*
    - chemo/rad/surgery

PEARL: peau d'orange (thickened, indurated, salmon colored skin) is a hallmark of ***inflammatory breast cancer*** (not in the blueprint, but should be) which is a lethal carcinoma; if the question says "peau d'orange" immediate referral to surgeon is indicated (you can treat for infection; but that is not the main issue here --- mortality is high!

Paget's Disease of the Breast – *Again, not in blueprint, but can't be missed*

- *Etiology*
    - Cancer of duct underneath nipple, causing just flaking of skin of areola
- *H & P*
    - Looks like eczema of nipple (very benign appearance)
    - Unilateral
- *Labs & Diagnostics*
    - Needs a breast biopsy
- *Clinical Intervention*
    - Could treat for one week with steroid cream if bilateral
    - ***But*** any "eczematous" change of the nipple that does completely cure, needs to be biopsied, so followup is the most important intervention

Mastitis

- *Etiology*
    - Infection of a portion of the breast
    - Due to staph aureus
- *H & P*
    - Pink, slightly warm, exquisitely tender quadrant of breast
    - If axillary node, then very tender axillary node
    - High fever, shaking chills, myalgias
- *Labs & Diagnostics*
    - None needed; treatment is empirical
- *Formulating Most Likely Diagnosis:*
    - In breastfeeding mom = nipple irritation, use emollients and treat for staph aureus (Dicloxacillin x 10 day)
    - In non-breastfeeding or menopausal woman = cancer; treat for staph aureus, and get mammogram after treatment
- *Complication*
    - Breast abscess
        - Fluctuant distinct mass
        - Will need I & D and follow up

NIPPLE DISCHARGE ***(only galactorrhea is in blueprint, but bloody discharge warrants a topic too)***

Galactorrhea

- *Etiologies*
    - Most typically due to pregnancy
    - Depo-Provera
    - Psychotherapeutic medications
    - Prolactinoma
    - Hypothyroidism

- *H & P*
  - LMP?
  - Pain?
  - Blood?
  - Mass?
- *Labs & Diagnostics*
  - SHCG
  - TSH
  - PRL (prolactin level);
  - Pap smear of fluid
  - +/- mammogram or ultrasound
- *Intervention depends on cause:*
  - If pregnant, no intervention
  - If hypothyroidism, treat thyroid
  - If elevated PRL, see endocrine section about prolactinomas
- *Scientific concept*
  - Usually the etiology of galactorrhea is benign

Bloody Nipple Discharge

- *Etiologies*
  - Most often a benign papilloma in the duct
  - Intraductal carcinoma
- *H & P*
  - Same as galactorrhea
- *Labs & Diagnostics*
  - Pap smear of fluid
  - Mammogram/US
- *Clinical Intervention*
  - GYN/surgical referral

Obstetrics

First Trimester Issues

ANTENATAL CARE GUIDELINES IN PREGNANCY

1st Visit Screening

- Screen for underyling diseases (hypertension, autoimmune disease, DM, etc.)
- Manage "already known" disease states in early pregnancy
- Prenatal vits (folate supplementation, 400 mg minimum, 1 gm is typical)

16-20 Weeks

- Fundal height checks begin; Quad screen-AFP, US

28 Weeks

- One hour glucose; H & H
    - 140mg/dL or higher on one hour glucose = order 3 hour glucose tolerance test (GTT)

34-36 Weeks

- Strep Group B screen from rectum and vagina

SPONTANEOUS ABORTION

Definitions of spontaneous abortion:

Threatened Ab

- Bleeding or cramping with closed cx

Inevitable Ab

- Bleeding or cramping with dilatation of cx

Complete Ab

- All products have been expelled

Incomplete Ab (missed)

- Products of conception (POC) remain in uterus

Anembryonic pg

- Blighted ovum (no embryo ever develops)
- Usually discovered in first trimester; inevitable that abortion follows.
- Can wait for "natural" abortion or D & C

Habitual abortion

- Three or more Ab's in succession
    - Think (lupus) SLE, thyroid, eating disorder

Spontaneous Abortion

- *Etiology/Epidemiology*
    - 20% of pregnancies terminate in abortion
    - Majority occur prior to 8 weeks
    - 60% result from major chromosomal abnormalities
- *H&P*
    - Pelvic is usually normal (uterus may feel small for dates)
    - Bleeding is typical, but not absolute
    - May have pelvic cramping
    - No fetal heart tones will be heard on Doppler or seen on US.
    - Sometimes no embryo at all (anembryonic pregnancy)
    - No fever, no focal left or R sided pain
- *Diagnostics*
    - HCG may be needed; may need to be "serial"
    - HCG should double within 48-72 hours if viable pregnancy

    - Ultrasound is done to confirm demise or anembryonic pregnancy
- *Scientific Concepts*
    - Most spontaneous abortions occur very early in pregnancy
    - Having a single (or two) SAb's does NOT increase your risk for a third (it's just bad luck)
    - ***However,*** having three in a row constitutes "habitual abortion", and may indicate maternal problem or chromosomal abnormalities.
    - ***Remember to give Rhogam to all Rh neg moms within 72 hours of Ab of any type***

Ectopic Pregnancy

- *Etiology*
    - Risk factors
        - Previous ectopic
        - H/o tubal ligation
        - IUD
        - H/o PID
        - Tubal surgery
        - Infertility
- *H & P*
    - Sudden onset unilateral pelvic pain
    - Vaginal spotting in a patient who is 4-8 weeks pregnant
- *Labs & Diagnostics*
    - Quantitative HCG
    - OB Rh
    - *Ultrasound with no evidence of IUP (intrauterine pregnancy)*
- *Formulating the Most Likely Diagnosis*
    - Have a high index of suspicion in any pregnant patient with pelvic pain
- *Clinical Intervention*
    - Referral to GYN for either medical or surgical management
    - Surgical emergency
- *Therapeutics*
    - Methotrexate is often used to abort the pregnancy from the tube in an early ectopic (if early in gestation, if no significant pain)
    - Requires patient who will be compliant with follow up
- *Scientific Concepts*
    - More than 90% of ectopics occur in the distal end of the Fallopian tube
    - Rhogam for Rh negative patients

Rh Incompatibility

- *Etiology*
    - RBC's either have or do not have D antigen
        - If Rh positive, patient has Rh D
        - If Rh negative, patient has no Rh D.
- *Labs & Diagnostics*
    - OB-Rh and antibody screen
- *Clinical Intervention*

    - If Rh negative mother, and ANY concern for bleeding (where fetal RBC's with antigen D may have crossed placenta); give Rhogam
- *Therapeutics*
    - Rhogam (Immunoglobulin that will bind any fetal D antigen on RBC's that may have gotten into mom's blood stream)
- *Health Maintenance*
    - Prophylactic Rhogam in all Rh negative mothers at 28 weeks, and up to 72 hours post-Ab or significant uterine bleeding of any type
    - And again at birth if baby is Rh positive
- *Scientific Concepts*
    - Not a concern for the fetus of a first pregnancy
    - If the fetus is RhD positive, it is *after* birth that mom will be sensitized, and will now have antibodies to D.
    - When she is pregnant with her second fetus (if it has RhD)
        - The antibodies in mom's blood stream will attack the fetus' RBC's and cause profound anemia and hydrops fetalis.

Gestational Trophoblastic Disease (Hydatidiform Mole)

- *Etiology*
    - Abnormality of fertilization
- *H & P*
    - Hyperemesis gravidarum (excessive vomiting)
    - Large for dates uterus
    - Vaginal spotting
- *Labs & Diagnostics*
    - HCG is higher than expected
    - US reveals hydropic tissue ("grape clusters" with or without fetus)
- *Formulating the Most Likely Diagnosis*
    - Differential includes twins or triplets
    - *US makes the diagnosis*
- *Clinical Intervention*
    - D & C must be done; tissue sent to lab for evaluation for invasive mole
- *Therapeutics*
    - Usually none except reliable birth control for a full 12 months
- *Health Maintenance*
    - A full year without pregnancy so that we can be sure there is no trophoblastic tissue growing in lungs
- *Scientific Concepts*
    - Trophoblastic tissue in a molar pregnancy can "metastasize" if it invades the uterus and uterine artery and gets to lungs.
    - To make sure this is not happening, we must check a pregnancy test every week until 0, and then monthly to make sure it stays at 0.
    - That is why the patient cannot get pregnancy again for a year.

Second Trimester Issues

Gestational Diabetes

- ***Definition***
  - Abnormal glucose tolerance in pregnancy
  - 50% of women with GDM will develop overt diabetes at later date
- *H&P*
  - Asymptomatic
- *Labs & Diagnostics*
  - 24-28 weeks of gestation
    - One hour GTT (50 gm. load)
    - If result is ≥ 140, then
  - Three hour GTT (100 gm. load)
    - Two levels elevated = GDM
    - Either two of the 1 hr; 2 hr; or 3 hr.
  - *If FBS is elevated – no glucose is given, GDM diagnosis is made*
- *Clinical Intervention*
  - Formal dietary counseling
  - Diabetic exchange diet
  - Blood glucose monitoring
    - Fasting and one hour after each meal
- *Therapeutics*
  - Insulin for persistent elevated FBS (mainstay for years)
  - Glyburide and metformin have been used recently with few fetal issues

    No well controlled studies; so I will not use it on exam yet
- *Health Maintenance*
  - Careful glucose control has been proven to decrease risk of:
    - Shoulder dystocia
    - Macrosomia
    - Preeclampsia
  - 6 12 weeks postpartum mom should have a 2-hr. GTT with 75 g. glucose load

HELLP Syndrome *(see preeclampsia in third trimester section below)*

- *Etiology* - unknown
- *Epidemiology*
  - An early and severe form of preeclampsia
  - Occurs in about 10% of patients with preeclampsia
  - Develops early in gestation, putting fetus at risk
- *H & P*
  - High BP (> 30 mm Hg above baseline SBP;or > 20 mm above baseline DBP)

    - If baseline 100/60; then 130/xx would constitute elevated BP!)
  - Most important clue: *hyperreflexia with clonus*!
  - Can have blurry vision/ r/o papilledema
  - Can have RUQ discomfort
- *Labs & Diagnostics*
  - To r/o preeclampsia, perform all of the following:
  - H = hemolytic anemia (get CBC)
  - E L= elevated L = liver enzymes (AST/ALT)
  - L P = low platelets (on CBC)
  - Urine – for protein (2+ or greater is too high)
- *Formulating the Most Likely Diagnosis*
  - Have a high index of suspicion in any pregnant or postpartum woman on the test that presents with elevated BP.
- *Therapeutics*
  - Magnesium sulfate 2 – 4 gm. IM or IV; may need a drip
  - Methyl Dopa (Aldomet), Hydralazine and Beta Blockers are most commonly used for BP (explanded info on therapeutics below)
- *Clinical Intervention*
  - ADMIT
  - DELIVER

Incompetent Cervix

- *Etiology*
  - Mostly unknown;
  - ***But*** consider in patient who has had multiple LEEP procedures for cervical dysplasia
- *H & P*
  - Effacement (thinning) of the cervix in the second trimester
- *Labs & Diagnostics*
  - Transvaginal US to measure cervical thickness (>2.5 cm length is good!)
  - Fetal fibrinectin
    - Swab of the cervix; fetal fibrinectin is secreted just prior to delivery or effacement
    - If positive, does not tell you when
    - ***But*** if negative, fairly good predictor of no delivery in next week
- *Formulating the Most Likely Diagnosis*
  - May be very vague symptoms so look for clue that there was a preterm delivery with last infant
  - Even mild vague symptoms warrant an US to check cervical length.
- *Clinical Intervention*
  - Bed rest
  - Cervical cerclage (stitch through cervix to prevent it from opening)
- *Therapeutics*
  - If delivery is imminent, give dexamethasone to hasten fetus' lung maturity.
- *Health Maintenance*
  - Regular pap smear screening to prevent cervical dysplasia treatments
  - Vaccine for HPV

Premature Rupture of Membranes (PROM)

- *Etiology*
  - Can be idiopathic
  - Can be from too much fluid (polyhdramnios)
  - Can be due to intrauterine infection
- *H & P*
  - Patient feels a "gush of fluid" which may, or may not be amniotic fluid.
- *Labs & Diagnostics*
  - Sterile speculum exam (no fingers in the vagina)
  - Check for "pooling" – fluid that pools in the posterior fornix
  - Check pH – alkaline with amniotic fluid, but also with urine and semen
  - Slide of fluid for "ferning" – a fern-like frond pattern on a slide that air dries with amniotic fluid – confirmatory
  - *Ultrasound to quantify fluid in uterus*
- *Formulating the Most Likely Diagnosis*
  - May be urine or semen – so check for ferning
- *Clinical Intervention*
  - If PROM – (premature) – referral to OB – usually admission since many deliver in the next couple of hours.
  - Steroids (dexamethasone) are used to help with fetal lung maturity.
  - Magnesium sulfate sometimes used to stop contractions.
    - Smooth muscle relaxation

Third Trimester Issues

Hypertension Disorders in Pregnancy *(this is the blueprint topic)*

PEARL: There are many ways in which hypertension (HTN) may manifest in pregnancy.

- First, the patient may have essential hypertension or secondary hypertension prior to becoming pregnant. This will be a concern for the fetus if not controlled adequately.

- Second, hypertension may be provoked by the pregnancy due to multiple known and unknown issues. Below you will see discussion of hypertension in pregnancy that will include all three known causes including PIH; pre-eclampia/eclampsia and HELLP syndrome.

- In all instances where there is increased blood pressure, there is systemic vascular resistance to blood flow. The placenta is a peripheral organ and will receive less blood flow with higher SBP levels. This will reduce the amount of nutrients, but more importantly, oxygen, to the fetus resulting in hypoxia, growth restriction, and could result in death.

Hypertension is defined differently in pregnancy, because peripheral resistance is usually lower in the pregnant state than in the non-pregnant state. Therefore, SBP and DBP are lower in pregnancy. There is normally a physiologic drop in BP to 28 weeks, with a return to pre-pregnancy BP levels starting at 28 weeks and to term.

<u>Hypertension variously defined as:</u>

- BP>140/90 on two occasions, six hours apart
- Rise in 30 mmHg systolic or 15 mmHg diastolic from 1st trimester values

<u>All patients with any of the hypertensive problems described below are at increased risk for:</u>

- Poor fetal growth (IUGR)
- Fetal prematurity/loss
- Placental abruption
- Pre-eclampsia/eclampsia

PIH (Pregnancy induced hypertension) now called Gestational Hypertension

- ***Definition***
    - BP elevation that occurs transiently in the latter half of pregnancy and resolves with delivery
        - *Must* occur > 20 weeks gestation
        - *Must* r/o pre-eclampsia
- *Labs & Diagnostics*
    - CBC (decreased platelet count)
    - Electrolytes (Na, K)
    - BUN/Creatinine (should be VERY low in normal pg)
    - LFT (transaminases should be normal)
    - U/A dip for protein (trace to 1+ is acceptable)
    - If U/A dip is > 1+ get 24 hour urine to quantitate protein
    - Uric acid (should be low)
- *Clinical Intervention/Therapeutics*
    - <u>Do Not</u> treat with:
        - ACEI/ARB's
        - Diuretics
    - Treat with:
        - **Methyldopa (Aldomet)**
        - **Labetalol (no IUGR)**
        - Nifedipine (can cause reflex tachycardia)
        - Hydralazine (many side effects)

Preeclampsia/Eclampsia

- ***Definition***
    - Preeclampsia is hypertension with proteinuria (>300mg/24 hrs or >3+ on dipstick on two samples >4 hours apart)
    - Any elevation in blood pressure during pregnancy should be evaluated carefully for pre-eclampsia
- *Epidemiology*
    - Occurs in 5% of *all* pregnancies
    - Occurs in 10% of nulliparous women
    - Occurs in 20-25% of patient who have chronic hypertension
- *Etiology*
    - Primary disorder of placental function resulting in:
    - Endothelial damage

  - Vasospasm
  - Placental insufficiency
  - Affects *all* maternal organs
  - Affects fetus secondary to decreased placental flow
  - Preeclampsia is categorized as mild or severe
- *Management of preeclampsia consists of careful maternal and fetal observation*
  - Mild pre-eclamptics are usually delivered at term.
  - Severe pre-eclamptics are usually delivered as soon as the diagnosis is made.
- *Severe pre-eclampsia definition:*
  - BP>160 /or 110
  - Proteinuria>5 grams/d (found on 24 urine collection)
  - Recall that 4+ is greater than 3000 mg/day
  - Elevated S. creatinine
  - Hyperreflexia (DTR's 4/4 with clonus)
  - Pulmonary edema
  - Oliguria (<500cc/24 hours)
  - IUGR
- *Acute treatment of severe preeclampsia*
  - **<u>Labetalol</u>**
    - **Drug of choice!**
    - **Selective alpha blocker & nonselective beta blocker**
    - **Vasodilatation with decrease in systemic vascular resistance**
    - **20 mg IV with repeat every 10 minutes up to 300 mg total**
    - **Slows HR, reduces myocardial oxygen consumption**
  - <u>Nifedipine</u>
    - Relaxes smooth muscle
    - *Should not be used with magnesium though*
  - <u>Hydralazine</u>
    - used to be the drug of choice
    - can cause maternal hypotension, detrimental to fetus
    - worse outcomes than labetalol and nifedipine
  - <u>Sodium Nitroprusside</u>
    - Significant and rapid vasodilation
    - Severe rebound hypertension can occur
    - Cyanide poisoning can occur
    - Only as last resort
- ***ECLAMPSIA – seizure occurring in the setting of pre-eclampsia***
  - <u>Seizure Prophylaxis</u>
    - Patients in labor and for 24 hours post partum are usually treated with Magnesium Sulfate, 4 grams IV loading dose
- *Scientific Concept*
  - Management of the BP does not alter the progression of preeclampsia
  - Management of the BP reduces incidence of cerebrovascular problems
  - Eclampsia can occur in the post-partum period
  - Delivery is still the answer!

Fetal Distress

- *Etiology*
    - Multiple:
        - Chromosomal disorders
        - Hypertension causing intrauterine growth restriction (IUGR)
        - Anything else causing IUGR
        - Gestational diabetes mellitus (GDM)
        - Maternal medical issues
        - Placental dysfunction

- *H & P*
    - Small for dates on fundus measurement
    - Decreased fetal movements reported by mom
- *Labs & Diagnostics*
    - Ultrasound
    - Fetal nonstress test
- *Clinical Intervention*
    - Prepare for delivery
    - Or if fetus in severe distress - DELIVER!
- *Health Maintenance*
    - Fetal kick counts should be measured in the third trimester by any mom at risk for fetal distress
- Scientific Concepts
    - When a fetus is "distressed" it will conserve energy and stop "breathing" and decrease its energy output (stop kicking)

Placenta Previa

- *Etiology*
    - Embryo implants in lower uterine segment and placenta grows across cervical opening to vagina
- *H & P*
    - Vaginal bleeding; painless
- *Labs & Diagnostics*
    - Ultrasound STAT
- *Formulating the Most Likely Diagnosis*
    - Always the most important cause of painless third trimester bleeding
- *Clinical Intervention*
    - No digital exam of cervix!
- *Health Maintenance:*
    - Should be identified on screening US at 20 weeks and prepared for with serial US to make sure it moves away from the cervix prior to active labor
- *Scientific Concepts*
    - If identified on very early US, likely that the placenta will "move" out of the way as the uterine neck elongates

Abruptio Placentae

- *Etiology*
    - Cocaine use
    - Poorly controlled hypertension
    - Bad luck
- *H & P*
    - Severe pain in uterus
    - Sudden onset painful vaginal bleeding (although can be occult with no blood, only pain)
- *Labs & Diagnostics*
    - Ultrasound STAT
- *Formulating the Most Likely Diagnosis*
    - Many benign causes of pain
    - But this severity, with any vaginal bleeding precludes any benign cause
- *Clinical Intervention*
    - Admission
    - High risk OB
    - Anticipate delivery
    - Manage as for any bleeding re: RH negative
- *Health Maintenance*
    - Drug history
    - Manage HTN

Postpartum Hemorrhage

- *Etiology*
    - Uterine atony
    - Retained placenta
    - Genital tract trauma (cervical or vaginal laceration)
    - Coagulopathy
- *H & P*
    - Uterine atony – no contraction, uterus "boggy"
    - Retained placent – no placenta passed, or only a portion
        - Look for bleeding site
    - Tachycardia; hypotension
    - Altered level of consciousness is bad sign.
- *Labs & Diagnostics*
    - Type and cross match
    - H & H (remember may not reflect blood lost rapidly)
- *Clinical Intervention – simultaneous:*
    - Correct reason for blood loss
        - Treat shock (replace fluids, blood when available)
    - Therapeutics
        - <u>Uterine Atony</u>
            - Oxytocin
            - Misoprostol (prostaglandin)
        - <u>Retained tissue</u>
            - manual exploration and removal
        - <u>Genital tract trauma</u>

                - Ssture bleeder
            - *Coagulopathy*
                - Fresh Frozen Plasma
- *Scientific Concepts*
    - Complication
        - *Sheehan's syndrome (pituitary hemorrhage causing hypopituitarism; can also cause adrenal hemorrhage causing acute adrenal crisis)*

Dystocia

- *Etiology*
    - Gestational diabetes (GDM) causing "large for dates" baby – shoulders get "stuck"
- *H & P*
    - Uterus is "large for dates"
- *Labs & Diagnostics*
    - Ultrasound to estimate fetal size
- *Clinical Intervention*
    - High risk OB to deliver (should already be there if known GDM)
- *Health Maintenance*
    - Good management of sugars

CHAPTER 16

Eye, Ear, Nose & Throat - 9%

Introduction to EENT

In the "old days", the eye was a separate section on the PANCE/PANRE and was 3%. ENT was covered separately as 6% of total questions.
Since the last update of the Blueprint, the two areas are now combined to be 9% of the total questions on your test.

My experience with reviewing the scores of my students and attendees at the review course is that EENT is notoriously a poor performance topic. I have come to understand that it is not because it is difficult information. There are few therapeutics to memorize, and these are disorders that are seen frequently in Family Medicine. In talking to attendees, it seems that this is a topic area that is felt by most of us to be "easy", and therefore we do not study it. Instead, we focus on topic areas like acid-base and coagulopathies that will represent only one or two questions on the entire test.

My advice to you is to study this section! It is weighted almost as heavily as all of GI; all of ortho *plus* rheum, and more than Women's Health. And, it is easier! So spend a little time on EENT, and score well and improve your score in general (remember, all you need is one question more than the cut-off to pass the test!)

The Eye

Eye Anatomy/Physiology Review

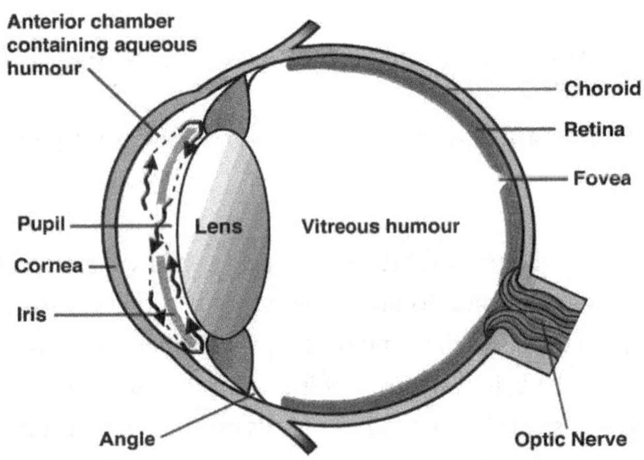

The cornea sits on top of the eye and there are many nerve endings; so corneal abrasions and corneal injuries hurt!

The iris sits in the anterior chamber, behind the cornea, and in front of the lens. It opens and closes like a camera aperture to let in light or decrease light, i.e. opens and closes the pupil.

Therefore, if the patient has iritis (used interchangeably often with the term uveitis), tetracaine for pain is not going to work for photophobia (it is a topical anesthetic and sits on top of the cornea; it is movement of the iris that hurts, so will not work for iritis pain/photophobia).

As the pupil opens, the iris becomes thicker (like an accordion that you squeeze) and "folds up" in the angle.

This angle is a tiny little opening covered with the trabecular meshwork which allows free flow of fluid around and around and around the anterior chamber.

The anterior chamber is filled with aqueous humour, thin and watery, and flows freely through the trabecular angle covered with the trabecular meshwork (there should be no cells in the anterior chamber, just fluid). This fluid needs to be able to drain and flow unimpeded.

Behind the anterior chamber, just behind the iris is the lens, suspended from ligaments that are connective tissue (recall, lens dislocation one of the "clues" that the patient may have Marfan's syndrome)

The lens is clear and the ligaments cause it to thin or thicken to focus on an object.

The older we get, the longer it takes for this to happen; so going from distance to reading takes minutes (or sometimes just does not happen anymore ☹).

The posterior chamber is filled with vitreous humour that is jelly-like – if you poke yourself in the eye with a stick, yellowish "jello" sticks out of the hole.

The older we get, the more "thin and watery" the vitreous becomes (much like our synovial fluid) --- this begins to happen at the ripe old age of 40 or so.

This watery change causes "floaters" – a few are always normal, they increase in number with age.

The retina is in the back of the eye; it receives light and sends the signals to the brain.

There are rods and cones: rods are all over the place and sense all vision; cones are concentrated in the macula and mainly produce color vision.

The cup and disk are slightly off center on the retina; there should be a 2:1 cup-to-disk ratio; and there should be crisp vessels coming out of it.

The macula sits in the direct center and provides central vision. *Remember* - it gets its arterial blood supply from other than the central retinal artery (so if central retinal artery occlusion, the entire retina is white except for the macula, causing a "cherry red spot or cherry red fovea") - I have no idea why there are always two or three names for the same thing...annoying.

PEARL: *VISUAL ACUITY* *must be obtained first* in the clinical intervention of any eye complaint. The only exception to this rule is the patient with liquid splashed in eye; then *first* wash the eye for at least 30 minutes before doing anything else (including visual acuity). Start with the eye chart, if the patient cannot distinguish any letters, then do fingers, if unable to see fingers, then document any light perception.

<u>Visual acuity evaluation is the only way to:</u>
1) Know how much vision was lost before you even got a chance to intervene.
2) Establish a baseline for the ophthalmologist in to use in a follow up visit.

BENIGN DISORDERS- NO VISUAL CHANGES

Blepharitis

- *H & P*
  - "Dandruff" of the eyelids
  - No or minimal conjunctival injection
- *Treatment –*
  - Sulfa shampoo (selsun blue)

Allergic Conjunctivitis (not infectious, so it belongs here)

- **Seasonal, contact (i.e, new cat)**
- *H&P*
  - Itching
  - Red conjunctiva
  - Normal visual acuity
  - Pale (bluish) palpebral fissures
- *Treatment*
  - Antihistamines
- *Clinical intervention*
  - Do not use antibiotics (they would not work anyway).

Hordeolum (Stye)

- *H & P*
  - Acute red "pimple" on inside or edge of eyelid – painful
- *Treatment*
  - Warm compresses
- *Clinical Intervention*
  - No need for antibiotics

Chalazion

- *Etiology*
  - Chronic "pimple" on inside or edge of eyelid – painless
- *H & P*
  - Not red, not warm
- *Clinical Intervention*
  - Warm compresses
  - If cosmetically unpleasant, or if irritating – refer to optho to remove
- *Scientific Concept*
  - <u>Do not</u> cut into the lid margin– this can cause permanent problem with closure.

CORNEAL ABNORMALITIES

Foreign Body (FB)

- *H&P*
  - History of foreign body
  - Most common in welders, wood workers, occupational involvement with grinding or sawing
  - Red eye, usually, with tearing
  - Can occur anywhere (under lid, on sclera) but most painful on cornea
  - Visual acuity normal unless central large FB
  - Stain with fluorescein after applying tetracaine (or anything-caine) for comfort
  - Look with slit lamp --- sometimes visible to the naked eye
  - Look for vertical "stripes" on the cornea, suggesting a FB under the upper eye lid

- *Clinical Intervention*
  - remove foreign body with eye spud, Q-tip
  - If metal, a rust ring forms within hours and will need to be drilled out.
  - If exam choices do not include drilling, then refer to ophtho for drilling- same day or next day at latest.
  - If central foreign body with significant defect – refer.

- *Treatment*
  - Antibiotics
    - Gentamycin drops
    - Erythromycin ointment
    - Tobramycin ointment
- *Health Maintenance*
  - Always have patient f/u with optho within 48 hours for recheck.

Corneal Abrasion

- *Etiology*
  - Most typical in contact lens wearers
  - Can happen from foreign body under lid, a "poke in the eye", or anything else that scratches the cornea
- *H & P*
  - Sudden onset of pain, redness and tearing
  - Normal visual acuity
  - Tetracaine and fluorescein
- *Clinical Intervention*
  - Slit lamp exam – look for uptake of stain
  - Treat with antibiotics
- *Therapeutics*
  - Gentamycin ophth. drops or ointment
  - sulfacetamide drops
  - Avoid ciprofloxacin ophth. drops so it can be used for corneal ulcer if needed.
- *Health Maintenance*
  - recheck in 48 hours – either you or ophthalmologist
- *Scientific Concept*
  - No pressure patches – may increase risk of infection.
  - No contact lenses until recheck shows complete healing.
  - most common complication --- corneal ulcer – in contact lens wearers

Corneal Ulcer

- *Etiology/Epidemiology*
  - Complication of corneal abrasion
  - Most common in contact lens wearers
  - Can cause permanent vision loss
- *H & P*
  - Persistent pain after 48 hours of treatment must be re-evaluated.
  - Slit lamp exam shows continued stain with fluorescein.
- *Treatment*

- Quinolone (cipro) eye drop (Ciloxan, Ocuflox, etc)
- *Clinical Intervention*
  - This must be seen by Optho!

INFECTIOUS DISORDERS

These are listed from least serious to life threatening; and can be a continuum, i.e. if bacterial conjunctivitis is not treated, may result in preseptal cellulitis and then orbital cellulitis

Viral Conjunctivitis

- *H&P*
  - Associated with upper respiratory disorder
  - Conjunctival injection with clear watery discharge
  - Usually bilateral
  - Visual acuity is normal.
- *Treatment*
  - None!
  - In our country, it has to be treated for the child to go back to day care, but it does not do anything; child is still contagious.

Bacterial Conjunctivitis

- *H&P*
  - Crusting of lashes
  - Purulent d/c from eyes
- *Treatment*
  - Antibacterial eyedrops
    - Sodium sulamyd (sulfa-based, watch for allergies)
    - Gentamycin
    - Tobramycin

Preseptal cellulitis

Eyelid infection

- *H&P*
  - Pink tender swelling of lid
  - Rye itself is fine – no conjunctival injection
  - Normal EOM's, normal PERRLA
  - Normal visual acuity
- *Treatment*
  - Cover for staph aureus
    - Dicloxacillin, Cephalexin

Orbital cellulitis

Infection of the orbit

- *H&P*
  - Decreased visual acuity
  - Pain with EOM's, may have abnormal EOM
  - Fever, malaise, "toxic" appearing patient

- *Scientific Concept*
  - Can cause infection which extends into the brain
- *Clinical Intervention*
  - Hospitalize
  - IV antibiotics
    - Broad spectrum to cover typical pathogens of head and neck infections
      - Strep *pneumoniae* (strep pneumo)
      - Hemophilus *influenza* (H. flu)
      - Moraxella *catarrhalis* (M. Cat)

CHRONIC LOSS OF VISION

Cataract

- *Epidemiology*
  - Very common as aging occurs
- *Risk Factors*
  - Congenital cataract is due to CMV infection and rubella
  - Cataract in adults is due to DM, corticosteroids, smoking, sun exposure
- *H & P*
  - Opacification of the lens
  - Painless
  - Slow, insidious blurring of vision
  - Glare in bright lights
  - Loss of red reflex
- *Clinical Intervention*
  - Refer for surgical replacement of the lens when poor vision interferes with activity
  - es of daily living.
  - OP surgery; topical anesthetic
    - Tiny, sutureless incision; few complications
- *Health Maintenance*
  - Yearly exam (not preventable)
  - Sunglasses/sun protection

Chronic Open Angle Glaucoma

- *Etiology/Epidemiology*
  - Slow, insidioius, and preventable cause of blindness.
  - It must be *screened for*, as the patient is asymptomatic until vision is lost.
  - It is familial, so look for a positive Family Hx in the question.
  - It is more common in African–American patients, and increases with age.
- *Diagnosis*
  - Made with the "puff of air" test or with Tonopen pressure measurements
  - Normal is around an even dozen (12), up to 20. Once >20, treat with eye drops.
- *Therapeutics (eye drops)*
  - Beta-blockers (Betagan, Betopic – look for a drug ending in "olol" as the chemical name)
    - Same SE profile as all BB's
  - Prostaglandin drops (tranaprost, i.e. Travatan)

- *Scientific concept*
    - "cupping" is the result of chronic compression on the nerve
    - To see cupping go to: http://www.glaucoma.org/treatment/optic-nerve-cupping.php
- *Health Maintenance*
    - This is preventable with dilated eye exam and pressure testing
        - Low risk – every 3 -5 years after age 50
        - High Risk – every year after age 50

Macular Degeneration

- *Epidemiology*
    - Most common cause of blindness in patients > 65 years of age.
    - Familial occurrence
    - Slow destruction of the central vision
- *Types*
    - Atrophic (dry) and neovascular (wet) types
        - Dry
            - Slow, gradual loss of central vision
            - Bilateral
        - Wet
            - More rapid, progressive loss of vision
            - Usually bilateral
            - Proliferation of choroidal vessels
            - Hemorrhage, fibrosis
- *H & P*
    - Blurring of central vision
    - Retinal exam (dilated), slit lamp only sees anterior chamber without device to change focus.
    - If decreasing visual acuity – refer to optho (many reasons for decreasing VA).
    - Positive family history
- *Treatment*
    - None; vitamins; experimental meds being tried
- *Clinical Intervention*
    - Amsler grid – boxed lines – patient looks at it each morning and if significant waviness
    - if waviness or blurriness of the lines
        - Urgent referral to optho
- *Health Maintenance*
    - yearly dilated exam by ophthalmologist in patient with risk (family history) or symptoms (central vision blurriness)

RETINOPATHY

This is the topic in the blueprint, but there are *two* different etiologies:

- **Diabetes**
- **Hypertension**

PEARL: Chronic elevation of glucose or blood pressure causes neovascularization, i.e. new vessel development (tiny blood vessels that don't function well and leak all over the place), causing chronic deposition of "stuff" onto the retina (cotton wool spots, flame hemorrhages, etc), with eventual destruction of the retina and resultant blindness over time. This pathophysiology results in either diabetic retinopathy or hypertensive retinopathy.

- Retinopathy must be screened for yearly by an ophthalmologist in *all* diabetics with dilated retinal exam.
- The only treatment is to do pan-retinal photocoagulation (PRP) to destroy the new tiny vessels.
- As in everything else, there are acute abnormalities and chronic; particularly in the case of blood pressure:
    - Acute (malignant) hypertension may result in papilledema
        - Acute retinal venous occlusions and blindness
    - Chronic uncontrolled blood pressure results in "copper wiring" light reflects off the dilated arterioles
        - "AV nicking" and flame-shaped hemorrhages and exudates

Diabetic Retinopathy

- *Epidemiology*
    - Occurs in 40% of Type 2 diabetics
        - Type 1 diabetics usually have changes noticeable after three years or more.
        - 20% of Type 2 diabetics having evidence already at the time of diagnosis.
- *H & P*
    - Neovascularization (small thin blood vessels proliferating over retina)
    - Exudates over entire retinal background, not just at macula
    - Flame-shaped hemorrhages (this bleeding can lead to vitreous hemorrhage, which then can result in retinal detachment from clot retraction)
- *Clinical Intervention*
    - Good glycemic control (A1C <7)
    - Yearly dilated exam by ophthalmologist
    - Emergent referral in sudden loss of vision
    - Urgent referral in proliferative retinopathy (significant change from prior exam)
- *Treatment*
    - PRP (pan retinal laser photocoagulation)
    - Done hopefully before vitreous hemorrhages and retinal detachment

Hypertensive Retinopathy

- *Epidemiology*
    - As above in diabetic retinopathy but due to chronically elevated BP causing neovascularization
    - Same thing for treatment: PRP

Emergent Referral to Ophthalmologist

Acute Angle Closure Glaucoma

- *Risk Factors*
    - Near sightedness
- *History*
    - Sudden pain unilaterally in eye
    - Associated HA
    - Associated nausea/vomiting
    - Halos around lights
- *Onset is sudden*
    - Mydriasis
    - Dark movie theatre
    - Sleeping
    - Iatrogenic cause = mydriatic drops placed in optho or FP office for eye exam
        - When the "pupil" is dilated, (in the dark) the iris "opens" and thickens in the corners of the angle – pinching off the angle and causing increased pressure and trouble with the fluid flowing through the angle (see diagram on first page of this section for visual)
- *Physical exam findings*
    - Injection of conjunctiva
    - Cloudy cornea ("steamy")
    - Mid, fixed dilated pupil
    - Very high Tonopen pressures (normal is up to 20 mm, this patient will be >40-60)
    - Globe is firm and painful to palpate
- *Clinical Intervention*
    - *Immediate* consultation with optho
    - Anterior chamber drainage (by optho)
- *Therapeutics*
    - Acetazolamide (osmotic diuresis to get fluid off)
    - Pilocarpine drops

PEARL: *Glaucoma:* The angle between the cornea and iris narrows such that the two structures are touching, blocking aqueous humor from reaching the "drain" known as the trabecular meshwork. This results in a significant increase in intraocular pressure, damaging the optic nerve.

The most common reasons for an acute angle closure glaucoma "attack" is that the iris is open (pupil is dilated) – think of it as "folding up" in the corner of the angle like an accordion. This then "pinches off" the angle and now fluid cannot flow. Severe pain with increase in pressure; the anterior chamber becomes firm and even protrudes forward. This is a sight-threatening emergency!

Acute Loss of Vision

Retinal Vein Thrombosis/Occlusion

- *Epidemiology*

  - Diabetes
  - Hypertension
  - Hypercoagulable state
- *H & P*
  - Sudden monocular loss of vision
  - No pain or redness
  - Retinal hemorrhages over either entire retinal background (central vein) or a sector of the background (branch vein)
  - Dusky dark background (remember, there is blood going in to the retina, the obstruction to flow is back out; so there will be engorgement, hemorrhage and lots of dark blood in the retinal background)
- *Clinical intervention*
  - Urgent referral to ophthalmologist
  - Intra=vitreal injections of several substances has been known to help
- *Scientific concept*
  - If vision is very poor (20/200) at presentation there is a high risk of neovascular glaucoma with very poor prognosis for regaining sight.

Retinal Artery Occlusion

- *Epidemiology*
  - In patients > 50 years old – think Temporal Arteritis (Giant Cell Arteritis).
  - Can occur as a result of carotid or cardiac embolism from:
    - Carotid plaque
    - Atrial fibrillation or patent foramen ovale
- *H & P*
  - Audden profound monocular vision loss
  - Island of vision only in temporal field
  - Pallor of retinal background with “cherry red spot” or cherry red fovea
  - Fovea receives its blood supply from other than the central retinal artery so flow is Preserved to the fovea with the rest of the retina turning “white”.
- *Clinical Intervention*
  - ***Emergent referral*** to optho
  - Ocular massage; patient flat; high flow oxygen, anterior chamber paracentesis
  - If temporal artery tenderness, begin high dose steroids.
- *Health Maintenance*
  - If vision recurs, think TIA (discussed next) and get Carotid Dopplers.

Amaurosis Fugax (Transient Monocular Blindness)

Subset of retinal artery occlusion above

- *Epidemiology*
  - Transient Ischemic Attack (TIA of the retinal artery)
  - Retinal embolism from either the carotid artery or the heart (atrial fibrillation)

- *H & P*
  - Emboli are rarely seen
  - May have carotid bruits
  - May have “irregular irregular rhythm”
  - Do complete neurologic exam

- *Clinical Intervention*
    - Carotid artery duplex ultrasonography
    - Echocardiogram
    - TEE – (trans-esophageal echo) if atrial fibrillation on PE and EKG

Vitreous Hemorrhage

- *Epidemiology*
    - Diabetic retinopathy
    - Retinal vein occlusion
    - Blood dyscrasias (bleeding abnormalities; and anticoagulant therapies)
- *H & P*
    - Sudden shower of "floaters"
    - Loss of visual acuity
    - On fundoscopic exam, difficulty seeing the retina due to blood in the posterior chamber

PEARL: A vitreous hemorrhage in the posterior chamber is a problem. Blood will clot. When it does, there is clot retraction; this may "tug" on the retinal wall and cause a small tear leading to vitreous detachment, which can be relatively benign, but dangerously can result in retinal detachment - much more serious.

Vitreous Detachment

- Similar to above
- Gel-like vitreous and watery vitreous are in the posterior chamber
- "Chunks" of the gel can break away from the retinal and cause a vitreous detachment with increase in floaters
- The danger is not in the vitreous detachment – the patient can still see – but this can then tug on the retina and cause a retinal detachment, much more serious for the patient.
- *H & P*
    - "Flashes of light" in the vision
- *Clinical Intervention*
    - *Emergent referral* to optho

Retinal Detachment

- *Epidemiology*
    - Can be spontaneous due to naturally occurring changes in the vitreous (recall that as we age the vitreous becomes more thin and watery
    - Near-sightedness is a risk factor
    - May result from a vitreous hemorrhage
    - Trauma
- *H & P*
    - "Curtain" coming down over vision
    - No pain, no red eye
    - Detachment is visible with ophthalmoscopy.
- *Clinical Intervention*

- *Emergent referral* to Ophthalmologist
- Intra-vitreal gas injection (patient must remain face down, and must not fly in an airplane (gas will expand)
- Scleral banding (like a rubber band put around the eyeball that forces the fluid back against the retina and pushes it back)

Urgent Referral to Ophthalmologist

Optic Neuritis

- *Etiology*
    - Inflammatory neuropathy
    - Most often is a hallmark for Multiple Sclerosis
- *H & P*
    - Unilateral mild to moderate visual loss over 2-3 days
    - Pain with EOM's
    - Loss of color (most say dullness of colors)
    - May have disk swelling, may be normal
- *Clinical Intervention*
    - *Urgent* referral to Ophtho
    - IV prednisone – high dose
    - MRI
- *Scientific Concept*
    - MS develops within 15 years in 50% of patients
    - Visual recovery prognosis is very good.

Uveitis/Iritis *(not in the Blueprint, but should be)*

Almost always due to autoimmune disease (HLA-B27 diseases).

- *H&P*
    - Severe and profound photophobia
    - Tearing and pain
    - Reduced visual acuity (hard to obtain due to pain)
    - Pain not relieved with tetracaine (not a corneal problem)
    - Pain with both direct and consensual light response
        - **<u>If L eye is effected:</u>**
            - L eye hurts both with light (iris moves as pupil closes and causes pain); and with taking light away (pupil opens and iris moves)
            - Pain in L eye *also* with direct and consensual light in R eye (when light is shone in R eye, both pupils close, L eye hurts; and when taken away from R eye, L eye hurts)
- *Clinical Intervention*
    - <u>No vision loss</u>
        - Oral steroids (high dose)
        - *Urgent* referral to optho
    - <u>Vision loss</u>
        - Admission
        - IV steroids
- *Health Maintenance*

  - careful history for rheumatologic symptoms
  - warrants lab testing if joint arthralgias
- *Most commonly associated with*
  - Ankylosing spondylitis
  - Reactive arthritis (formerly Reiter's syndrome)
  - Psoriatic arthritis
  - Colitic arthritis
  - Behcet's syndrome
  - I have seen it with SLE and RA as well

Hyphema

- *Etiology*
  - Secondary to trauma
- *H & P*
  - Painful eye; +- decreased visual acuity (depends on how much blood in anterior chamber)
  - RBC's in the anterior chamber
- *Scientific Concept*
  - Can cause acute angle closure glaucoma (RBC's block the flow of aqueous humor through the channel.

Blowout Fracture

- *Etiology*
  - Trauma to eye and tissue/bone around orbit
- *H & P*
  - Severe contusion, swollen bruised lids, pain with palpation of facial bones
  - Check for cranial nerve entrapment (make sure EOM's (extraocular movements) are intact)
- *Diagnostics*
  - CT of the facial bones
- *Clinical Intervention*
  - Referral to ENT or oral maxillofacial surgery

Elective Optho/Surgical Referral

- **Ectropion**
  - Lids droop out
  - Eyelids don't close properly
  - Elderly, connective tissue diseases
- **Entropion**
  - Lids droop inward
  - Lashes scratch cornea
  - Elderly, connective tissue diseases
- **Pterygium**
  - Thick membrane grows over conjunctiva and onto cornea
  - Due to sun and wind exposure

- Comes in from "nasal side" and can obscure vision when covers cornea

- **Pingueculum**
    - Thick membrane grows over conjunctiva
    - From sun and wind exposure
    - Does not encroach on cornea; so usually just a cosmetic issue

---

The Ear, Nose and Throat (adult)

THE EAR

Cerumen Impaction

- *Epidemiology:*
    - Self-induced from using Q tips improperly
- *H & P:*
    - Unilateral conductive hearing loss
    - Should not cause pain
- *Labs & Diagnostics:*
    - Look in ear and see the wax.
- *Clinical Intervention:*
    - Ear lavage
- *Health Maintenance:* education
- *Scientific Concepts:*
    - **Note:** you are not supposed to lavage a TM that is perforated
        - How can you tell if it is perforated if you cannot see it? You cannot.
        - So, if the patient has cold symptoms, fever and ear pain, do not irrigate.
    - In a blind patient, cerumen impaction can cause gait abnormalities and ataxia.

Otitis Externa

- *Epidemiology*
    - Result of water in ear or mechanical trauma
- *H & P*
    - Pain with movement of pinna
    - Tragal tenderness
    - Red inflamed auditory canal
    - No fever, not toxic appearing
    - Foul smelling green slimey discharge suggests pseudomonas
- *Labs & Diagnostics*
    - None needed
- *Clinical Intervention*
    - Ear wick if canal very swollen, otherwise antibiotics will not get to the entire canal

- *Therapeutics*
  - Directed at pseudomonas
  - Ciprodex drops
  - (When I say water, you say.....pseudomonas....and then you say "cipro")
- *Health Maintenance*
  - Protection of the ear from moisture (ear plugs while swimming)
  - Drying agent (alcohol and vinegar)
- *Scientific Concepts*
  - (Remember, Cipro HC is contraindicated in TM perforation (it is not a sterile solution), so make sure you can see the entire TM before prescribing, or just avoid)

Malignant Otitis Externa *(not in blueprint!)*

- *Epidemiology*
  - Immunocompromised older adult
  - Most commonly diabetics
- *H & P*
  - Pain with movement of pinna
  - Tragal tenderness
  - Red inflamed auditory canal
  - High fever, toxic appearance
  - May have cranial nerve palsies; if so, severe illness
- *Labs & Diagnostics*
  - Get a culture!
- *Clinical Intervention*
  - Usually need admission.
  - IV antibiotics
  - CT to r/o osteomyelitis
- *Therapeutics*
  - IV antibiotics directed toward pseudomonas (quinolones)
- *Scientific concept*
  - Can result in osteomyelitis of the ear canal and lead to infectious spread to CNS.

Acute Otitis Media

- *Epidemiology*
  - Most common in children due to short, wide Eustachian tubes.
  - Very common in Down syndrome for the same reason.
- *H & P*
  - Red, bulging TM
  - No vibration with insufflation
- *Labs & Diagnostics:* none needed
- *Clinical Intervention*
  - Observation vs. treatment --- debatable lately (in U.S., we usually treat)
- *Therapeutics*
  - Amoxicillin 80-90 mg/kg/day in divided doses
- *Scientific Concepts*
  - Same pathogens as acute sinusitis and community acquired pneumonias (because it is all connected)

- Amoxicillin 20-40 mg/kg/day can still be used, but higher dose will cover dose dependent strep pneumo resistance and is most commonly used in younger kids.

Serous Otitis Media/Otitis Media with Effusion

- *Epidemiology*
    - Common
    - Due to prolonged eustachian tube dysfunction
    - Viruses
    - Allergic rhinitis
- *H & P*
    - No fevers, nontoxic
    - Conductive hearing loss is common
    - Popping and crackling with yawning
    - Serous fluid in middle ear
    - TM is not red!
    - Sluggish or no vibration with insufflation
- *Labs & Diagnostics:* none, clinical diagnosis
- *Clinical Intervention*
    - Decongestants are no longer used in children.
    - OK to try in adults (with no hypertension or heart disease)
    - Referral to audiology for testing hearing if small child (to preserve normally developing speech patterns)
    - Tympanostomy tube placement referral
- *Therapeutics*
    - If you use antibiotic, direct it empirically at the most common pathogens for the ears, nose and throat (s. pneumo, H. flu, M. catarrhalis).

Chronic Otitis Media

- *Epidemiology*
    - Those with decreased access to health care as children
    - Those with frequent acute otitis media infections
- *H & P*
    - Main finding: chronic TM perforation
    - Otorrhea when water gets into middle ear
    - Conductive hearing loss
- *Labs & Diagnostics*
    - Culture discharge if chronic to identify fungus and other more unusual pathogens.
- *Clinical Intervention*
    - Ideally, TM perforation repair would be done, however, most of these patients have no insurance and are unable to have surgery performed.
    - Avoidance of water in the ear
- *Therapeutics*
    - Directed at pseudomonas, staph aureus, proteus and mixed anaerobes
        - Ciprofloxacin x 2-6 weeks
- *Scientific Concepts*
    - _Reminder:_ acute pathogens are usually very different from chronic pathogens
        - As a general rule: acute infection are treated empirically, chronic infections should have culture performed

      - How many antibiotics does it take to cure a fungal infection? Exactly!

Cholesteatoma

- *Epidemiology*
  - Result of chronic otitis media/prolonged Eustachian tube dysfunction
- *H & P*
  - Retraction pocket filled with keratinous material
  - May retract back and disrupt ossicles and invade bone
  - Conductive hearing loss
- *Labs & Diagnostics:* none
- *Clinical Intervention*
  - Refer to ENT, needs surgical removal
- *Therapeutics:* no medication

Mastoiditis *(surgical mastoiditis is the topic in the blueprint)*

- *Epidemiology/Etiology*
  - Recurrent AOM (acute otitis media) infections, treated incompletely, or untreated
- *H & P*
  - Mastoid redness
  - Swelling
  - Warmth and pain
  - May cause swelling behind pinna
- *Labs & Diagnostics*
  - CBC
  - CT of mastoids
  - Culture via myringostomy
- *Formulating Most Likely Diagnosis*
  - Recurrent/persistent AOM with mastoid swelling/pain on percussion of the mastoid bone and fever
- *Clinical Intervention*
  - Admission if "toxic"
  - ENT referral (I & D)and IV antibiotics
- *Therapeutics*
  - Ceftriaxone IV
- *Health Maintenance:*
  - Appropriate treatment of ear infections (access to healthcare for children)
- *Scientific Concepts*
  - Same pathogen in middle ear as in mastoid air cells
  - Because the mastoid communicates with the middle ear;, most AOM includes some infection/inflammation of the mastoid
  - If mastoid develops suppurative infection, removal of mastoid process itself may be indicated.

Barotrauma

- Those with serous otitis media, acute otitis media, and Eustachian tube dysfunction should not dive or go up in unpressurized airplanes.
    - Acute vertigo may result if round window ruptures due to pressure.
    - Emesis can be very dangerous when 50 feet below the water surface.
    - May cause a hemotympanum (looks like blood bulging behind the TM) must be drained! Usually myringostomy tube is placed for drainage.

Evaluating Hearing Loss

PEARL: *Hearing loss evaluation:*

There are two types of hearing loss: conductive and sensorineural

Most questions have to do with:

- Distinguishing between the types by physical examination
- Identifying the type of hearing loss associated with each

THE TUNING FOR TESTS EXPLAINED

Recall how hearing works:

Conduction of the sound:

- Sound (vibrations in air) arrives at the pinna, swirls around those cool folds, and gets concentrated at the opening to the canal
- Sound waves (vibrating air) goes down the canal and strikes the tympanic membrane
- This makes the TM vibrate (if it can)
- The vibrating TM then vibrates the ossicles
- The vibrating ossicles stimulate the cochlea and labyrinth

Sensorineural conduction to the brain

- The cochlea and labyrinth are stimulated and are connected to the acoustic nerve (CN VIII)
- CN VIII "converts" this vibration to nerve conduction and that is transmitted to
- The acoustic centers of the brain

Therefore, the following would cause a conductive hearing loss:

- *Missing a pinna*
    - Recall that sound travels in a straight line, the pinna allows sound from 180 degrees entire the canal
    - Without a pinna you can only hear sound coming directly at you
- *Wax in the canal*
    - Sound, carried in air, cannot get to the TM to vibrate it
- *TM perforation; fluid in the middle ear; TM scarring; cholesteatoma*
    - TM cannot vibrate and therefore vibrate the middle ear ossicles
- *Fusion or damage of the ossicles*
    - They cannot vibrate and therefore transmit that vibration

The following would cause a sensorineural hearing loss:

- Cochlear damage/developmental abnormality
- Vestibular neuritis
- Acoustic neuroma/Vestibular Schwannoma
- Presbyacusis (age-related hearing loss)
- Noise induced hearing loss (damages CN VIII)

THE WEBER TEST

The point of the Weber test is to vibrate CN VIII through the skull (and therefore bypass the conductive system entirely!)

A conductive hearing loss with the Weber test:

- The tuning fork is vibrated and placed in the center of the skull
- If you have a ball of wax in your L ear (cerumen impaction), no air will get to your TM and you will have a conductive hearing loss (i.e. you are deaf in your L ear)
- When the tuning fork vibrates, a miracle occurs!! you can hear in your L ear!
    - Because your CN VIII was always ok, yes?
    - And the problem was just that sound couldn't get through the wax
- This is called by "Bates" lateralizing to the "bad ear"
- The bad ear can now hear, and it suggests to you that the patient has a conductive problem
    - Look in your five choices for a conductive cause of hearing loss!

A sensorineural hearing loss with the Weber test:

- Tuning fork is vibrated same as above
- There is damage to your L acoustic nerve (CN VIII)
- So no matter where you put that tuning fork, the nerve is still not working well
- "Bates" would say it lateralizes to the "good ear"
- Because the bad ear has a bad nerve
    - Look in your five choices for a SN hearing loss cause!

THE RINNE TEST

This test is checking the normal air > bone conduction of our hearing system.

- The reason we all have giant pinnas on the sides of our heads is to improve the conduction of sound to the acoustic nerve.
- If the system is working well
    - Air should always be greater than bone conduction (otherwise, we would not need our pinnas at all!)
- In this test, the tuning fork is put on the mastoid (bone conduction), then when the sound stops, it is put in front of the pinna (air conduction) and the sound is present again.

  - If you have a conductive hearing loss (ball of wax in your ear), air conduction would not work at all, yes? so the bone conduction would now be greater than the air conduction
  - If you have an acoustic nerve that is damaged and only has 50% function, you would still be hard of hearing in that ear but
    - Air conduction would still be > the bone conduction

Tinnitus

- *Epidemiology*
  - Very common after loud noise
  - Occur spontaneously for no known reason
  - Due to ototoxic agents (gentamycin, tobramycin, aspirin)
- *H & P:* Normal
- *Labs & Diagnostics*: None
- *Clinical Intervention*
  - Distraction techniques
- *Health Maintenance*
  - Avoid loud noises
  - Ear protection
- *Scientific Concepts:*
  - Pulsatile tinnitus (listening to your own heartbeat) may signify a carotid bruit, AVM, or other vascular problem.

Vertigo (Peripheral)

- *Epidemiology*
  - Acute labyrinthitis (secondary to upper respiratory infection)
  - Benign positional vertigo (due to otolith)
- *H & P*
  - Acute onset
  - Severe vertigo lasting several days to weeks
  - Hearing loss/tinnitus
  - Horizontal nystagmus, easily fatigable
- *Labs & Diagnostics*
  - If recurrent or not resolving – get MRI
- *Clinical Intervention*
  - Physical therapy – "Epley maneuver" movement of head to "reset" the otolith
- *Therapeutics*
  - Diazepam
  - Meclizine (antivert)
- *Scientific Concepts*
  - In any questions about vertigo – makes sure you distinguish it from central vertigo which could have a much more serious etiology

Vertigo (Central)

Central vertigo is the most worrisome; peripheral is self-limited and covered below.

- *Etiology*
    - Cerebellar dysfunction (due to multiple reasons – see scientific concepts below)
- *H & P*
    - Complete neuro exam on all patients with vertigo!
    - Milder, more gradual onset of vertigo (than peripheral)
    - Vertical or horizontal nystagmus (unlike horizontal of peripheral)
    - Vertigo does NOT fatigue (peripheral does)
    - Other neurologic signs and symptoms
- *Labs & diagnostics*
    - MRI of brain indicated if above or concern for stroke
- *Formulating Most Likely Diagnosis*
    - Neurologic abnormalities are the most important clues, i.e.
    - Vertical and rotator nystagmus
        - Vertigo does not fatigue!
- *Clinical Intervention:* Imaging of the brain
    - CT if emergent
    - MRI for more specific information
- *Therapeutics*
    - Meclizine may help (antihistamine, like Benadryl) trade name Antivert
- *Scientific concept*
    - Causes (from the brain):
        - Cerebellar stroke/ischemia/hemorrhage/tumor
        - Meniere's disease
        - Migraine
        - Multiple sclerosis

THE NOSE AND SINUSES

Viral Rhinitis

- *Etiology:* Virus
- *H & P*
    - Viral symptoms
    - Red turbinates
    - Clear rhinorrhea
- *Labs & diagnostics:* None
- *Clinical Intervention:* Symptomatic
- *Therapeutics:* None

Allergic Rhinitis

- *Etiology:* Allergens
- *H & P*
    - Itching/sneezing; seasonal or daily; or with contact
    - Pale, blue boggy turbinates
    - Clear rhinorrhea

  - Often concomitant eye symptoms (itching, redness, watering)
- *Labs & diagnostics:* None
- *Formulating most likely diagnosis*
  - From the history above of allergen reaction
  - From the physical exam above of itching and pale blue boggy turbinates with clear rhinorrhea
- *Clinical Intervention:* Avoid allergens if possible; antihistamines
- *Therapeutics*
  - OTC antihistamines (diphenhydramine)
  - Non-sedating antihistamines (loratadine)
  - Nasal steroids (fluticasone; budesonide)
- *Health Maintenance*
  - Avoidance when possible
  - If starting nasal steroids
    - Start two weeks before spring bloom or fall ragweed

Acute Bacterial Sinusitis

- *Etiology*
  - Strep pneumoniae/h. influenzae/m. catarrhalis
  - Most common in smokers and diabetics
- *H & P*
  - 7-10 days after onset of upper respiratory infection (cold)
  - Purulent sinus drainage
- *Labs & diagnostics*: None
- *Formulating most likely diagnosis*
  - Timing (at end of cold symptoms)
  - Change in mucous from clear to dark yellow/green/brown
  - Fever (?)
- *Clinical Intervention:* Treat empirically with antibiotics for normal pathogens
- *Therapeutics*
  - Amoxicillin x 10-14 days
  - Bactrim (if Pen allergic)
- *Health Maintenance*
  - Smoking cessation

Chronic Sinusitis

- *Etiology*
  - Completely different pathogens than *acute*
    - Fungal
    - Staph aureus
- *H & P*
  - Sinus symptoms over 3 months
  - Or failed appropriate treatment x 2 or 3
- *Labs & diagnostics*
  - CT indicated after failed appropriate therapy
- *Clinical Intervention*
  - Imaging

  - Biopsy if needed
  - Referral to ENT if polyp or tumor on CT
- *Therapeutics*
  - Directed at culture results, e.g., antibiotics will not work if it is a fungus!
- *Health Maintenance*
  - Smoking cessation
  - Diabetic control

PEARL: Note again the difference in pathogens between acute sinusitis (s. pneumo, h. flu, m. catarrhalis) and chronic sinusitis (staph aureus, fungal infections)

Epistaxis (Anterior Bleeds)

- *Etiology*
  - Trauma to Kiesselbach's triangle (nose-picking)
- *H & P*
  - Since anterior, the blood runs out of the nose and is obviously visible
  - Patients usually present before hemodynamic compromise (because of obvious bleeding)
  - PE shows lesion, in anterior 1/3 of nasal septum
  - Orthostatics should be normal unless massive blood loss
- *Labs & diagnostics*
  - None needed **unless**:
    - If on warfarin, get INR
    - If heavy bleeding or abnormal orthostatics, get H & H
- *Clinical Intervention*
  - Nasal clamp on anterior nose
  - Neo-synephrine nasal spray + topical anesthetic (tetracaine/pontocaine)
  - AgNO3 cautery (silver nitrate on a Q-tip like swab, "roll" it on the area)
  - If unable to stop flow with above, insert a "nasal tampon"
  - If you insert nasal tampon: *be sure to cover with antibiotics* (occlusion of ostia with tampon will cause sinusitis)
- *Health Maintenance*
  - Patients on warfarin should not pick their noses

Epistaxis (Posterior Bleeds)

- *Etiology*
  - Most often in elderly
  - Warfarin; clopidogrel
- *H & P*
  - Hematemesis
  - Blood streaming down posterior pharynx
  - Asymptomatic otherwise
  - May or may not be orthostatic
- *Labs & diagnostics*
  - If on warfarin, get INR.

  - CBC
- *Formulating Most Likely Diagnosis*
  - Includes all hematemesis, but when you examine the mouth, you see blood coming down from the nasopharynx
- *Clinical Intervention*
  - Nasal clamp (probably won't work, too posterior)
  - Neosynephrine to vasoconstrict blood vessels
  - Place anterior packing; check posterior pharynx; if still bleeding:
    - Posterior packing – if placed:
    - Patient will need overnight admission as packing may suppress the nasopulmonary reflex and patient will stop breathing (particularly in the elderly)
- *Health Maintenance*
  - Maintain INR levels
  - Humidify air in winter
  - No nose picking!

Nasal Polyps

- *Etiology*
  - In neonate, think cystic fibrosis
  - Otherwise more common with aging
- *H & P*
  - Fleshy growth between turbinates protruding from them
- *Labs & diagnostics*
  - CT of sinuses may document additional polyps
- *Formulating Most Likely Diagnosis*
  - May be encephalocele (unlikely)
- *Clinical Intervention*
  - Refer to ENT PA for removal

PEARL: Meconium illness + nasal polyps in infant = cystic fibrosis

THE MOUTH

Dental Pain/Dental Abscess

- *Etiology*
  - Infection that spreads from dental nerve abscess from a mandibular tooth
- *H & P:*
  - Pain typically in a specific tooth
  - hHot/cold sensitive
  - Tender to percussion
  - +/- swelling of face on that side
  - No trismus; no drooling; no adenopathy unless abscess

    - If abscess, soft tissue swelling along gumline or on palate
- *Labs & diagnostics:*
    - None usually needed
- *Formulating Most Likely Diagnosis*:
    - No signs or symptoms of Ludwig's angina (see below)
- *Clinical Intervention:*
    - I & D if abscess
    - Dental block
- *Therapeutics:*
    - Pen VK/Clindamycin
    - Pain medications
- *Health Maintenance:*
    - Good dental hygiene

Ludwig's Angina

- *Etiology*
    - Infection that spreads from dental nerve abscess from a mandibular tooth
- *H & P*
    - Very ill, fever, toxic-appearing
    - Trismus
    - Contraction of masseter muscle causes grimace
    - Induration to skin of anterior neck
    - Swelling; pain base of tongue
- *Labs & diagnostics*
    - CBC with differential
    - CT of neck with contrast
- *Formulating Most Likely Diagnosis*
    - Poor dentition with severe cellulitis of head and neck
    - Base of tongue swelling
- *Clinical Intervention*
    - Admission
    - Manage airway
- *Therapeutics*
    - IV antibiotics to cover normal oropharyngeal pathogens
- *Health Maintenance*
    - Treat all dental infections with Pen VK or Clindamycin (if pen allergic)
    - Need for good dental management

THE THROAT

Pharyngitis/Tonsillitis

- *Etiology*
    - 15-30% due to group A strep; rest are viral
- *H & P*
    - Fever
    - Pharyngeal erythema (both strep and viral)

- Tonsillar enlargement (symmetrical) if assymetric, think peritonsillar abscess
- Exudative tonsillitis (this can be either viral or bacterial, equally)
- Adenopathy
  - Anterior cervical adenopathy with strep group A
  - Preauricular adenopathy with adenovirus specifically
  - posterior cervical adenopathy with infectious mono
- With URI symptoms, likely viral
- With no URI symptoms, more likely Group A strep

- *Labs & diagnostics*
  - Rapid strep screen (90% sensitive)
    - Not necessary if classic symptoms
    - Do culture on child if rapid is negative to improve sensitivity.
  - Monospot
    - Remember, this may be negative early in process.
  - Always r/o strep in kids
- *Clinical Intervention*
  - If classic strep symptoms; treat with penicillin VK
  - If not classic; symptomatic treatment as viral
  - If large tonsils, concern for airway or not able to drink, consider prednisone.

Peritonsillar Abscess

- *Etiology*
  - Group A strep
  - Bacteroides
- *H & P*
  - Swelling of one tonsil larger than the other
  - Pushing of the soft palate to the opposite side; "deviation of the uvula"
  - Trismus' "hot potato voice"
  - Trouble handling secretions
- *Labs & diagnostics*
  - Rapid strep screen; culture of throat
  - CT of neck usually not needed; clinical diagnosis
- *Formulating Most Likely Diagnosis*
  - It's all about uvula deviation and assymetrical swelling of the tonsil
- *Clinical Intervention*
  - ENT referral if airway compromise – STAT
  - Usually attempt at PO medications with close f/u by ENT – next day
  - I & D can be attempted; but careful of carotid!

- *Therapeutics:*
  - Amoxicillin/clavulanate (Augmentin)

Retropharyngeal Abscess *(not in blueprint)*

- *Epidemiology*
  - Uncommon
  - Increasing in incidence in adults (uncommon now in children)

- *H & P*
    - Sore throat
    - Stridor
    - Fever
    - Stiff neck; neck pain
    - Very toxic/ill appearing
- *Labs & diagnostics*
    - CBC = leukocytosis
    - Soft tissue lateral neck - if shows soft tissue swelling, then:
        - CT neck (with contrast)
- *Formulating Most Likely Diagnosis*
    - Similar in presentation to tonsillitis or peritonsillar abscess
    - But, sicker in appearance; tonsils not inflamed; no uvula deviation; instead:
    - Fullness in the posterior pharynx; severe pain in anterior neck space
- *Clinical Intervention*
    - Oxygen and airway management
    - Blood cultures prior to starting antibiotics
    - Emergent ENT consult; may need drainage of abscess
- *Therapeutics*
    - Antibiotics IV
- *Scientific Concept:*
    - Antibiotic selection directed at beta hemolytic strep and staph aureus with anaerobic coverage

Oral Candidiasis

- *Etiology*
    - Candida albicans
- *H & P*
    - Curdy "thrush" on mucous membranes
    - Scrapes off with tongue depressor
- *Labs & diagnostics*
    - KOH = hyphae
- *Formulating most likely diagnosis*
    - *Not* leukoplakia (only on surface, NOT in epidermis)
- *Clinical intervention*
    - *No* biopsy necessary if it wipes off!

- *Therapeutics*
    - Topical nystatin is cheapest
    - Can use PO fluconazole if esophageal
- *Health Maintenance*
    - Good glycemic control

Oral Herpes Simplex

- *Etiology*
    - Herpes simplex virus (type 1 or 2 can be present in the mouth)

- *H & P*
    - Gingivostomatitis is most common presentation
    - Painful, multiple oral ulcers along gingival ridges
    - May have constitutional symptoms (feel sick generally)
- *Labs & diagnostics*
    - Tzanck smear – "multinucleated giant cells"
- *Formulating Most Likely Diagnosis*
    - Painful ulcers is clue
- *Clinical Intervention*
    - None needed
    - But often treatment is given if within 48-72 hours of onset
- *Therapeutics*
    - ------cyclovir
- *Health Maintenance*
    - Hand washing
- *Scientific concept*
    - Tzanck smear unable to distinguish between herpes simplex or zoster.

Aphthous Ulcers

- *Etiology*
    - Unknown
- *H & P*
    - Painful ulcer – usually singular not multiple like HSV
- *Labs & diagnostics:* None
- *Formulating Most Likely Diagnosis:*
    - Single, not associated with constitutional symptoms
- *Clinical Intervention:* None
- *Therapeutics:* None
- *Scientific Concept*
    - Canker sores are one of the criteria for autoimmune disease
    - As a singular symptom canker sores are very inconsequential, but if multiple other symptoms (including arthritis), then consider autoimmune problem.

THE LARYNX

PEARL: Acute and Chronic laryngitis are as dissimilar as most acute and chronic medical conditions.

Acute laryngitis is viral, self-limited, and no big deal; there is no treatment except to have the patient stop talking and wait for the virus to go away.

Chronic laryngitis is either due to:

- *A mass or irritation of the vocal cord*
    - In which case it would move just fine during phonation on indirect or direct laryngoscopy

        - Most likely is due to a polyp, a tumor, or inflammation from something like GERD, or alcohol, or cigarette smoke
            - Concern here is for laryngeal cancer.
- *Or stretching of the recurrent laryngeal nerve*
    - Recall that the nerve leaves the brain; enters the anterior mediastinum, wraps around the thoracic aorta and then goes back up to the hypopharynx (larynx).
    - If anything is enlarged, growing, or present in the anterior mediastinum and stretches the nerve, the patient develops chronic laryngitis
    - Therefore, indirect or direct laryngoscopy, the vocal cords *will not move* during phonation.
        - Many of these diagnoses are life-threatening (see below).

Laryngitis (Acute)

- *Etiology*
    - Vocal cord inflammation
    - Viral etiology; self-limited
- *H & P*
    - Laryngitis
    - Scratchy sore throat;
    - *No stridor*
    - *No drooling*
- *Labs & diagnostics:* None
- *Formulating Most Likely Diagnosis*
    - Acute = < 4-6 weeks
- *Clinical Intervention*
    - Vocal cord rest (no talking!!)
- *Therapeutics*
    - Humidity; lozenges
- *Health Maintenance:*
    - May be due to overuse; voice "hygiene" referral to occupational therapy if speaker/singer, etc.

Laryngitis (Chronic)

- *Etiology*
    - Vocal cord nodules, tumor, inflammation
    - Paralysis of the left recurrent laryngeal nerve
- *H & P*
    - Chronic hoarseness (>6-8 weeks)
    - Indirect or direct laryngoscopy shows
        - <u>Movement of cords with</u>
            - Nodule, tumor or erythema
            - Indirect or direct laryngoscopy shows
        - <u>No movement of cords meaning</u>
            - Anterior mediastinal issue
- *Labs & diagnostics*
    - Indirect laryngoscopy (spray anesthetic in back of mouth; pull out tongue, look at cords with dental mirror, have patient phonate

    - Direct laryngoscopy (done by ENT PA with endoscope; can visualize directly, obtain biopsies if needed)
- *Formulating Most Likely Diagnosis*
    - Must determine if cords are moving or not moving
- *Clinical Intervention:*
    - Referral to ENT if cords are moving.
    - Not an ENT problem if cords not moving:
        - CXR to start
        - Image the chest (? Chest CT)
- *Therapeutics*
    - None; *diagnosis is key*
- *Health Maintenance*
    - Smoking and alcohol are major risk factors for laryngeal cancer.
        - Can also cause benign nodules; inflammation
        - Can cause tumors in chest that can stretch laryngeal nerve too!
    - Smoking cessation!!!

HEAD AND NECK CANCERS

PEARL: When answering a question about a lesion in the oropharynx; benign lesions will tend to be painful and acute (few days); while cancer will be chronic and painless.

Cancer of the Head & Neck

- *Etiology*
    - Chronic inflammation secondary to:
    - Smoking, ETOH, HPV infection
- *H & P*
    - Leukoplakia/erythroplakia
    - Painless
- *Labs & diagnostics*
    - Biopsy
- *Formulating Most Likely Diagnosis*
    - Leukoplakia can look like candida but yeast scrapes off;
    - Erythroplakia can look like canker sores, but cancer is painless, and canker sores hurt
- *Clinical Intervention*
    - Refer to ENT for biopsy.
    - Refer to oncology for management.
    - Surgery is needed and then usually radiation therapy
- *Health Maintenance*
    - Education about smoking cessation
    - ETOH moderation
    - Screening in patients with history of HPV infection
- *Scientific Concept*
    - Squamous cell carcinoma

Leukoplakia

- *Etiology*
  - Smoking
  - Irritation from dentures or bruxism (grinding teeth)
  - Inflammation of mucous membrane (HPV has been implicated)
- *H & P*
  - White patch (does not scrape off like yeast)
  - Painless, non-itchy
- *Labs & diagnostics*
  - Biopsy (KOH would be negative)
- *Formulating Most Likely Diagnosis*
  - Smoker with white patch in mucosa needs biopsy
- *Clinical Intervention*
  - Biopsy
- *Health Maintenance*
  - Smoking cessation
  - Early intervention by oral exam

Erythroplakia

- *Etiology*
  - Smoking products
  - Alcohol
- *H & P*
  - Small painless velvety red patch on mucosa (>90% malignancy rate)
- *Labs & diagnostics*
  - Biopsy
- *Formulating Most Likely Diagnosis*
  - The description gives it to you!
- *Clinical Intervention*
  - Biopsy (referral to ENT)

Salivary Gland Tumors

- *Risk Factors*
  - Smoking and alcohol (like all squamous cell cancers)
- *H & P*
  - Mass in one of the salivary glands
  - Firm and *painless*
- *Formulating Most Likely Diagnosis*
  - Cancer until proven otherwise
- *Clinical Intervention*
  - Biopsy
- *Health Maintenance*
  - Regular examination of all glands
- *Scientific concept:*
  - 80% of all tumors are in the parotid and 80% of them are benign.
  - Tumors (even tiny) in smallest glands have highest rate of malignancy.

        - These tumors do not hurt, so do not be fooled by the seemingly benign nature of a tiny little pea in a submandibular gland – it is likely malignant!
        - The marble in the parotid is likely benign!

Sialadenitis (Salivary Gland Inflammation/Infection)

- *Etiology*
    - Usually an infection or inflammation due to an obstructing stone in duct
    - If from stone, likely staph aureus
    - Historically was a viral infection (mumps – parotitis)
- *H & P*
    - Swelling, redness and pain in a salivary gland
- *Labs & diagnostics*
    - Usually not needed
    - If I & D, obtain wound culture
- *Formulating Most Likely Diagnosis*
    - Differentiate from tumor
    - Cancer is painless
    - Sialadenitis is painful! (may have fever)
- *Clinical Intervention*
    - I & D if abscess or if external to face – refer!
        - Remember, laceration of facial nerve if you I & D externally on face would be bad.
    - Warm compresses
    - Sialogogues (lemon drops, pickles to make patient salivate)
- *Therapeutics*
    - If staph – typical drugs, i.e. dicloxacillin, cephalexin
    - If suspect MRSA – Bactrim (TMP/SMX)

Parotitis

(not sure why this is listed separately by in the blueprint as parotitis is certainly a sialadenitis!)

- *Etiology:* same as above

- *H & P*
    - Mumps-like swelling of cheeks
    - Painful!
- *Labs & diagnostics:* None
- *Formulating Most Likely Diagnosis*
    - Not likely to be cancer if painful
    - Cancer would be a firm painless mass.
- *Clinical Intervention*
    - Antibiotics
    - Warm compresses
    - Sialagogues (lemon drops, pickles to make the patient salivate and hopefully push stone out)
- *Therapeutics*
    - None needed unless infected
    - Antibiotics if infected (to cover staph aureus)

CHAPTER 17

Neurology - 6%

Vascular Problems

Ischemic Stroke

- *Epidemiology*
    - 3rd leading cause of death worldwide (1st = ischemic heart disease, 2nd = cancer)
- *Etiologies*
    - (Ischemic stroke) atherosclerosis in the vessel itself
    - (Ischemic stroke) embolism from remote source (left atrial clot, ventricular clot, carotid plaque)
    - (Ischemic stroke) inadequate perfusion (hypotension/hypovolemia, etc)
    - (Hemorrhagic stroke) rupture of arteriovenous malformation (AVM), aneurysm
- *Risk Factors*
    - <u>Non-modifiable</u>
        - Aging
        - Gender (men > women)
        - Ethnicity (African-American > Hispanic > Caucasian)
        - Family history
    - <u>Modifiable</u>
        - Hypertension – single most important modifiable risk factor for stroke
        - High cholesterol
        - Smoking
        - Diabetes
        - Atrial fibrillation
- *H & P*
    - <u>History</u>
        - Time last seen normal
        - Risk factors for CAD
            - More likely ischemic stroke
        - No risk factors (young, healthy)
            - More likely hemorrhagic stroke
        - Headache
            - Very severe HA is more likely hemorrhagic stroke
    - <u>Anterior circulation problem</u>
        - Aphasia (difficulty finding words; can be expressive or receptive)
        - Monocular visual loss
        - Hemiparesis

    - Hemisensory deficit
  - Posterior circulation problem
    - Bilateral visual loss; diplopia; nystagmus
    - Ataxia, vertigo, syncope
    - Dysarthria (able to say the words, but abnormal phonation)
    - Nausea/vomiting
- *Labs & Diagnostics*
  - STAT Head CT acutely
  - Swallow study (before any PO fluids or meds are given)
  - MRI after stabilization and to evaluate extent
  - Carotid Imaging (Doppler ultrasound)
  - TEE (trans-esophageal echo) looking for clots in atria or ventricles
- *Formulating Most Likely Diagnosis*
  - In most cases a true anterior circulation stroke is easy to distinguish on PE
  - If vertigo, see ENT section about distinguishing peripheral (benign, ENT cause) vs. central (CNS cause)
  - Always keep stroke in the differential of any abnormal neuro presentation as it is very common
- *Clinical Intervention*
  - Tissue plasminogen activator (t-PA) – "dissolves" clot
  - Within 3 hours for consideration for t-PA and no blood on stat head CT
  - If symptoms are resolving or no definite onset, not a candidate
  - Contraindications to t-PA must be sought (see list below)
  - Manage BP
  - Most strokes present hypertensive
    - Avoid hypotension in ischemic stroke; keep the brain perfused! lowest BP ~ 160/100
    - Lower BP, elevate head in hemorrhagic stroke
- *Therapeutics*
  - T-PA (streptokinase)
- *Health Maintenance (chronic stroke management)*
  - <u>No best therapy has been established</u>
    - Aspirin 81 mg- 325 mg. daily
    - Clopidogrel (Plavix) 75 gm. daily
    - Dipyridamole (Aggrenox)
  - <u>Control risk factors</u>
    - BP management (ACEI & thiazide)
    - A1C control <6.5 (or some sources say <7)
    - Lipids (statins)
    - Smoking cessation
    - Alcohol moderation
- *Scientific Concepts*
  - <u>Amaurosis fugax</u>
    - Sudden unilateral vision loss that restores within minutes = TIA of retinal artery (same concern as TIA's in general)
  - <u>Carotid stenosis (ipsilateral to stroke) 70-99% luminal defect should undergo endarterectomy (total occlusion, not a candidate...too late)</u>

Anatomy **PEARL:**

- Anterior brain circulation supplied by the carotids
- Posterior brain circulation supplied by the vertebral and basilar arteries

Transient Ischemic Attack

- *Etiology*
  - Same risk factors as ischemic stroke
- *H & P*
  - Same as stroke in distribution patterns
- *Labs & Diagnostics*
  - Carotid Doppler US
- *Therapeutics*
  - Aspirin
- *Health Maintenance*
  - Risk factor management
- *Scientific Concepts*
  - ** Amaurosis fugax is a TIA of the optic artery --- TIA of the eyeball

PEARL: Contraindications to thrombolytic therapy in acute ischemic stroke (and any other reason you may want to use it i.e. pulmonary embolism; peripheral artery embolism, coronary artery occlusion, carotid artery occlusion, etc):

- Previous intracranial bleeding at any time
- Stroke in less than 6 months
- Closed head or facial trauma within 3 months
- Suspected aortic dissection
- Ischemic stroke within 3 months (except in ischemic stroke within 3 hours time)
- Active bleeding diathesis,
- Uncontrolled high blood pressure (>180 systolic or >100 diastolic)
- Known structural cerebral vascular lesion, arterio-venous malformations
- Thrombocytopenia
- Known cogulation disorders
- Brain tumors (of any kind)

PEARL: Please note that instead of memorizing this list, just recognize that all the absolute contraindications are to avoid bleeding into the brain (or from the aorta). Those two structures must not hemorrhage, or the human will die.

Hemorrhagic Stroke

- *Etiology*
  - Intracerebral
- *Risk Factors*
  - #1 – hypertension
  - Aging

- Ethnicity (African-American>Hispanics>Caucasians)
- Cocaine/amphetamines
- Hemodialysis
- Warfarin use
- *H & P* - same as above
- *Labs & Diagnostics*
  - STAT head CT
- *Clinical Intervention*
  - Lower blood pressure only if needed (SBP>200) – don't lower too much, needed to perfuse the brain!
  - Elevate head of bed to 30- 45 degrees
  - Neuro ICU admission; observation; surgery only if deteriorating
- *Health Maintenance*
  - BP management!

Subarachnoid Hemorrhage

- *Etiology*
  - Cerebral aneurysm
  - AVM (arteriovenous malformation)
- *Risk Factors*
  - Hypertension
  - Smoking
  - Family history (screening only if two first degree relatives have history)
- *H & P*
  - "Thunderclap" "worst HA of my life"
  - CN III palsy (lid droop)
  - Meningismus (without fever)
- *Labs & Diagnostics*
  - STAT head CT (does not rule out SAH!) – 90-95% sensitive
  - if high suspicion, LP (lumbar puncture) is needed looking for xanthochromasia
- *Clinical Intervention*
  - Admit to neuro ICU
  - Swallow test
  - Surgical intervention if needed
- *Therapeutics*
  - Seizure prophylaxis
  - CCB (nimodipine) – but do not cause hypotension!

Subdural Hematoma (Acute, subacute, chronic)

- *Etiology*
  - Closed head trauma (in elderly, may be minor bump on the head!
  - Especially if on warfarin, clopidogrel, dabigatran
  - Tearing of subdural bridging veins (slow venous bleed, typically)
- *H & P*
  - HA (headache)
  - AMS (altered mental status)
  - *Period of lucency from time of trauma to time of symptoms --- hours (acute) to weeks (chronic)!

- *Labs & Diagnostics*
  - Noncontrast head CT for acute bleed
  - MRI for subacute or chronic
- *Clinical Intervention*
  - Observation
  - Serial CT's
  - Surgical management only if severe
- *Health Maintenance*
  - Prevent falls

Epidural Hematoma

- *Etiology*
  - Closed head injury
  - Always acute (no subacute or chronic arterial bleeding issues)
- *H & P*
  - Very short (if any) lucid interval
  - Arterial bleed so rapid onset of symptoms after injury
- *Labs & Diagnostics*
  - Head CT
- *Clinical Intervention*
  - As subdural

Infections

Meningitis (Bacterial)

- *Etiology*
  - S. pneumoniae most common pathogen
  - Neisseria meningitides (college age)
  - Listeria (infants)
  - H. flu (very rare now because of vaccine)
- *H & P*
  - Fever
  - Nuchal rigidity
  - Kernig (resistance to flexing hip) &
  - Brudzinski signs (flex patient's neck; hip will automatically flex due to stiffness)
- *Labs & Diagnostics*
  - LP= >1000 WBC's (pmns)
  - Low glucose (cells using it for fuel);
  - High protein (due to dead WBC & bacteria)
  - Elevated CSF opening pressure
- *Clinical Intervention*
  - Rapid LP and rapid onset of antibiotics is imperative
- Therapeutics
  - Ceftriaxone (rocephin)
  - And vancomycin; tailor to culture results

Meningitis (Viral)

- *Etiology*
  - Enterovirus is most common
- *H & P*
  - Similar to bacterial menigitis
- *Labs & Diagnostics*
  - LP=only a few WBC (lymphs)
  - Normal glucose
  - Only modest protein
  - Normal CSF opening pressures
- *Clinical Intervention*
  - Always start treatment for presumptive bacterial meningitis --- can stop later

Encephalitis

- *Etiology*
  - Viral = HSV, West Nile,
  - ***BUT**** if HIV positive, then toxoplasmosis
- *H & P*
  - Fever
  - Photophobia
  - Altered mental status
  - May have meningismus
- *Labs & Diagnostics*
  - See CSF fluid chart below
    - CSF may have cells, but < 1000
    - Mostly lymphocytes and monocytes
    - Gram stain and culture negative
- *Clinical Intervention*
  - Admit to the hospital
  - Antibiotics are begun immediately until culture is negative

---

Seizure Disorders

Generalized Convulsive Disorder

- *Etiology*
  - 1% of kids
  - Can be a symptom of tumor/ infection also
  - Increased risk in developmental delay
- *H & P*
  - Absence – "staring" episodes – brief LOC but no loss of postural tone
    - Ethosuximide
  - Tonic-clonic – LOC – incontinence – postictal drowsiness
    - Valproic acid/ phenytoin/ topiramax /tegretol
- *Labs & Diagnostics*
  - MRI

    - EEG
    - Consider LP if new-onset or if fever
- *Therapeutics* – as above
- *Health Maintenance*
    - ** No driving – until controlled (each State has its own laws re: seizures and driving)
- Scientific Concepts
    - All antiepileptics have black box warning about suicide risk

Status Epilepticus

- *Epidemiology/Etiology*
    - Seizure greater than 5 minutes or repeatedly so patient doesn't return to baseline in between
    - 20% mortality
- *Labs & Diagnostics*
    - EEG
- *Therapeutics*
    - Ativan
- *Scientific Concept*
    - ***Remember!*** If seizure in pregnant woman due to eclampsia, do not use benzodiazepines, use magnesium sulfate 4 gm IV!!!

Absence seizures & febrile seizures are covered in Pediatrics

---

Distinguishing Headaches

Primary Headaches – Headaches that originate in the brain and are due to probably vascular abnormalities; not due to another medical disorder

- Migraine
- Cluster
- Tension-type

Clues that it is a primary headache:

- onset about puberty; migraines frequently occur with menses or ovulation
- triggers apparent
- no systemic symptoms or PE findings (no fever, papilledema, neuro impairment)
- often associated with anxiety, depression, fibromyalgia and other functional disorders

Secondary Headaches – The headache is due to an abnormality within the brain, infection, inflammation, or something

- Brain tumors (benign and malignant)
- Temporal arteritis
- Intracranial hemorrhages (AVM's, others)
- Meningitis

Clues that it is a secondary headache

- onset of HA after age 50
- systemic symptoms (fevers, myalgias, weight loss)
- Very sudden onset
- Increases with valsalva, exertion, having a bowel movement, cough
- Worse when lying down (vomiting if supine)
- Papilledema on fundoscopic exam

PRIMARY HEADACHES

Migraine

- *Etiology*
    - 17% of women
    - Vascular HA
- *H & P*
    - Unilateral, throbbing, with (Classic) or without aura (Common); lasts > 4 hours, usually 24-72
    - Photophonophobia, nausea, vomiting
    - Vertigo is common
- *Labs & Diagnostics*
    - Usually a normal neurologic exam
    - If abnormal; transient and resolve with onset of HA
    - Imaging (CT) if sudden onset; or change in pattern, intensity
- *Clinical Intervention*
    - Abortive therapy for acute HA
    - Prophylactic prevention
- *Therapeutics*
    - <u>Abortive</u>
        - Triptans --- * not in hypertension; coronary vasospasm (Prinzmetals'), basilar migraines, pregnancy
        - Sumatriptan; rizatriptan; etc.
    - <u>Prophylactic</u>
        - BB's; CCB's; amitryptiline; valproic acid; topiramate
- *Health Maintenance*
    - Identify and avoid triggers
- *Scientific Concepts*
    - Basilar migraine (avoid triptan) = vertigo, diplopia, hyperacusis

Tension Headache

- *Etiology*
    - Stress
    - Straining at reading, computer
- *H & P*
    - "Band-like", squeezing HA across entire top of head – like a tight "swimming cap"
- *Labs & Diagnostics*
    - None needed
- *Therapeutics*

- NSAID's

Cluster Headache

- *Etiology*
  - Men:women , 4:1
- *H & P*
  - Severe, unilateral HA, lasting 15 min to 1 hour; recurs daily for weeks, then gone for months-years
  - Ipsilateral lacrimation; conjunctival injection; ptosis
- *Labs & Diagnostics*
  - None if typical;
  - If atypical, get CT
- *Therapeutics*
  - High flow oxygen : 10 liters in nonrebreather mask
  - Subcutaneous (SQ) triptan (sumitriptan)

Alzheimer's Disease

- *Epidemiology*
  - 50% by age 85 are afflicted
- *H & P*
  - AD is a clinical diagnosis
  - Short term memory loss is first significant finding
- *Labs & Diagnostics*
  - There is no lab or diagnostic that will diagnose AD
  - Imaging and labs are done to r/o another organic cause of the neurologic symptoms
  - MRI to r/o vascular disease
  - R/O B12 deficiency (most common cause of preventable dementia)

Advances have been made in diagnosis to allow identifying the patient earlier and beginning treatment.

- It is now understood that the clinical appearance of AD happens decades before the patient has developed symptoms that are distinct.
  - There are three classifications of AD:
    - probable AD
    - possible AD
    - possible AD with evidence of AD pathophysiologic process. Really??
- In addition, there is now an identified asymptomatic preclinical phase; and a symptomatic predementia phase
- *Therapeutics*
  - Acetylcholinesterase inhibitor – most common side effect is GI upset and diarrhea
  - Donepezil (Aricept)
  - Memantine (Namenda)

PEARL: *Alzheimers Disease*

- The most definitive clinical abnormality that suggests AD is the inability to learn new information or retain information (called episodic memory).
- Initially, there is the functional ability to do tasks like paying bills, shopping, but with mild difficulties
- This becomes more difficult over time as short term memory is impaired
- All organic causes of abnormal cognitive function must be ruled out in order to consider AD (MRI, labs are all needed)

Multiple Sclerosis

- *Etiology*
    - Probably immune mediated
    - Inflammatory demyelination and axonal injury in the brain and peripheral nerves
- *Epidemiology*
    - Most common in women who were born and lived 8 years or more north of the Mason-Dixon line (northern U.S.)
    - Men are affected too; and usually more severely and more rapidly progressive in men
    - Onset usually between ages 20-50 years
- *H & P*
    - Very vague initial symptoms; many visits before diagnosed
    - **Optic neuritis (must always consider diagnosis of MS) – 60%
    - Weakness
    - Paresthesias (numbness, tingling) – more common in upper extremities
    - Spasticity, clumsiness in upper extremities initially
    - Symptoms are worse in heat
- *Labs & Diagnostics*
    - MRI – multifocal lesions in cerebral white matter
    - CSF – increased immunoglobulin levels – oligoclonal bands
    - Visual and sensory evoked potentials - slowed velocity and blocked conduction
- *Clinical Intervention*
    - Optic neuritis should be seen by ophthalmologist STAT ; prednisone PO or IV
- *Therapeutics*
    - Mainstay of treatment are the "Disease-modifying agents"
    - They are not curative but delay disease progression and severity
        - Immunomodulators: CRAB (Copaxone, Rebif, Avonex, Betaseron) are pretty much equally effective overall, offering about one-third reduction in relapses when compared to a placebo over two years in people with relapsing-remitting MS
    - Treatment of symptoms
        - <u>Diazepam or baclofen for spasms</u>
        - Carbamazepine or phenytoin for painful posturing
        - IV steroids (high dose) are useful for flares

- *Health Maintenance*
  - Often bladder hypotonia – frequently get UTI, and UTI worsens their symptoms
  - Immunomodulator treatments increase the patient's susceptibility to opportunistic infections
- *Scientific Concepts*
  - Relapsing-remitting (RRMS) 85-95%= stable between flares of attacks (most common)
    - Secondary-progressive = second phase of RRMS, suggests progression
  - Primary progressive 10-15%= gradual, steady accumulation of symptoms from onset
  - Progressive-relapsing = progressive course with flares (less common)
  - Malignant = rapidly progressive course (less common)

- *Treatment may help RRMS most with increasing areas of remission, and may delay progression to secondary-progressive*

Movement Disorders

Parkinson's Disease

- *Etiology*
  - Relatively common in north America; average age 70
- *H & P*
  - Classic "pill rolling" rest trmor
  - Cogwheel rigidity (tension in a muscle which gives way in little jerks when the muscle is passively stretched)
  - Akinesia (loss of control of voluntary muscle movements)
  - Bradykinesia (slow voluntary muscle movements, i.e. slow to get started)
- *Labs & Diagnostics*
  - Clinical diagnosis
  - But MRI indicated
- *Clinical Intervention*
  - PT/OT/speech/Swallow study
- *Therapeutics*
  - Sinemet (Carbidopa/Levodopa)
    - Dose dependent side effects, i.e. too much = dyskinesias and on-off periods
    - Dyskinesia = sudden, involuntary jerking movements
    - On-off periods = sudden, unpredictable changes in movement, varying from typical Parkinson's movements to a complete lack of movement ("freezing").
- *Health Maintenance*
  - Fall prevention
- *Scientific Concepts*
  - Acronym to remember the symptoms:
    - **T** - tremor
    - **R** -rigidity
    - **A** -akinesia
    - **P** –postural impairment

- Neurologic abnormality is felt due to dopamine depletion in basal ganglia (substantia nigra, subthalamic nucleus and thalamus).
- Treatment, therefore, aimed at increasing dopamine (dopaminergic drug, i.e. levodopa)
- Just educated recently about this little tidbit: in patients presenting with Parkinsonian symptoms who are < 40 years old – rule out Wilson's disease (order a serum ceruloplasmin which would be DECREASED in Wilson's disease)

Essential Tremor (Benign Familial Essential Tremor)

- *Etiology*
  - Autosomal dominant
- *H & P*
  - Postural action tremor of hands
    - (Vs. Parkinson's which is a rest tremor)
- *Labs & Diagnostics*
  - None needed if family history and typical tremor
- *Therapeutics*
  - Propranolol
  - (Or an ounce of alcohol every hour – has its problems!)

Huntington's Chorea

- *Epidemiology*
  - Autosomal dominant disease
    - Men and women affected equally
    - If you have it, one of your parents must have had it.
    - If you have it, 50% of your children are at risk.
- *H & P*
  - Healthy until age 30 or so when choreiform movements begin
  - Chorea (rapid, jerking movements of limbs initially, then diaphragm and larynx)
  - Progression to akinesia that leads to death from immobility
  - Dementia – if patient lives long enough
- *Labs & Diagnosis*
  - None needed; usually family history is well known, so onset of chorea makes the diagnosis
- *Clinical Intervention*
  - PT/OT/social support
- *Therapeutics*
  - Tetrabenazine (new FDA approved dopamine depletion drug)

Neuropathies

Bell's Palsy

- *Etiology*
  - Viral infection (herpes)
  - Idiopathic

- *H & P*
    - Sudden onset of unilateral facial weakness with entire half of facial muscles paralyzed
    - If vesicles = Ramsay-Hunt syndrome (HZV infection causing CN VII palsy)
    - **If forehead wrinkles are "spared", meaning the forehead "wrinkles" – get imaging to r/o stroke**
    - If other cranial nerve abnormalities – get imaging
- *Labs & Diagnostics* - None
- *Clinical Intervention*
    - Protect eye (lid doesn't close) with lubricant ointment and patching eye at night
- *Therapeutics*
    - Debate about efficacy of steroids and –cyclovirs
    - Most treat with both
- *Scientific Concepts*
    - With or without treatment with medications, most people have significant improvement and few sequelae (90-95%); but may have permanent deficit; may take 3-6 months before sure of resolution

PEARL: Parotid gland tumors can cause facial nerve paralysis too – so be aware if they give you a mass in the parotid – don't pick Bell's Palsy!

Diabetic Peripheral Neuropathy

- *Etiology*
    - 50% of diabetics after 25 years of disease
- *Risk Factors*
    - Hyperglycemia
    - Smoking
    - Hypertension
    - Hypertriglyceridemia
    - Obesity
- *H & P*
    - Vibratory sense is MOST sensitive
    - Pinprick
    - Temperature
    - Proprioception
    - Decreased reflexes
    - Poor balance/gait ataxias
- *Labs & Diagnostics*
    - EMG gold standard (usually not done)
    - R/o other causes: B12 deficiency; autoimmume disease
- *Clinical Intervention*
    - Foot care by podiatrist
- *Therapeutics*
    - Duloxetine (Cymbalta)

  - Pregabalin (Lyrica)
  - Amitryptiline
  - Gabapentin (Neurontin)
- *Health Maintenance*
  - Falls are common; examine frequently for foot ulcers (socks off during office exams)

Guillain-Barre Syndrome

- *Etiology/Epidemiology*
  - Quite rare 2/100,000
  - Campylobacter is most common infectious agent
  - Also common in HIV patients
- *H & P*
  - Distal, symmetrical ascending muscle weakness
  - Decreased or absent reflexes
  - Paresthesias
  - Progressive over 3-4 weeks
  - Eventually respiratory failure (30%)
  - Dysautonomia (70%)
- *Labs & Diagnostics*
  - Elevated CSF protein but no WBC's
  - Demyelination on nerve conduction studies
- *Clinical Intervention*
  - Supportive care (respiratory, autonomic, neuropathic pain)
- *Therapeutics*
  - *Do not use steroids!*
  - Immunoglobulin or plasmapheresis
- *Health Maintenance*
  - *Hold all vaccines* for one year after G-B infection
- *Scientific Concepts*
  - 65% of patients walk again at 6 months
  - 80% recover completely

Myasthenia Gravis

- *Etiology*
  - 10:100,000 (not common)
- *H & P*
  - Fatigue of the muscles occurs at end of day
  - Weakness of skeletal muscles (*not fatigue*)
  - Ocular muscles are most common – diplopia; ptosis
  - Dysarthria
  - Chewing
  - Weakness of respiratory muscles late; may need intubation
- *Labs & Diagnostics*
  - Acetylcholine receptor antibodies
- *Therapeutics*
  - Pyridostigmine
  - Steroids
  - Cyclosporine

    - Azathioprine
- *Health Maintenance*
    - These agents may cause worsening symptoms:
        - Aminoglycosides
        - Beta blockers
        - Quinidine
        - Dilantin
- *Scientific Concepts*
    - Antibodies bind to acetylcholine receptors (prevents muscle contraction)
    - *All patients should have CT or MR of thymus gland
    - If thymoma, should have thymectomy

CHAPTER 18

Psychiatry – 6%

Introduction to Psychiatry

Pyschiatry and Behavioral Medicine is mostly about formulating the most likely diagnosis, clinical intervention and therapeutics. Focus on these three knowledge & skills areas as you go through this chapter. Psych therapeutics are covered in much more detail in the Clinical Therapeutics Chapter 4.

THE PSYCHIATRIC EXAMINATION

- ***General Appearance*** – Dressed appropriate for weather? situation? grooming/hygiene; stated age?
- ***Speech*** – Pressured, volume, coherent, slurred
- ***Insight*** – Ability to understand what is happening in a given situation
- ***Mood*** – Euphoric, anxious, paranoid; depressed
- ***Affect*** – Flat; appropriate?
- ***Thought Process*** –Content; halting/blocking
- ***Thought Content*** – Hallucinations, delusions, obsessions
- ***Orientation*** – To person, place, date, situation
- ***Memory*** – Short and longterm
- ***Attention*** – Able to maintain attention long enough to answer questions
- ***Knowledge*** – Reading ability, writing ability
- ***Suicidal Ideation/Homicidal Ideation***

THE AXIS CATEGORIES

Axis I – Major Psychiatric Disorders

Axis II – Personality disorders

Axis III – Medical conditions

Axis IV – Psychosocial/environmental disorders

Axis V – Global assessment of functioning

Mood Disorders

Major Depressive Disorders– DSM IV – Unipolar Disorder

- *Distinguishing Features*
    - Loss of interest with 5 of 8 present most days for two weeks:
    - Sleep changes
    - Loss of interest
    - Feeling of guilt/worthlessness
    - Loss of energy
    - Difficulty concentrating
    - Change in appetite or weight
    - Psychomotor slowing
    - Thoughts of death or suicide
- *Labs & Diagnostics*
    - R/o thyroid disease; other medical illnesses
- *Clinical Intervention*
    - Referral to psychiatrist when: risk of suicide; severe psychomotor retardation; psychosis; vegetative symptoms (weight loss, lack of sleep)
- *Therapeutics* – both work together better than either alone:
    - Cognitive therapy (psychotherapy)
    - **Medications**
        - SSRI's
            - Any OK
            - Fluoxetine is preferred in pregnancy, but questionable in nursing and concentrated in milk.
        - Tricyclic Antidepressants
            - Nortriptyline is safest in pregnancy
        - ECT (electroconvulsive therapy) – safe in pregnancy!

Dysthymic Disorder

- *Distinguishing Features*
    - Unipolar disorder of depressed mood but lasting more than 2 years
    - Loss of interest, but not severe enough to be major depressive (lack of vegetative sx)
    - Lifelong history of "feeling depressed", low self esteem
- *Labs & Diagnostics*
    - *TSH/free T4*
- *Therapeutics*
    - Psychotherapy is more effective than drugs
    - SSRI's may be indicated

Bipolar Disorder

- *Distinguishing features – three types:*
    - Bipolar I
        - Male=Female
        - Onset in 20's, single manic episode signals onset

        - Depression follows without euthymic (normal) period
        - High incidence of suicide during depressive state
    - Bipolar II
        - Female > male
        - Hypomania
    - Bipolar III
        - Patients who become manic when treated with antidepressants for depressive disorder
- *Labs & Diagnostics*
    - hyperthyroidism; hypothyroidism (TSH/free T4)
    - drug induced mania (toxicologyscreens)
- *Therapeutics*
    - Acute Mania
        - Antipsychotics/benzodiazepines
    - Chronic mood stabilizer
        - lithium

Anxiety Disorders

Panic Disorder

- *Distinguishing Features*
    - Females < 30 y.o
    - Recurrent, unexpected panic attacks
        - Palpitations
        - Sweating
        - Chest pain/shortness of breath
        - Dizziness
        - Fear of dying
    - Typical presentation
        - Sudden onset; lasts 5-20 minutes
        - Soncern about future attacks
        - Significant change in behavior related to fear of attacks
- *Labs & Diagnostics*
    - TSH/freeT4 to r/o Grave's disease
    - Obtain history to r/o risk factors for pulmonary embolism. (is she on BC pills?)
        - D-Dimer might be warranted
    - Drugs screen for : cocaine, amphetamine, ADD drug abuse
- *Therapeutics*
    - Cognitive-psychotherapy
    - ***Medications***
        - Tricyclic Antidepressants
            - Amitryptiline, Nortriptyline
        - SSRI's
            - Fluoxetine, Sertraline, Paroxetine
        - Benzodiazepines (long acting better i.e. clonazepam)
            - For acute panic lorazepam is drug of choice

Generalized Anxiety Disorder

- *Distinguishing Features*
  - 20's; Male = Female
  - Daily (and all day long) worry with symptoms of anxiety
  - May interfere with sleep, work, relationships
  - No panic attacks
- *Labs & diagnostics*
  - TSH/free T4
- *Therapeutics*
  - Clonazepam
  - Buspirone
  - Beta-blockers (?)
  - Relaxation therapy

Adjustment Disorders (Situational stress disorder)

- *Distinguishing Features*
  - Change in emotional state or behaviors due to an identified psychosocial stressor
  - Divorce, death of a child, loss of a job
  - Resolves within 6 months of the stressor
- *Labs & Diagnostics*
  - Check TSH/free T4
- *Clinical Intervention*
  - Psychotherapy is most effective
  - Patient may self-medicate; question alcohol, drugs, caffeine, OTC meds
- *Therapeutics*
  - Very careful (judicious) use of sedatives for anxiety
    - Lorazepam 0.5 BID or TID, but for short length of treatment

Acute Stress Disorder

- *Distinguishing Features*
  - Traumatic event precipitates syndrome
  - Lasts < 1 month
- *Labs & Diagnostics*
  - None indicated
- *Therapeutics*
  - Psychotherapy
  - If needed, judicious use of lorazepam for acute stress

Posttraumatic Stress Disorder

- *Distinguishing Features*
  - Traumatic event precipitates syndrome
  - Re-experience event through flashbacks
  - Difficulty sleeping
  - Detachment from others
  - Lasts > 1 month
  - 75% of patients have comorbid depression and panic attacks

- *Labs & diagnostics*
    - Includes thyroid testing
- *Therapeutics*
    - Propranolol for "anxious arousal"
        - Helps to blunt the sympathetic symptoms of rapid heart rate, tremors
    - SSRI's for treatment of associated depression
        - Sertraline and paroxetine are approved by FDA for PTSD
    - Psychotherapy

Phobic Disorder

- *Distinguishing Features*
    - Intense fear of a particular thing or event (spiders, heights)
    - Has to interfere with daily functioning
    - Patient notes that it is unreasonable
    - *In kids, often disappears spontaneously with age
- *Labs & Diagnostics* - none
- *Therapeutics*
    - Desensitization (exposure) therapy

Delusion/Psychosis

Delusional Disorder

- *Distinguishing Features*
    - Delusions that are not bizarre (may have basis in fact) but are not actually happening
    - Disrupts patient's life
    - Female> Male; in mid to later life
- *Therapeutics*
    - Psychotherapy is primary treatment
    - Most medications are not effective

Schizophrenia

- *Distinguishing Features*
    - Men>Women; onset early 20's male; late 20's female
    - Familial
    - Psychotic symptoms for 6 months or more
    - High risk for suicide
    - H/o depression/ recent hospital discharge
    - Abnormal functioning in society; poor social skills; unusual behavior and thinking
        - Positive symptoms
            - Hallucinations
            - Delusions
              Bizarre behaviors
        - Negative symptoms
            - Decreased expression of emotion
            - Poverty of speech

        - Few friends; no interests or activities; occupational issues
- *Labs & Diagnostics*
    - Drug screening
    - Thyroid screening
    - Basic health screening
- *Therapeutics*
    - Psychotherapy
    - Vocational training
    - Antipsychotic agents
        - <u>Typical</u>
            - Thioxanthenes
            - Phenothiazines
        - <u>Atypical (neuroleptics)</u>
            - Clozapine
            - Risperidone
            - Quetiapine
            - Aripiprazole
            - Olanzapine
    - *One large trial compared atypicals and typicals; and while no tremendously wonderful findings, the drug best tolerated and with similar efficacy to the others was olanzapine (Zyprexa). Patients stayed on it, tolerated it well, and patient compliance is the biggest problem with schizophrenia*

Schizoaffective Disorder

- *Distinguishing Features*
    - Both a thought disorder and a mood disorder
    - Psychotic episodes coupled with a major mood disorder, i.e., manic/depressive disorder
- *Labs & Diagnostics*
    - As above
- *Therapeutics*
    - Mood stabilizer (lithium) combined with:
        - <u>Antipsychotic drug</u>
            - Clozapine is most effective; but has side effects
        - *Any antipsychotic (see schizophrenia list) could be used*

Somatoform Disorders

- *Distinguishing Features*
    - Positive review of systems without clinical evidence of illness (look for physical signs of autoimmune disease or rheumatologic disease before selecting somatoform disorder)
- *Labs & Diagnostics*
    - Usually has had multiple workups, "doctor shopper"
    - Pain in four different organ systems
        - Two GI complaints
        - Sexual symptom
        - Pseudoneurologic symptom
    - All occurring before age 30 and persistent despite numerous normal evaluations

Personality Disorders

Basic tenets about personality disorders:

- Onset in adolescence (sometimes childhood)
- Maintain normal reality (do not hallucinate)
- Enduring pattern; difficult to change
- Often "treated" with substances (alcohol)

ODD AND ECCENTRIC

Paranoid

- *Distinguishing features*
    - Suspicious
    - Anticipates deception, betrayal
    - Must have some basis in reality (otherwise psychotic

Schizoid

- *Distinguishing features*
    - Emotionally detached
    - Avoids relationships
    - Difficulty with expressing emotions

Schizotypal

- *Distinguishing features*
    - Unusual thought patterns, beliefs
    - Has some paranoia, some schizophrenic attributes
    - Less severe; no continued psychotic symptoms

DRAMATIC AND EMOTIONAL

Antisocial

- *Distinguishing features*
    - Complete disregard for societal rules; mores
    - No remorse for actions
    - Lies frequently
    - Poor impulse control
    - Alcohol abuse is common

Borderline

- *Distinguishing features*
    - H/o unstable relationships
    - Poor self-image
    - Fear of abandonment
    - Unsafe behaviors

Histrionic

- *Distinguishing features*
  - Excessive emotionality
  - Seductive and inappropriate behaviors

Narcissistic

- *Distinguishing features*
  - Self-centered
  - Demands excessive attention
  - Lack of empathy for others
  - Envious and jealous of others

ANXIOUS AND FEARFUL

Avoidant

- *Distinguishing features*
  - Anxiety prevents development of relationship
  - Overly sensitive to criticism
  - Fear of rejection

Dependent

- *Distinguishing features*
  - Needy
  - Unable to make decisions without other's approval
  - Submissive and clinging
  - Terrified of abandonment

Obsessive-compulsive

- *Distinguishing features*
  - Perfectionistic
  - Excessive need to control environment
  - Requires order at all times
  - Cold and rigid

Substance Abuse

In general, substance abuse is a maladaptive pattern of substance use that leads to clinical impairment and physical disease:

- Failure to maintain occupation/obligations/school functioning
- Recurrent uses of substances despite obvious dangers
- Legal problems with illegal substance use
- Continued use despite social and personal problems directly related to the substance use

Dependence is defined as:

- Tolerance of the drug
- Withdrawal if the drug is stopped
- Repeated excessive use
- Persistent failed attempts to stop use

- Reduction in other important activities due to drug intoxication
- Continued use despite illness and other social problems related to use

ALCOHOL ABUSE

CAGE Screening

Cut down – have you made attempts (and failed) to limit your drinking?
Annoyed – do you get annoyed when someone asks or comments on the amount you drink?
Guilty – do you feel guilty when you drink too much, or too often?
Eye opener – do you need to have a drink when you wake up to "calm your nerves"?

Acute Alcohol Intoxication

- *Alcohol is a sedative-hypnotic drug*
  - Signs and symptoms for alcohol are similar to that of benzodiazepines, and muscle relaxants
- *Life-threatening alcohol intoxication can occur in much lower levels than seen in chronic alcoholics*
  - Chronic alcoholic with blood alcohol level of 0.57 was talking to me!
  - Acutely comatose 19 year old had BAL of only 0.3, and had to be intubated
  - Remember this acute vs. chronic presentation for questions about alcohol intoxication
- *Activated charcoal can be given if the patient is protecting the airway*
  - Otherwise management is supportive; airway, fluids, monitoring
- *Flumazenil is a benzodiazepine antagonist but does not work on alcohol or others*
  - It has actually been found to do more harm than just observation and respiratory support in a patient with benzodiazepine overdose!

Treatment for Alcohol Dependence

- *Disulfiram (Antabuse)*
  - Interfered with the metabolism of alcohol
  - Slows the conversion of acetaldehyde to acetyl coenzyme A
  - Buildup of acetaldehyde causes nausea, vomiting, headache and low BP
  - Similar to metronidazole in structure (so when giving Flagyl, remember, no alcohol!)
- *Interesting fact:* Some patients of SE Asian ancestry specifically lack an enzyme needed for conversion of acetaldehyde to CoA – many think they are "allergic" to alcohol

ALCOHOL WITHDRAWAL

- *Life threatening emergency from delirium tremens*
- *H & P*
    - History of seizures during periods of abstinence increases risk of DT's
    - Anxiety & tremulousness
    - Increased HR & BP
    - Hyperthermia
        - "Shaker, baker"
    - Begins within 8 hours of abstention, can last 3 days
- *Delirium Tremens*
    - Usually occurs within 24-72 hours after last drink
        - But can occur as late as 7 days
    - AMS
    - Tremor, *visual hallucination* (hence name, delirium tremens)
    - Diaphoresis, dehydration, hypokalemia, hypomagnesemia; seizures
    - Often occurs unexpectedly during hospitalization (patient may not even be aware of danger)
    - Suspect in every delirium which is unexplained, particularly with VS abnormalities
- *Treatment*
    - Hospitalize
    - Thiamine 100 mg. PO or IV for all AMS (Wernicke-Korsakoff syndrome)
    - Prevent seizures and help with symptoms
        - Ativan
        - Magnesium replacement
        -

OPIATE DEPENDENCE AND WITHDRAWAL

Opiate Intoxication

- *H & P*
    - Somnolence
    - Euphoria
    - Nausea
    - Miosis (pinpoint pupils)
- *Treatment*
    - Support airway
    - Naloxone, 2 mg IV
        - Dramatic results within minutes
        - Short half-life, dose may need to be repeated
        - Hospitalize to manage airway if concern

Management of Opiate Withdrawal

- *Early symptoms of withdrawal include:*
    - Agitation
    - Anxiety
    - Muscle aches
    - Increased tearing
    - Insomnia
    - Runny nose
    - Sweating
    - Yawning
- *Late symptoms of withdrawal include:*
    - Abdominal cramping
    - Diarrhea
    - Dilated pupils
    - Goose bumps
    - Nausea
    - Vomiting
- *Clonidine (Catapres)*
    - A centrally acting antihypertensive
    - Useful in acute withdrawal
    - Orally QID or transdermal patch
    - Helps with symptoms; does not help with anxiety, muscle aches, but does help with cardiovascular hypertension and tachycardia

Unlike alcohol and benzodiazepine withdrawal, opioid withdrawal reactions are very uncomfortable but are not life threatening. Symptoms usually start within 12 hours of last heroin usage and within 30 hours of last methadone exposure.

Treatment for Opiate Dependence

- *Suboxone (naltrexone) – special certificate for dispensing needed!*
    - Must be withdrawn and free of narcotics for 7-10 days
    - Opiate antagonist (blocks HIGH of heroin use)
    - Main complication = liver failure
- *Buprenorphine – special certificate for dispensing needed!*
    - Partial agonist
    - OP therapies, combined with group therapy
- *Methadone – special certificate for dispensing needed!*
    - Used to prevent withdrawal, both acutely and chronically
    - In acute; give 10 mg every 4-6 hours until relief
    - This replaces the opiate, is a Band-Aid, so goal should be to then wean from methadone (a step many forget about!)

DRUG ABUSE OF PRESCRIPTION DRUGS

- Death rate from prescription drug overdose has exceeded accidents in adults < 30 years old.
- Often the drugs are the parents'; roommates', or purchased on the street, but legally prescribed drugs.

SMOKING CESSATION

PEARL:

- Smoking is the most important preventable cause of all cancer.
- Treating tobacco abuse is a primary prevention of cancer.
- Clinical intervention for tobacco abuse should be given to all patients in whom it would benefit their health.
- Ask at every visit
- Outcomes improve when counseling is added to medications although each is effective alone.

Five steps:

- *Ask* – Identify ALL users (repeat at every visit)
- *Advise* –Urge every user to quit
- *Assess* – Check for willingness at every visit
- *Assist* – Offer pharmacotherapy and counseling
- *Arrange* – Follow up is CRUCIAL to success

In addition, studies have shown:

- Simple information from a clinician can yield smoking cessation rates of 10-20%.
- Intensive follow up and counseling improves outcomes.
- Social contact intervention
    - Framingham showed 67% cessation rate if spouse stopped as well.
    - Smoking cessation by a friend resulted in 36% cessation rate.

Smoking Cessation Agents

- Drugs should not be given without counseling, follow up, "quit plan":
    - nicotine replacement
        - stimulant effects in overuse
    - bupropion (Wellbutrin)
        - lowers seizure threshold; (so don't give it to anyone with seizure history)

        - helps with weight gain (patients typically lose weight on Wellbutrin)
    - varenicline (Chantix)
        - 7/2009 – Black box warning about increased risk of suicide and depression
        - 6 & 7/2011 – study in US and one in Canada found increase in serious cardiovascular events in patients on Chantix

---

Eating Disorders

Anorexia Nervosa

- *Distinguishing Features*
    - Severe loss of weight which is intentional (BMI<18.5) and refusal to gain weight
    - Excessive exercise
    - Restricts food intake
    - Purging/ Laxative abuse
    - Female>Male (although occurs in males); average age 17
    - Preoccupation/distorted body image
- *Clinical manifestations*
    - Metabolic disturbances (hypokalemia, hypoalbuminemia)
- *Labs*
    - Electrolytes/albumin, TSH/free T4
- *Treatment*
    - Medications do not work well
    - Inpatient supervised meals, individual and group therapy, weight monitoring

Bulimia Nervosa

- *Distinguishing Features*
    - Binging and purging with maintenance of normal weight
    - Females:Males; 10:1
- *Clinical manifestations*
    - Not as profound unless severe vomiting (hypokalemia)
- *Labs*
    - Electrolyte evaluation & albumin level (CMP – comprehensive metabolic panel)
- *Treatment*
    - Psychotherapy
    - Management of behaviors
    - SSRI's are effective
        - Best results with fluoxetine, but other SSRI's work well too

Obesity

- *Epidemiology*
    - Second leading cause of preventable death in U.S.
- *Distinguishing features*
    - BMI >31 (overweight 25-30)
    - Morbid obesity > 40
- *Clinical manifestations*
    - Type II DM
    - Gall bladder disease

- Breast and colon cancer increased risk
- Risk factor for ischemic heart disease

- *Labs*
    - A1C or FBS x 2
    - Fasting lipid panel
    - TSH/FREE T4
    - Consider Cushing syndrome
- *Treatment*
    - Dietary referral for evaluation of dietary and exercise habits
    - Manage DM and lipids if abnormal
    - Consider anti-obesity meds
        - Orlistat
        - Lorcaserin (approved 7/2012)
        - Phentermine/topiramate
        - Bariatric surgery
            - Lowers A1C levels
            - Decreases CV risk
            - Diabetes remission is seen with weight loss post-op

---

Abuse

Abuse takes multiple forms in each of the categories:

- *Physical Abuse*
    - Physically harming the person through frustration and aggression
- *Psychological Abuse*
    - Demeaning; verbally abusive, controlling behaviors
- *Sexual Abuse*
    - Pedophilia, elder sexual abuse, rape and incest
- *Neglect*
    - A less obvious form of abuse; many times not even intentional
        - (You can imagine a 90 year old woman caring for her 93 year old husband, and just being weary; yet he is not cared for and suffers from neglect)

Child Abuse

- *Clues*
    - The child's story does not match the parent.
    - The parent does not let the child say what happened.
    - The child is xrayed and other fractures of other ages are found.
    - The injury does not match the mechanism described.
    - Burn marks, ligature marks, fingernail scratches are found.
- *Remember that Hemophilia A presents with multiple joint hemarthroses and can look like child abuse.*

Psychological Abuse

- *Bullying; name-calling; verbal abuse*
- *Clues*
    - Poor performance in school

- Social ineptitude
- Multiple somatic complaints

Sexual Abuse

- *Clues*
  - Sexual precociousness
  - Acting out sexual actions
  - Physical signs of sexual abuse of the vagina and rectum

Neglect

- *Clues*
  - Child is not attending school
  - Patient is missing doctor appointments
  - Patient's serum drug levels are not appropriate
  - Patient is losing weight
  - Patient (adult or child) is not dressed appropriately for the weather
  - Patient has poor hygiene
  - Remember that often this is not intentional, but due to poor ability by the caregiver
  - All must be investigated

In addition to the above; Child Abuse has a special form:

- *Munchausen by Proxy*
  - A parent (usually the mother, who is a health care professional) creates an illness in a child so that the parent can maintain a relationship with clinicians and be perceived as a caring parent.
- *Clues*
  - Multiple visits
  - Moving frequently
  - "Doctor shopping"
  - Real symptoms
  - Abnormal results with no diagnosis found
  - Over protective

Elder Abuse

- Everything above in child abuse is almost identical to elder abuse; possibly even including Munchausen's by proxy

Domestic Violence (Now called Intimate Partner Violence)

- *Prevalence 4-18%; often not reported*
- *Abusive behavior by a person in an intimate relationship with the victim*
- *Physical, sexual, emotional*
- *Neglect, i.e. economic deprivation*
- *Risk factors*
  - Victim under age 35
  - Pregnancy
  - Single, divorced, separated
  - Alcohol or drug abuse in victim or partner

- *Low socioeconomic status*

Attention Deficit Disorder --- Covered in pediatrics, Chapter XX

CHAPTER 19

Endocrinology – 6%

Introduction to Endocrinology

- **If the patient has a completely positive ROS, consider the following etiologies:**
  - *Psychiatric problem*
  - *Autoimmune problem*
  - *Endocrine problem*
- If you are concerned that the patient has hormone excess, order the suppression test.
- If you are concerned that the patient has hormone deficiency, order the stimulation test.
- A primary endocrine disorder is one in which the patient's symptoms are due to a "sick" gland, i.e. most thyroid diseases are actually a problem with the thyroid, therefore, a primary disorder.
- A secondary endocrine disorder is one in which the patient's symptoms are actually due to the hypothalamus (uncommon) or pituitary, i.e. most cortisol excess is not due to the adrenal, but rather a tumor on the pituitary that stimulates the adrenal. The adrenal is just doing "what it's been told to do", therefore, a secondary disorder.

In a problem of cortisol excess (the toughest one to understand), pay attention to whether the disease is ACTH dependent or ACTH independent:

- *ACTH dependent* = the cortisol excess is due to ACTH being secreted somewhere in the body (again, the adrenal is just doing what it is supposed to do!)
  - Cushing disease – ACTH secreting pituitary tumor – *most common*
  - Small cell carcinoma of the lung – Much less common
  - Ovarian tumors – Even more rare
- *ACTH independent* = the cortisol excess is due to the adrenal secreting too much cortisol (it is independent of the amount of ACTH from the pituitary)

- Adrenal adenoma
- Adrenal cancer
- Exogenous steroids (patient is taking cortisone for some reason) – this is the *most common*

THE NEGATIVE FEEDBACK LOOP

The normal negative feedback loop begins in the hypothalamus with:

- Release of hypothalamic releasing factors
- These releasing factors stimulate the pituitary to release its stimulating hormones.
- These pituitary stimulating hormones act on the target endocrine organ causing it to release its hormone.
- This organ hormone "feeds back" to both the pituitary and hypothalamus, and "shuts them off".
    - This happens constantly throughout the day, week, or month to adjust hormones quite precisely.
    - For this reason, if a serum level is just a wee bit high, or at high limits of normal, you may be catching it as it is adjusting, and the test should be repeated.
    - If result is markedly out of the normal range, then believe it!

Normal function of hypothalamic-pituitary-adrenal axis

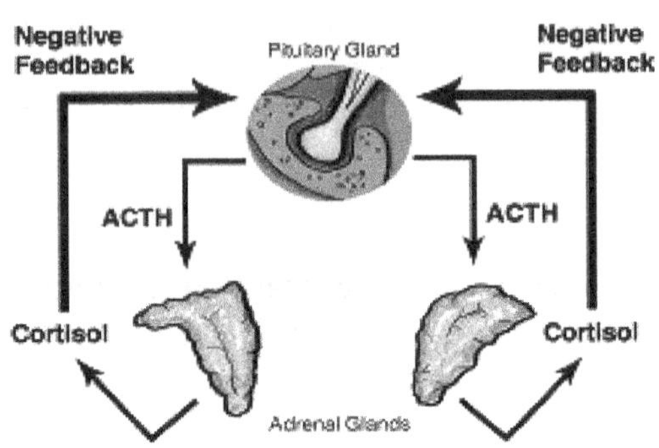

The Hypothalamus Secretes:

- CRF –Corticotropin Releasing Factor
- TRF – Thyrotropin Releasing Factor
- GnRH – Gonadotropin Releasing Hormone
- GHRH – Growth Hormone Releasing Hormone
- Dopamine
- Somatostatin

This stimulates the anterior pituitary to secrete:

- ACTH (adrenocortical hormone)
- TSH (thyroid stimulating hormone)
- FSH/LH (follicle stimulating hormone/luteinizing hormone
- GH (growth hormone)
- Prolactin (PRL)

The posterior pituitary gland secretes only two hormones (independently from the hypo-thalamus)

- Antidiuretic hormone (ADH) –which is also called vasopressin
    - As the name implies
        - ADH causes the kidney to hold water
        - And also causes peripheral vasoconstriction (as vasopressin)
- Oxytocin (stimulates active labor)

The Pituitary Gland

Pan-hypopituitarism

- *Etiology/Epidemiology*
    - Uncommon
    - Due to a benign adenoma most often
    - Can be secondary to surgery, trauma, bleed, etc.
    - Can be due to Sheehan's syndrome
        - Bleed into the pituitary stalk after a massive postpartum hemorrhage
- *H & P*
    - Multiple hormone deficiencies
    - *Symptoms related to hypogonadism, hypothyroidism, hypoadrenalism*
- *Diagnostics*
    - Low TSH with low T4
    - Low ACTH with low cortisol
    - Low FSH with low testosterone/estradiol
    - MRI
    - Transphenoidal resection of tumor (usually damages pituitary though)
- *Therapeutics*
    - Replace all hormones
        - Thyroxine
        - Cortisol
            - Given twice a day; full dose in a.m. and half dose in p.m.
        - Testosterone; must be given IM or transdermally
        - Estradiol is fine PO

            - GH replacement mainly if pre-pubertal
                - *If adult very symptomatic; IM injection of GH*
- *Health Maintenance*
    - Just like any person with adrenal insufficiency, stress dosing is needed. *(See adrenals below)*

Acromegaly

- *Etiology/Epidemiology*
    - Pituitary tumor
- *H & P*
    - "Gigantism" if pre-pubertal when tumor starts secreting GH
    - Acromegaly after growth plates have closed
    - Enlargement of forehead, jaw, tongue, feet and hands
    - Enlargement of tongue (macroglossia) causes obstructive sleep apnea.
    - Cardiomegaly
    - Hypertension (50%)
    - Insulin resistance
- *Labs & Diagnostics*
    - Random serum IGF-1 for screening
        - Insulin-like growth factor is increased with increased GH
    - If normal, acromegaly is ruled out
    - MRI
- *Clinical Intervention*
    - Pituitary microsurgery is treatment of choice.
- *Scientific Concept*
    - GH causes secretion of IGF-1; therefore the insulin resistance

Hyperprolactinemia

- *Epidemiology*
    - Women > Men
- *Etiology*
    - Prolactin secreting tumor
    - Centrally acting drugs (too many to list)
        - Psychotropics
        - Antiemetics
- *H & P*
    - Women
        - Amenorrhea & Galactorrhea
    - Men
        - Decreased libido
    - Mass Effects
        - Bitemporal hemianopsia

        - Headache
        - Vomiting when supine (from increased CSF pressures)
- *Labs & Diagnostics*
    - Women
        - Check serum HCG
    - Men & Women
        - Serum prolactin (PRL)
            - Normal level is about 10-14
            - Drug-induced usually 40
            - Most are small with PRL < 100
            - Rarely > 200 – 300
    - MRI
    - Formal peripheral field testing on all tumors
- *Clinical Intervention*
    - Stop offending drug and recheck serum prolactin.
- *Therapeutics*
    - Dopamine agonists if fertility desired
        - Cabergoline
        - Bromocriptine
    - If large
        - Treat with cabergoline to decrease size of tumor.
        - pituitary microsurgery
- *Health Maintenance*
    - If patient does not desire fertility, no need to treat.
    - However, increased PRL can cause decreased estrogen and resulting osteoporosis.

PEARL: *Diabetes Insipidus:* A hundred years ago or more, a physician would see a patient with polyuria and polydipsia and would taste his urine to see if it was tasteless or sweet.

- The Greek word "diabetes" means siphon or excessive discharge of urine.
- The Greek word "insipidus" means tasteless.

When a patient had polyuria, the only way to figure it out was to taste the urine. Fortunately for us today, we have urine dipsticks that can tell us what the specific gravity of the urine is, and if there is glucose in the urine.

Recall that specific gravity as it relates to urine has to do with the number of particles in the fluid. The specific gravity of water is 1.000 (no particles in the fluid); a high specific gravity is > 1.030 indicating many particles in the fluid.

- If the patient has polyuria and the specific gravity is 1.002, he likely has DI.
- If the patient has polyuria and the specific gravity is 1.030, he likely has DM.
- It also helps to know if there is glucosuria, which the dip will also tell you.

ADH was put in our bodies to preserve extracellular fluid volume (like aldosterone, and angiotensin). If the body is dehydrated, or if there is decreased perfusion to the brain, ADH is secreted; and the renal Loop of Henle will retain water and send it back to the body to perfuse the brain.

- In diabetes insipidus, there is no ADH.
- Head trauma, anoxia or brain surgery may damage the posterior pituitary and no ADH is secreted.

So, what happens when there is no ADH secretion?

Answer: The body loses water. The patient has polyuria. This makes the patient have polydipsia, (if the patient is alert and awake, that is). If the patient is unconscious, the patient will be losing water, and become hypernatremic.

In addition, there are two types of DI:

- Central DI, due to lack of ADH as discussed above
- Nephrogenic DI due to lithium therapy in which ADH is produced, but the renal tubule "ignores" it.

Diabetes Insipidus

- *Etiology/Epidemiology*
  - Central DI = Due to head trauma; anoxia; surgery
  - Nephrogenic DI = Lithium
- *H & P*
  - Polyuria/Polydipsia
- *Diagnostics*
  - Urine is very dilute (like water) with specific gravity of < 1.005
  - No glucose in urine; and normal serum glucose
  - Hypernatremia (if the patient is unable to drink extra water)
  - Desmopressin (DDAVP) is given intranasally or I.V. to see if urine output goes down
    - This is a clinical diagnosis - you cannot do a serum ADH (cannot measure it directly)
- *Clinical intervention*
  - Water replacement (I & O's)
  - Stop Lithium (if patient has nephrogenic DI due to it) and change to a different medication
- *Therapeutics*
  - I.V. DDAVP drip, or scheduled nasal spray
- *Health Maintenance*
  - Maintain adequate fluid intake

The Adrenal Gland

Cushing's Syndrome

- *Etiology*
    - Latrogenic
        - Due to giving the patient cortisone for extended period of time (exogenous excess steroid)
- *H & P*
    - Looks just like any other "cushingoid" patient – you cannot tell the difference from looking at the patient
        - Moon facies
        - Supraclavicular fat pads
        - Dorsal fat pad (buffalo hump)
        - Truncal obesity
        - Purple striae
        - Hyperglycemia/glucose intolerance
        - Hypertension
        - Dyslipidemia
- *Diagnostics*
    - None needed if you know the patient is on steroids
- *Clinical intervention*
    - None if the patient needs the full replacement dose, nothing much you can do about it - if on excess doses, wean slowly
- *Health Maintenance*
    - Stress dosing is necessary if the patient is ill, febrile, has traumatic injury, etc.
- *Scientific Concepts*
    - This is the most common cause of Cushing Syndrome (*not Cushing Disease)* in the U.S.

Cushing Disease (Pituitary Adenoma)

- *Etiology/Epidemiology*
    - This is the most common *endocrine* cause of cortisol excess.
    - It is a secondary endocrine disorder, i.e., it is *not* due to an adrenal problem.
- *H & P*
    - The same as all "cushingoid" patients – memorize that list above
- *Diagnostics*
    - Recall one of my basic tenets --- If you are looking for cortisol excess, order the suppression test.
    - Overnight dexamethasone suppression test
    - 24 hour urine free cortisol *or*
    - Late night salivary cortisol (should be low late at night, that's why you sleep ☺)
- *Clinical intervention*

- MRI is best, CT if the patient cannot have MRI, even plain film could be done, but not best test
- Surgical removal

- *Therapeutics*
  - Cortisone replacement if removal damages pituitary (check ACTH levels)
- *Health Maintenance*
  - Lifelong replacement; stress dosing; medic alert bracelet
- *Scientific Concepts*
  - This is the most common cause of primary adrenal excess. (in patients not on steroids)

Adrenal Adenoma

- *Etiology/Epidemiology*
  - "Incidentaloma"
  - Discovered incidentally on an imaging study looking for something else
  - Most commonly occurs in adults
    - Usually a common benign tumor
    - Not considered to have the potential for malignant transformation
  - But must r/o potential metastatic tumor
- *H & P*
  - Asymptomatic
- *Diagnostics*
  - Further imaging is needed to r/o malignancy
- *Clinical Intervention*
  - Nonfunctional adrenal cortical adenomas are not premalignant, and surgical excision is not indicated.
  - If hormonally active, adrenal tumor surgery is necessary.
  - The treatment for a malignancy depends on the cell type, spread, and location of the primary tumor.

Corticoadrenal Insufficiency (*Acute* Adrenal Crisis)

- *Epidemiology*
  - Common *in those who are dependent on steroids*
- *H & P* – vague symptoms
  - Vomiting, diarrhea
  - Hypotension
  - Fatigue
- *Therapeutics*
  - Hydrocortisone IV if needed, PO if stable
- *Health Maintenance*
  - Patient must have medic alert bracelet that states they are cortisone dependent.
  - They must be educated about the need to seek attention immediately if unable to take their usual PO dose.

  - They must be educated about "stress dosing", i.e. increasing their dosage if they become ill, or performing heavy physical exertion.

Corticoadrenal Insufficiency (Chronic Adrenal Insufficiency, i.e., Addison's Disease)

- *Etiology/Epidemiology*
  - Uncommon
  - Autoimmune destruction of the entire adrenal glad
- *H & P*
  - Vague symptoms as above, but insidious in onset
  - Chronically increased ACTH causes hyperpigmentation
  - Gingival mucosa and hard palate, then palms and soles, then general skin
- *Diagnostics*
  - Low plasma cortisol at 8 a.m. is diagnostic
  - Get a cosyntropin (synthetic ACTH) stimulation test
    - It will not stimulate the adrenals (because they are dead!)
- *Therapeutics*
  - Cortisone replacement therapy
    - Hydrocortisone is the drug of choice.
      - Two divided doses (2/3 in a.m., 1/3 in p.m.)
  - Fludrocortisone acetate for sodium retention
    - Usually only given in patients with postural hypotension
    - Most of us get more sodium in our diets than we need
- *Health Maintenance*
  - Medic alert bracelet warning of dependence on cortisol
  - Stress dosing for this patient should he/she become ill, febrile, have trauma, etc.

PEARL: *ACTH causes melanocyte production, hence the hyperpigmentation.*

  - Hyperpigmentation is first noticeable on the gingiva, hard palate, then palms and soles

- *Loss of adrenal function includes the mineralocorticoid function, i.e. Aldosterone*
  - Angiotensin II is responsible for the release of aldosterone.
  - Aldosterone is secreted in response to the kidneys sensing 'decreased perfusion', whether that is really true or just perceived as true, i.e. in a lousy heart pump, there may be plenty of fluid, it just isn't getting to the kidneys.
  - Aldosterone causes the renal tubules to hold *sodium*, because "where sodium goes, so goes water".
    - If your kidneys are not getting enough fluid, the assumption is that extracellular fluid volume (ECF) is decreased, and the human needs more fluid, and more sodium.
- *Sometimes, that cannot be farther from the truth:*
  - Remember Mr. Jones, my sausage eating, beer drinking man with EF < 20%?
  - His kidneys are underperfused, but he certainly does not need more sodium or water.

- This system has been in place for millions of years, and has not adapted to our new lifestyles yet.

If aldosterone is there to make our caveperson retain sodium during a period of drought, and no salt licks are available, what happens if our caveperson has loss of aldosterone production due to Addison's disease?

Answer: He loses sodium – it is lost in the urine, and volume will go down.

Discussion: The truth about the U.S. of A. is that most of us get 10 times more sodium than a body needs, so many patients with Addison's do not need fludricortisone to maintain sodium balance. Someone on a Na restricted diet due to CHF might however.

Primary Hyperaldosteronism (Conn syndrome)

- *Epidemiology*
    - Not common
    - But most common cause of refractory hypertension (a secondary hypertension cause) in youth and middle-aged adults
        - May be as high as 20%
- *H & P*
    - Hypertension
    - Retention of sodium
    - Therefore retention of water
    - Therefore hypertension
- *Labs & Diagnostics*
    - Electrolyte panel
        - *The hallmark is hypertension in the setting of high sodium and low potassium*
    - Elevated plasma aldosterone and urine aldosterone
    - Low plasma renin levels
    - CT of abdomen
- *Clinical Intervention*
    - Laparoscopic adrenalectomy (if single tumor)
    - If hyperplasia of both adrenals
        - Spironolactone or eplerenone
- *Scientific Concepts*
    - Uncommon cause of secondary hypertension

Pheochromocytoma

- *Epidemiology*
  - Rare incidence
  - Occurs in some autosomal dominant syndromes
    - MEN 2 (*multiple endocrine neoplasia)* – not in blueprint
- *H & P*
  - "Classic" Presentation = Paroxysms of:
    - Headache
    - Palpitations
    - Diaphoresis
    - Severe hypertension
    - Hyperdynamic PMI (increased contractility of heart)
    - Cardiac dysrhythmias (a fib, V tach)
    - Pulmonary edema, dilated myopathy
  - Can cause hypertensive crisis
  - *No exophthalmos*, if eye symptoms are present, choose Grave's disease!
- *Diagnostics*
  - Plasma metanephrine testing has sensitivity of 96%, but lower specificity (85%) than:
  - 24-hour urine collection for catecholamines and metanephrines (87% sens; 99.7% spec)
  - MRI is preferred (almost 100% sensitivity)
  - CT *only done if above is positive* (85%) and MRI not able to be performed
- *Clinical intervention*
  - Surgical resection
  - Pre-op treatment with BOTH alpha blockers AND beta blockers (to block both parts of the sympathetic nervous system)
- *Therapeutics*
  - Alpha blockers (started 7-10 days before surgery)
  - Beta blockers (started after appropriate alpha blockade)
  - Fluid expansion with liberal salt prior to surgery
- *Health Maintenance*
  - Plasma metanephrines 2 weeks post op = should be in reference range yearly for 5 years
  - BP monitoring
- *Scientific Concepts*
  - Catecholamine secreting tumor, usually in adrenal gland (90%), but can be elsewhere (98% in abdomen)
  - 10% are malignant
  - Secretes both epinephrine and norepinephrine

Adrenal Cancer

- *Epidemiology*
  - Incredibly rare, so I am surprised this is in the blueprint, but pheochromocytoma is not!
  - 1 per million
  - Very aggressive
  - Bimodal occurrence
    - Children < 5 years
    - Adults 30-40 years
- Very hormonally active tumor causing
  - Cushing syndrome
  - Conn syndrome
  - Virilization
    - Clitoromegaly in a female infant is suspect (but can be normal too)

The Thyroid Glands

Hyperthyroidism

- *Epidemiology*
  - Grave's disease is most common cause of hyperthyroidism- 80%
  - Women>men, 10:1
  - Peak incidence 20-40 years
- *Etiology*
  - This is a *primary* endocrine disease – the thyroid is the problem
  - Autoimmune disorder
- *H & P*
  - *Exophthalmos* is pathognomonic for Grave's disease
  - Diffuse goiter
  - Weight loss
  - Sweating
  - Heat intolerance
  - Palpitations, tachycardia, hypertension
  - High output congestive heart failure
    POsteopenia
  - psychiatric presentation of panic disorder, panic attacks, psychosis
- *Diagnostics*
  - High FT4 (free T4), therefore a low TSH (high FT4 feeds back to pituitary and shuts off TSH)
  - Thyroid-stimulating immunoglobulin, anti-thyroid peroxidase (anti-TPO) and antithyroglobulin (anti-TG)

- *Clinical intervention*
    - For exophthalmos – ophthalmology referral and maintenance – lubrication and patching
- *Therapeutics*
    - Propranolol is the drug of choice for the cardiac manifestations *(except in patients with asthma).*
        - It decreases peripheral conversion of T3 to T4 in tissue
        - It also functions like any other BB to lower HR and BP
    - Radioactive iodine
        - Effective, safe, but slow in response (sometimes PTU or methimazole are used until response)
        - Destroys the thyroid, hypothyroidism is the expected goal of therapy
        - *Category X in pregnancy and lactation– DO NOT EVER USE*
        - *Avoid in patients with exophthalmos, worsens it especially in smokers*
    - PTU (propylthiouracil) has been used since 1940's and is the drug of choice in first trimester pregnancy
        - Please note that *both PTU and pregnancy begin with the letter "p"*
        - After 12 weeks, switch to methimazole
    - Methimazole – safer than PTU in patients who are not going to have iodine but not in first trimester of pregnancy
        - Often used to control symptoms until iodine can be done
        - Side effect = agranulocytosis (present with fever and sore throat) and liver injury
    - Thyroidectomy
        - Reserved for special cases, rarely used anymore
        - Most common SE is hypoparathyroidism (from inadvertent destruction of the parathyroids during thyroid removal)
- *Health Maintenance*
    - Once controlled on levothyroxine at TSH around 1-2, yearly TSH, FT4 checks should be done.
- *Scientific Concepts*
    - Exophthalmos is pathognomonic for Grave's – protein deposits behind the eyeball in the orbit and forces the globe forward, the eyelid no longer closes around the protruding globe (proptosis); surgical correction removing the eye, scraping out protein, and putting it back is possible, but not usually selected by the patient as treatement
    - Radioactive iodine, a very good treatment for Grave's, may significantly worsen exophthalmos.
    - Atrial fibrillation with a rapid ventricular response occurring in a young woman (without cardiac disease) is Grave's disease until proven otherwise.

Thyrotoxicosis (Subacute Thyroiditis)

- *Etiology*
    - Viral damage causes release of preformed thyroid hormone from the thyroid.
    - Common postpartum
- *H & P*
    - Same symptoms as Grave's disease
    - *No* exophthalmos (only in Grave's disease)
- *Diagnostics*
    - TSH, reflex FT4
- *Clinical intervention*
    - Observation
    - Sometimes it is self-limited, sometimes results in Grave's and sometimes in hypothyroidism

Hypothyroidism (Hashimoto's)

- *Etiology/Epidemiology*
    - Autoimmune; female:male 9:1
- *H & P*
- *Diagnostics*
    - FT4 (free T4) would be low (it's HYPOthyroidism)
    - Therefore, TSH would be high
- *Therapeutics*
    - Levothyroxine
    - The only Category A drug in the U.S. in pregnant and nursing women
    - <u>In patients with good cardiac function:</u>
        - Start full replacement dose (0.10; 0.112; 0.125) in healthy adult
            - *Wait 6 weeks, recheck TSH*
    - <u>In patients with poor cardiac function:</u>
        - Start low and titrate up, once or twice a week, until you get to 0.10,
        - Then wait 6 weeks and recheck TSH
        - To prevent high output cardiac failure
- *Health Maintenance*
    - Levothyroxine should be taken on an *empty* stomach
    - Yearly TSH; needs change with aging/ weight gain/ etc.
- *Scientific Concepts*
    - Hashimoto's is most common cause of hypothyroidism in US.
    - Iodine deficiency is most common cause worldwide.

Thyroid Cancer

- *Etiology/Epidemiology*
  - Relatively low incidence overall
  - Mean age 50 – more common in women
  - Risk factor – radiation to head and neck
    - Radiologists and radiology techs before neck shielding
    - Patient with external radiation (squamous cell, laryngeal, Hodgkins or other lymphomas, skin cancer treatment)
- *H & P*
  - *Painless* palpable solitary nodule
  - Always presume cancer until evaluated
- *Diagnostics*
  - Fine needle aspirate biopsy (FNA)
- *Clinical intervention*
  - Surgical
  - Thyroidectomy
  - Iodine ablation to destroy remainder of gland
  - Over suppressive doses of levothyroxine to suppress thyroid function
- *Therapeutics*
  - Levothyroxine
- *Health Maintenance*
  - Yearly thyroid exam
  - Daily thyroid medication
- *Scientific Concepts*
  - *Papillary* cancer is most common (80%) and has the best prognosis.
  - Medullary less common, aggressive tumor
  - Oversuppressive thyroid maintenance increases risk of osteoporosis.
  - Thyroid replacement is the only Category A drug in the USA.

The Parathyroid Gland

PEARL: *Understanding parathyroid gland function:*

- The parathyroids do not "associate" with the pituitary or hypothalamus. (they take care of themselves)
- The four glands sitting on the thyroid sense the concentration of "free" calcium.
- If too low, the parathyroid secretes PTH (this is a quick response).
- If too high, the parathyroid will "shut off" PTH (also quickly).

<u>If the patient has low calcium (for any reason), PTH is secreted:</u>

- It stimulates osteoclast activity
    - Osteoclasts go to bone to get calcium and sends it into bloodstream...
    - (Remember that osteoporosis causes loss of *trabecular* bone (hip, pelvis, thoracic spine), and PTH causes loss of all bone including *cortical* bone (radius, ulna, tib, fib, and carpals and metacarpals)
- It causes the renal tubule to hold any calcium that arrives, and send it into bloodstream...
- It also causes the renal tubule to get rid of phosphorus (so it doesn't bind to calcium, therefore, would not be available for the action potential of the heart and the nervous system)
    - So, if you are low in calcium, you would now be resorbing your bone (bad); and holding calcium and dumping out phosphorus (good for the heart and nervous system). As soon as that calcium level gets to the normal range (use your pull down menu), then the PTH will *shut off*!

This is the premise for all parathyroid diseases. Read the above until you really understand it, then go on to the bullet pointed content topic areas for hyper- and hypo- parathyroidism.

Primary Hyperparathyroidism – *(the blueprint does not distinguish between primary and secondary, but I will...)*

- *Epidemiology*
    - Fairly common
    - Women > Men; generally > 50 y.o.
- *H & P*
    - Bones (from PTH being secreted all day long and resorbing bone = osteopenia)
    - Stones (from PTH making the kidney hold calcium = calcium oxalate stones)
    - Groans (from PTH increasing calcium which deposits in the pancreas and can cause pancreatitis)
    - Moans ("psychic moans" – I don't know what these are, but can cause somnolence and depression)
    - ****Most importantly, almost all patients are actually asymptomatic!**
- *Diagnostics*
    - *Hypercalcemia* – #1 sign of primary hyperparathyroidism
    - Hypophosphatemia
    - PTH (will be normal or high) <recall, this should be SHUT OFF)
- *Clinical intervention*
    - Surgical parathyroidectomy *(if indicated – see example Q below)*
- *Therapeutics*
    - Fluid hydration
    - Bisphosphonates will not "cure" this disease and has lots of side effects
- *Health Maintenance*
    - Monitor calcium levels
- *Scientific Concepts*

- This is a PRIMARY disorder – due to an adenoma on the gland that produces PTH all day long --- this is the most common cause of hypercalcemia
- Please distinguish this from *secondary* hyperparathyroidism (next topic)

PEARL: *Secondary* *Hyperparathyroidism* – I do not like this title, but no one asked me. As already discussed in the beginning of the chapter, secondary disorders occur when the problem is not actually in the gland.

- In this case, the problem is that the calcium is *low.*
- If the normal parathyroid gland is doing its job, it will secrete PTH.
- If that becomes a chronic issue, it will cause problems for the patient.
- This is termed "secondary hyperparathyroidism".
- *This is nothing like Primary Hyperparathyroidism.*

HYPOCALCEMIA

PEARL: *The most common cause of hypocalcemia is chronic renal failure.* When a patient has chronic renal failure, they often have hypoalbuminemia. Calcium is bound to albumin and when you obtain total calcium (on a CMP, for example), it is this "bound" calcium level that you get. Therefore, the calcium must be "corrected" for the patient's albumin level (there's an app for that!)

The most common cause of hypoparathyroidism (which does, incidentally cause hypocalcemia, but is incredibly rare) is inadvertent destruction of the parathyroids during thyroidectomy.
Which is more common, renal failure or thyroidectomy? Yep – renal failure.
So, here is a tricky question:

If the patient has renal failure, and because of that, develops hypocalcemia, will the PTH be high or low?

Answer: The PTH should be high (stimulating osteoclasts to go get some calcium from the patient's bone). They call this "secondary hyperparathyroidism":

Secondary Hyperparathyroidism

- *Etiology*
  - Most common cause is *chronic renal failure*
- *H & P*
  - Due to hypocalcemia
  - Twitching/spasms/tingling

  - Chvostek's (tap cheek and spasm occurs)
  - Trousseaus's sign (pump up BP cuff and carpal spasm occurs)

- *Diagnostics*
  - Hypocalcemia *(so cannot be primary hyperparathyroidism!)*
  - High phosphorus (CRF patients have trouble getting rid of phosphorus anyway, but if no calcium to bind to, the phosphorus level is really high)
  - High PTH
- *Clinical intervention*
  - Treat the renal disease
- *Therapeutics*
  - Vitamin D analogues
  - Phosphate binders
  - Calcimimetics (cinacalcet)
- *Health Maintenance*
  - Manage your diabetics and hypertensives to prevent them from developing CRF!

If the patient has hypoparathyroidism because of inadvertent destruction of the parathyroids, his calcium will be low. What will his PTH be?

Answer: it will be low, because he has no functioning parathyroids at all!
Be very careful on the test to read the words carefully, hypocalcemia and hypoparathyroidism are due to completely different etiologies.

Diabetes

Type 1 Diabetes Mellitus

- *Etiology/Epidemiology*
  - Immune mediated
  - Pancreatic B cell destruction
  - Peak in children and young adults
- *H & P*
  - Polyuria/polydipsia/polyphagia with weight loss with random BS > 200 mg/dL
  - FBS >126 mg/dL on two occasions
  - Most kids present in DKA with an acute infection
  - Hgb A1c is still controversial in diagnosis (patient may be too early in course)
- *Diagnostics*
  - As above
  - Serum ketones and urine ketones are present
    - Due to fat metabolism
    - The sugar is out in the serum instead of in the cell

        - The cell utilizes fat for fuel, metabolic breakdown product of fat is ketoacids
- *Clinical intervention*
    - Insulin & fluids
    - *see PEARL below for management of DKA*
- *Therapeutics*
    - <u>Insulin</u>
        - Regular
        - Rapid acting insulin analogues
        - Long-acting insulins
        - NPH
        - Insulin glargine (Lantus)
        - Insulin detemir (Levemir)
- *Health Maintenance*
    - Dilated eye exam every year
    - Microalbumin (or creatinine: albumin ratio) every year

PEARL: *Diabetic Ketoacidosis*

A child with Type I DM does not develop that disease suddenly, even though it often appears that way. Autoimmune destruction of the pancreatic islet B cells takes weeks and months to occur. While this is happening, the child has polyuria and polydipsia, and is losing weight despite having polyphagia. This is because as his islet cells die, insulin decreases. Insulin is needed to carry glucose to the cell for fuel. It also is used to carry potassium into the cell where it is utilized. The glucose levels in serum are slowly increasing and the cells have no glucose for fuel. They breakdown fat for fuel instead; the breakdown product of fat is ketoacids (ketones). Therefore, the child is slowly developing hyperglycemia, ketosis, and hyperkalemia.

<u>When a child becomes ill, stressed, or has a traumatic injury, DKA occurs.</u>

- When one is ill for any reason (infection, stress, trauma), cortisol is secreted by the adrenal gland.
- Cortisol causes gluconeogenesis by the liver. This increases glucose levels to help cells fight the illness. The glucose is transported into the cell where it can be utilized.
- In the case of an ill diabetic, all this blood glucose remains in the blood due to the lack of insulin. The potassium also remains in serum due to lack of insulin.
- Ketones accumulate due to the body's need to utilize fat for fuel.
- The glucose in the serum causes an increase in osmolarity; as the body tries to get rid of the glucose, body water is lost and the patient becomes profoundly dehydrated.
- The diabetic is now in DKA.
- The ketoacids in the serum cause an acidic pH – a metabolic acidosis. The ketones create an anion gap.
- The lungs quickly respond by hyperventilating to blow off CO_2 (an acid) to try to normalize pH (this is called Kussmaul's respirations).

The treatment of DKA consists of fluids, insulin, and replacement of potassium *(if needed).*

Honeymoon phenomenon

A child with DKA and concomitant infection with very high blood sugars due to gluconeogenesis will receive treatment for the infection. The resolution of the infection will decrease cortisol and gluconeogenesis. The blood sugars will decrease due to treatment of the infection. In many cases, there are still some functioning pancreatic islet cells, and a "honeymoon" period can occur at the time of discharge from the hospital wherein the child does not need insulin for a short period of time.

Your clinical intervention is to be proactive in explaining this to parents so they do not believe you have made an incorrect diagnosis, and so that they understand that blood sugars must be checked regularly throughout the honeymoon period, as sugars will eventually climb again, and insulin will again be needed.

Type 2 Diabetes Mellitus

- *Etiology/Epidemiology*
  - Genetic & environmental
  - Both a relative decrease in insulin levels and
  - Decreased sensitivity to insulin in tissues
- *H & P*
  - *Asymptomatic* at the time ideally diagnosed
  - Retinopathy or neuropathy or renal disease may be presenting symptom
- *Diagnostics*
  - Hgb A1c approaching 6.5 needs therapeutic intervention
  - FBS ≥126 mg/dl on TWO separate occasions
  - 2 hour oral glucose test ≥ 200 mg/dl
  - Random BS ≥ 200 mg/dl with symptoms
- *Clinical intervention*
  - Behavior modification
    - Weight loss; exercise; stop smoking; manage lipids
  - Formal dietary instruction
- *Therapeutics*
  - Oral hypoglycemic agents
    - <u>Secretagogues</u>
      - Sulfonylureas
      - Glyburide & glipizide
  - Reduces insulin resistance in tissue
    - <u>Biguanides</u>
      - Metformin
  - Activates PPAR which increases insulin sensitivity
    - <u>TZDs (thiazolidinediones)</u>
      - Rosiglitazone & pioglitazone

        - **Rosiglitazone is no longer available as a new prescription since 9/2010. Patients who were already on it before then can remain on as long as they are informed and agree to be on it despite increased incidence of MI and death.*
    - Affect absorption of glucose
        - Acarbose & miglitol
    - Injectable Type 2 meds:
    - Incretin effects (incretin is good!) & boosts effects of insulin
        - Exenatide
        - Sitagliptin
    - Insulin – *see above in Type I*
- *Health Maintenance*
    - Lifestyle changes are superior to drug therapy in delaying onset of diabetes in patients with impaired glucose tolerance
    - Most have retinopathy and nephropathy already on presentation
    - Need dilated optho exam every year (or sooner if retinopathy)
    - If urine dip is positive in clinic for albumin, no need to do microalbumin (it's too late)
        - ACEI is indicated with positive albumin
    - If negative urine dip, microalbumin every year
- *Scientific Concepts*
    - The most common side effect of the oral hypoglycemic is – you guessed it! hypoglycemia.
        - The most common side effect of metformin is --- lactic acidosis, especially in patients with renal insufficiency
    - Type 2 diabetics can die of hyperosmolar nonketotic coma
        - Treatment is fluids, fluids, fluids and insulin

Hypoglycemia

- *Etiology/Epidemiology*
    - < 50 mg/dL is generally considered the threshold, although some patients report "symptoms" higher than that
    - Oral hypoglycemic drugs
    - Insulin
    - Idiopathic (alcohol intoxication, other drugs)
- *H & P*
    - Early warning symptoms are usually related to sympathetic activation
        - Diaphoresis
        - Palpitations
        - Tremors
        - Anxiety
        - Hunger
    - If not treated more severe symptoms develop
        - Confusion

        - Irritability
        - Hallucinations
        - Hemiplegia
        - Slurred speech
        - Coma/death
- *Diagnostics*
    - "Whipple" Triad =
        - Low blood sugar (documented)
        - Symptoms
        - Asymptomatic after treatment and BS normal
- *Clinical intervention*
    - Oral replacement of sugar is best
        - Followed by normal diet
    - If patient is unconscious and no IV established, give IM glucagon
    - If IV in place, give D50 (50% dextrose)
- *Scientific Concepts*
    - Beta blockers mask hypoglycemic symptoms in diabetics
    - Consider hypoglycemia in all patients who are diabetic with altered mental status (or who appear drunk)
    - All diabetics who are unconscious
    - Do not wait for a blood sugar; get IV access or give glucagon

PEARL: *ALL patients presenting with altered mental status need blood sugar done STAT. EMS will do one in the field in anyone who appears altered, drunk, under the influence of drugs, even without a diagnosis of diabetes.*

CHAPTER 20

Dermatology – 5%

Introduction to Dermatology Chapter

- *See therapeutic section at end of this chapter for drug information*
- *See Therapeutics chapter 4 for additional antimicrobial and antifungal information*
- *See Physical Exam Chapter 5 for more information on the dermatologic exam*
- *See the Labs & Diagnostics Chapter 6 for more information on diagnostic testing*

Rather than pictures, most dermatologic questions on a standardized exam will involve descriptions of lesions. For this reason, I am categorizing the content topics in derm according to their morphologic characteristics, the characteristic symptom associated with the rash, the characteristic morphology of the individual lesions, or the characteristic distribution of the rash that distinguishes each from the other. This allows you multiple ways to creat a differential diagnosis for each basic descriptive lesion, and then the specific "buzz words" that help you narrow to the "most likely" diagnosis.

PEARL: *To get dermatology questions correct quickly and easily:*

- Let the KOH guide you!
- Nummular eczema looks just like ringworm (tinea corporis)
    - If KOH is positive, give an antifungal, it is tinea.
    - If KOH is negative, give a steroid cream, it is eczema.
- Constitutional symptoms
    - *Is there a fever? Is the rash painful?*
        - Bacterial infection or viral exanthema are likely
        - Impetigo, erysipelas, cellulitis, herpes ulcers
    - *Is it itchy?*
        - Allergic, atopic
        - Poison ivy, eczema, urticaria
- Duration of rash
    - *If acute*
        - Bacterial infection or viral exanthema
        - Acute allergic or contact allergy
    - *If chronic*
        - Think all those chronic causes of rash
            - Tinea, dermatophytes, autoimmune diseases

- Distribution
  - *Sun exposed areas of body*
    - Drug reaction, lupus, malignancies
  - *Palms & soles*
    - Syphilis, Kawasaki's
  - *Specific locations (around neck, tummy)*
    - Nickle allergy, contact dermatitis
  - *Web spaces*
    - Scabies
- Benign vs. malignant
  - *Remember, benign lesions usually hurt.*
    - Canker sores, herpes zoster, herpes simplex, pimples
  - *Malignan lesions are typically painless, chronic and nonhealing.*
    - Look for "sun" as a risk factor, also "smoking"
    - Chronic nonhealing ulcer = cancer

Diagnosis by Symptoms

ITCHING- PRURITIC LESIONS

Eczema – Atopic Dermatitis

- *Cheeks on baby*
- *Antecubital fossa and popliteal fossa on older kids and adults*
  - KOH scraping is negative/ history of allergies, asthma
- *Treatment*
  - Corticosteroids
    - Use high potency only on thick areas (elbows, lichenified skin)
    - Very low potency on baby face, adult eyelids

Contact Dermatitis – *Treat with avoidance & Corticosteroid cream*

- *Poison Ivy – Rhus Dermatitis*
  - History of gardening or being outside
  - Linear scratches, blisters, severe itching
    - Only on exposed skin
- *Nickel Allergy*
  - Ear lobes (earrings)
  - Neck ringed rash (necklace)
  - Round circle on tummy (snap on pants)
- *Latex allergy*
  - Glove distribution (or shoe distribution)
  - Or where touched with latex
- *Treatment*
  - Corticosteroids

Fungal Infections

Distinguished by positive KOH scraping (positive for tinea, negative for eczema)

- Tinea Corporis – *Ringworm (looks exactly like nummular eczema)*
    - Treat with topical antifungal cream.
- Tinea Cruris – *Intertriginous zones (folds of groin, under pannus, under breasts, in axilla)*
    - Treat with topical antifungal cream.
- Tinea Capitus – *Scalp – Usually kids –*
    - "Kerion" is secondarily infected – needs antibiotics to cover staph and strep
    - Capitus must be treated with *oral griseofulvin.*

Lichen Simplex Chronicus

- *Unknown Etiology*
    - Hallmark is itching
    - Chronic thickening of the skin from scratching
- *KOH is negative – biopsy may be needed*

Lichen planus *(See below in Papules)*

- *The 5 P's*
    - Papules that are pruritic, purple, planar (flat-topped) and polygonal

Dyshidrosis

- *Tapioca blisters – webs of fingers and toes*

Lice, Scabies, Pinworms

- Covered individually below
- All itch like crazy!

PUPPP *(Pruritic Urticarial Papules and Plaques of Pregnancy)*

- on pregnant belly, buttocks, upper thighs, sometimes chest (not extremities, face, neck)
- pregnancy is the clue here!

Painful Rashes

NON-INFECTIOUS

Diaper Dermatitis

- Not yeast, not cellulitis
- This is from the urine causing irritation to the skin
- *Not* in the folds (that is yeast), will be on the chubbier parts, like the buttock and the thighs
- Treat with avoidance; frequent changes; occlusive ointment (Vaseline or desitin).

INFECTIOUS

Bacterial infections

Impetigo

- Honey colored crusts and erosions, tender, around nares and mouth; can be spread to body

Cellulitis

- Infection in deep dermis and subcutaneous fat layers
- Pink in color; mild discomfort
- Diffuse, unclear borders

Erysipelas

- Infection in superficial dermis and lymphatic system
- Bright red rash; extremely tender; usually on face and neck
- Very red, well demarcated borders
- Slightly raised

Hidradenitis Suppurativa

- Bacterial infection (skin flora) in inguinal and axillary sweat glands
- Abscess formation - needs I & D

Viral Infections

Herpes Simplex

- Oral or genital (little distinction any more)
- Vesicles, leading to ulcers, extremely painful
    - Located in areas, but not unilateral presentation as zoster
- When in the mouth, typical pattern of gingival ulcers ringing the whole mouth
- Pain only of blister, not in dermatome area
- Often fever, malaise if first occurrence
- Treatment
    - Acyclovir, Valacyclovir

Shingles (Herpes Zoster)

- Viral infection
    - Reactivation of varicella virus
- Vesicles in clusters on erythematous skin
    - Dermatome distribution
- Painful even in skin areas that are not blistered
- Must have had chicken pox to have zoster
- Treatment
    - Acyclovir, Valacyclovir
    - Higher doses than for HSV (simplex)

Diagnosis by Morphology

ACNEIFORM LESIONS (PUSTULES ARE PRESENT)

Acne Vulgaris (Teens and Young Adults) – *We all know what this looks like*

- Start with topicals drying agents (benzoyl peroxide)
- Then move to topical antibiotics
- Then oral antibiotics (minocycline)
- Then to isotretinoin (Category X in pregnancy)

Rosacea (Middle Aged Adults) – *Looks like the lupus "rash" over nose and cheeks*

- Treat with topical metronidazole (yep – Flagyl, but topical cream instead of vaginal)

Perioral Dermatitis

- Women
- Due to steroid use (anywhere on face) causes pimples around the mouth
- Stop the steroid !
- Can use topical metronidazole or topical erythromycin

PAPULAR LESIONS

Lichen Planus

- Five P's
- Planar (flat), pruritic, polyganol, purple, papules

PUPPP

- Pruritic urticarial pupules and plaques of pregnancy
- Pregnancy is the clue here!

SCALING LESIONS

Seborrheic Dermatitis

- Dandruff of the eyelids, eyebrows and scalp, mild erythema and scale
- Not itchy
- Treat like a dermatophyte with selsun blue (sulfur based shampoo)

Pityriasis Rosea

- Salmon colored oval patches with scaling in a Christmas tree distribution
- Look for buzz word "herald patch"
    - Which appears a few days before the rash

- No treatment (self-limited)
- *If sexually active, rules out secondary syphilis*

Psoriasis

- Purple plaques with a silvery scale on extensor surfaces, scalp, trunk
- Auschwitz's sign
    - Bleeding occurs when you pick off the scale from the plaque
- Koebner phenomenon
    - Any minor epidermal scratch causes "papules" along the scratch line (also seen in lichen planus)

DESQUAMATION- LOSS OF EPIDERMIS

Kawasaki's Disease *(Mucocutaneous Lymph Node Syndrome)*

- *(See also CV peds)*
- *Epidemiology*
    - Uncommon
    - Idiopathic (viral??) probably autoimmune
    - Occurs in children < 5 y.o.
    - Usually self-limited and mild course, but major complications rarely
    - Major complication is coronary artery vasculitis
    - Can cause a heart attack (in a 3 year old!!)
    - Can destroy the vessels in the heart
- *H & P*
    - High fever for one to two weeks or longer
        - (Does not respond to treatment with Tylenol or ibuprofen)
    - Rash on trunk
    - Swollen lips and throat ("strawberry tongue")
    - Swollen lymph nodes
    - Peeling hands and feet
- *Labs & Diagnostics*
    - Clinical diagnosis – no specific lab test
- *Clinical Intervention*
    - Hospitalize
    - Cardiology consult/ Rheumatology consult/ ID consult
- *Therapeutics*
    - IV immunoglobulin
    - Aspirin
- *Scientific concept:*
    - <u>To make the diagnosis clinically you need:</u>
        - Five days of high fever *plus* four of the following:
            - Red lips, strawberry tongue
            - Conjunctivitis
            - Adenopathy
            - Rash on trunk
            - Desquamation of hand
    - Strawberry tongue is seen also in Scarlet Fever (group A strep)

- Difference is:
  - Kawasaki – strawberry tongue; conjunctivitis; bloody blistered lips
  - Scarlet fever – strawberry tongue; exudative tonsillitis, cirumoral pallor, sandpaper rash

PEARL:

- Erythema multiforme (EM)
- Stevens-Johnson Syndrome (SJS)
- Toxic Epidermal Necrolysis (TEN)

It is thought that these are all on the same spectrum of hypersensitivity reactions, but in lesser to greater degrees across the continuum.

Many authors believe that SJS; also known as erythema multiforme major is a manifestation of the same process involved in TEN, with the latter involving more extensive necrotic epidermal detachment. TEN involves more than 30% of the body surface, whereas SJS involves less than 10%.

TEN is a clinical diagnosis, confirmed by histopathologic analysis of lesional skin. The mainstay of treatment is supportive care until the epithelium regenerates. Early transfer of patients to a burn or intensive care unit has been shown to reduce the risk of infection, mortality rate, and length of hospitalization.

Erythema Multiforme

- Target lesions
- No desquamation of skin in EM minor
- Desquamation in EM major (then it is called Stevens-Johnson syndrome)
- Rarely due to anything but a drug (see below)
  - Most often due to drugs
    - PCN
    - Sulfa
    - Tetracyclines
    - Phenytoin
  - Recurrent HSV infection – have never seen it
  - Mycoplasma pneumonia – I have seen two cases

Minor
No prodrome
centripetal spread
Major
Prodrome in 50%
Acral to central spread

Stevens-Johnson Syndrome

- EM major
- Almost always due to a drug
  - < 10% of body surface area desquamation
  - Most commonly begins on lips/hands

Toxic Epidermal Necrolysis

- Potentially life-threatening

- Widespread erythema, necrosis, and bullous detachment of the epidermis and mucous membranes, (> 30% body surface area)
- Mucous membrane involvement can result in gastrointestinal hemorrhage, respiratory failure, ocular abnormalities, and genitourinary complications

VESICULAR BULLAE

Bullous Pemphigoid

- Autoimmune relatively benign itchy small blisters
- Negative Nikolskys' sign (see below)
- Much milder form similar to pemphigus vulgaris (below)

Pemphigus Vulgaris

- Loss of the connection between the epidermis and dermis so the top layer of skin "slides off"
- Nikolsky's sign i= rubbing the skin and having the epidermis come right off
- Treated with immunosuppressives, i.e. methotrexate

Pigmentation Abnormalities - *(Macular Lesions)*

- Change in color of "normal" skin
- No itching, no pain, no symptoms except pigment change

Vitiligo

- Complete loss of pigment – no known etiology – autoimmune?

Tinea versicolor – *(this is not Vitiligo)*

- This is a change in the color of the skin
- Not complete loss of pigment due to a skin fungus which "coats" the skin and doesn't allow sun to cause tanning
- Symmetrical and uniform
- Treat with sulfur lotion (selsun blue shampoo)

Café au Lait Spots

- Hyperpigmented macule (can't palpate it)
- If many spots – think Neurofibromatosis
  - 95% incidence if many spots

Melasma/Chloasma

- Hyperpigmented macules on cheeks and upper lips in sun exposed areas
- Women on birth control pills, and pregnant women

Phytophotodermatitis

- Photo is the clue --- sun sensitivity
- Usually due to oral or topical drug (Bactrim, Cipro, Flagyl, Doxycycline are most common)

- Can also occur after a primary insult to skin (i.e. sun reaction after poison ivy)

Diagnosis by Specific Distribution Patterns

HAIR AND NAILS

- Alopecia areata
- Androgenetic alopecia
- Kerion (tinea capitus)
- Onycomycosis
- Paronychia

FACE

- Perioral dermatitis
- Rosacea
- Erysipelas (more commonly face, neck, ears – but can be elsewhere)
- Vitiligo (eventually involves bigger area)

TRUNK

- Pityriasis
- Secondary Syphilis *(also involves PALMS & SOLES)*

GROIN

- Tinea cruris
- Hidradenitis suppurativa

PRESSURE POINTS

- Decubitus ulcers (pressure ulcers)

VIRAL INFECTIONS

A viral exanthem is any kind of rash that occurs in the setting of a viral infection.

Herpes Simplex

- Painful discrete vesicles which ulcerate on an erythematous base
- Mainly genital or oral

Varicella-Zoster Virus Infections – Zoster

- Painful patches of vesicles in a dermatome distribution, pain can precede the blisters

Molluscum contagiosum

- Umbilicated papules on kids can be anywhere
- On sexually active adults, in groin area

Verrucae

- Warts due to HPV
- Can be plantar and palmar
- All treated with freezing, or topical TCA, duct tape --or time

Condyloma acuminatum

- Due to HPV 6,11
- Benign check
- Treat as for any warts, 6 & 11 do not cause cancer
- Cervix for 16, 18 (just in case)

BACTERIAL INFECTIONS

Painful not itchy helps to distinguish these:

Folliculitis

- Can be staph from a dirty razor
- Axillae, groin, beard
  - Treat for staph with cephalexin or Dicloxacillin
- If all over the body and the patient was anywhere near water, think pseudomonas
  - And treat with ciprofloxacin

Impetigo

- Honey colored crusts and erosions, tender, around nares and mouth; can be spread to body

Cellulitis

- Infection in deep dermis and subcutaneous fat layers
- Pink in color; mild discomfort
- Diffuse, unclear borders

Erysipelas

- Infection in superficial dermis and lymphatic system
- Bright red rash; extremely tender; usually on face and neck
- Very red, well demarcated borders
- Slightly raised

Hidradenitis Suppurativa

- Bacterial infection (skin flora) in inguinal and axillary sweat glands

- Abscess formation - needs I & D

Decubitus ulcer

- *H & P*
  - Acute
    - High fevers
    - Pain
  - Chronic
    - Low grade fevers
    - +/- pain
- *Labs & Diagnostics*
  - Labs (CBC, CMP, blood cultures)
  - Plain film (looking for bone loss, gas)
  - MR/CT/bone scan (any, all would be appropriate)
- *Most Likely Diagnosis – two criteria:*
  - Sterile probe easily enters wound to bone (no resistance)
  - Ulcer > 2 cm2
- *Clinical Intervention*
  - Surgical debridement
  - Antibiotics
- *Therapeutics*
  - Acute – ideally according to culture results
  - Chronic – Cipro 750 mg. BID x 8 weeks
- *Health Maintenance*
  - Wound care for decubitus ulcers
  - Aggressive treatment of wounds

Neoplasms

Remember these are all painless, and have been there a while! Sun is the risk factor for all!

Basal Cell Carcinoma

- Most common of the skin cancers
- Sun exposed areas (usually face, nose, cheeks)
- *H & P*
  - Pearly raised borders, usually circular lesion
  - Telangiectasias

Melanoma

- Most malignant of the skin cancers
- *H & P*
  - Back in males, legs in females, but can be any sun exposed areas
  - Rarely occurs in non-sun areas, like cervix, retina
- *ABCDE's*
  - **A**symmetry
  - **B**orders (irregular)

- **C**olor (variegated and dark)
- **D**iameter (>5-6 mm)
- **E**volution (changing)

Squamous Cell Carcinoma/Actinic Keratosis (AK)

- *AK is the precursor* – think of it as carcinoma in situ
  - Sun exposed areas
- *H & P*
  - Crusty, scaly, hyperkeratotic, painless lesions
- *Cannot distinguish from benign without biopsy*

OTHER

Seborrheic Keratosis

- *Epidemiology*
  - Most common of benign lesions
  - Old age (used to be called "old age barnacles" because of their "stuck-on" appearance
  - Not in areas of sun exposure – usually on the back, neck
  - Look at grandpa – he's got some!
- *Benign, no intervention needed*
- *Formulating the most likely diagnosis*
  - Distinguish it from melanoma, but these are discrete, "greasy" appearance, "stuck on"

Acanthosis nigricans

- Brown velvety stripe on back of neck or in pannus – may mean a variety of different problems
  - Diabetes mellitus is most common
  - Many different cancers
  - Medications

Burns

- *Etiologies*
  - Scald
  - Contact

- ○ Fire
- ○ Chemical
- ○ Electrical
- ○ Radiation

- *Burn Depth*
    - First Degree
        - Red skin
        - Painful
        - Treatment
            - Pain management
            - Emollients
    - Second Degree
        - Superficial partial thickness
            - Blisters
            - Usually no scar
        - Deep Partial Thickness
            - Thick Blisters
            - Scar Results
    - Third Degree
        - Full thickness
            - No bleeding
            - No pain
            - Skin Grafting
    - Fourth Degree
        - Involves fascia, muscle and bone
- *Estimating BSA*
    - Rule of 9's
        - 9% = Face and Neck (18% in a child)
        - 9% = Each UE is 9%
        - 18% = Anterior Trunk
        - 18% = Posterior Trunk
        - 18% = Each leg is 18%
        - 1% = Genitalia
        - (your palm is 1% as an estimate of BSA)
- *Clinical Intervention*
    - Major burns
        - Partial thickness > 25% BSA adult/>20% in child < 10 or adult > 50
        - Full thickness > 10% BSA
        - Involving face, ears, eyes, hands, feet
        - Involving caustic agent; electricity
        - Inhalation
        - Associated trauma
    - *Major burns need transfer to burn center*
- *Clinical Intervention*
    - Airway management
    - Cool skin
    - Parkland formula for fluid resuscitation

- Lactated Ringer solution (4 mL/kg/% TBSA burned) is administered intravenously in the first 24 hours, one half given in the first 8 hours, and the other half administered over the next 16 hours. Calculate fluid loss from the time of injury, and take into account the fluid administered by prehospital personnel for fluid replacement
- Over-replacement increases ARDS
  - Therefore, new push to use urine output as a guide instead

Lipoma

- *Description*
  - Benign tumor composed of adipose tissue
  - It is the most common form of soft tissue tumor
  - Usually movable, and are generally painless
  - Many lipomas are small (under one centimeter diameter) but can enlarge to sizes greater than six centimeters.
- *Epidemiology*
  - Commonly found in adults from 40 to 60 years of age
- *Clinical Intervention*
  - Do not need to be removed unless pain develops

Epithelial Inclusion Cysts

- *Epidemiology*
  - Most common of the cutaneous cysts
  - Usually in adults 40-60 years old
- *H & P*
  - Cyst of face, scalp, neck and trunk
  - Painless but frequently become infected
- *Clinicial Intervention*
  - None needed
  - If infected, then I & D is necessary
    - After I & D and resolution of infection
    - The cyst capsule itself must be removed, or it will recur

BUGS

Lice

- *Epidemiology*
  - Low socioeconomic conditions, but also the start of every school year
  - Parasites that live on the head, and body, at base of hair follicles
  - Easily seen by scratching off the "black dot" and watching it crawl away (eeew)
- *Treat with*
  - Permethrin (available OTC)

- Malathion lotion
  - Flammable (smokers, hair dryers, curling irons)
- Lindane (Kwell)
  - Issues with neurotoxicity
  - *Never* in infants or pregnant women

Scabies

- *Epidemiology*
  - Usually in patients in low socio-economic environments (but can be anyone)
  - Close contact is needed
- *H & P*
  - Itching and lesions develop 2-6 weeks after infestation.
  - That is why it is so contagious
  - Starts in web spaces of fingers and around waistband of underwear.
  - Very itchy
  - The mite burrows under the skin, causing little raised streaks that you can see.
  - The mite is not visible to the naked eye.
- *Treat with*
  - #1 - Permethrin cream
    - 2 months or older
    - Two applications, a week apart
  - Not recommended anymore --- Lindane (Kwell)
    - Neuroxocity issues
  - Ivermectin is FDA approved for worms
    - Often used by dermatology, but not FDA approved or indicated for scabies, so I would not choose it, even if it were what you do clinically.

BED BUG BITES

- *Epidemiology*
  - Epidemic in the country recently (not in blueprint)
  - This bug bites and then goes back into mattress.
  - No bug in skin, no treatment needed
- *Self-limited, but itches, so can use diphenhydramine (Benadryl) or steroid for itching*
  - Usually needs a new mattress; hot soapy water for clothing

SPIDER BITES

Brown Recluse Spider

- Causes severe local necrosis (loss of tissue)
- Very dependent on where bitten
  - Patient can lose an entire finger, a huge portion of skin, leaving terrible scars
- No treatment available

Black Widow Spider

- Antivenom is available
- Neurotoxin in venom

Secondary Lesions - *Skin Eruptions due to Scratching, Healing, etc.*

Atrophy

- Due to using *too potent a steroid cream*
- *Never* use a high potency ointment or cream on thin skin (like the face, eyelids)

Crusts

- Honey-colored = impetigo (the drying of serous draining)

Erosions

- From shallow ulcers – loss of the epidermis

Fissures

- Tears or breaks in the epidermis and dermis
- Eczema and dry skin on the hands in the winter with painful cracks is a good example

Lichenification

- The thickening and pronounced skin lines that occur from chronic scratching
- Antecubital and popliteal fossa in eczema
- Thickened skin of lichen planus

Purpura

- *Non-blanching* blood 'blister' under the skin --- may indicated a serious problem

Petechia

- Flat
- Teeny tiny little bruises
- Check platelet count

CHAPTER 21

Urology/Nephrology - 6% (combined)

Introduction to Urology

Urology and Nephrology are combined to make up 6% of the total questions.

Urology is mainly about cancers, and infectious diseases of the urinary tract; some anomalies; and clinical intervention. It is relatively easier material compared to Nephrology.

Nephrology is about osmolarity; and acid-base balance; and electrolytes, and really tough stuff.
But, it is weighted no more than urology.

So, should you re-learn acid-base balance if you never use it clinically? No!
That question (or two) is worth no more than the two easy questions about recognizing and treating cystitis or working up painless hematuria.

Acid-base is in the physiology chapter, and I would recommend that you review it for the basics of the concept, so that you can make an educated guess when a question pops up, then move on!

Urologic Cancers

OLDER PATIENTS

Prostate Carcinoma ***-#1 cause of cancer in men and #1 cause of GU cancer in men***

- *Risk Factors*
  - Risk increases with age
  - African ancestry
  - Family history
- *H & P*
  - Usually no symptoms of the cancer itself
  - Can have BPH-like obstructive voiding symptoms
  - On DRE
    - "Stony" prostate

        - Lump on prostate
        - Enlargement of the sulcus
        - Asymmetry of the lobes (one larger than the other)
- *Labs & Diagnostics*
    - Lab – PSA – see discussion below
    - Transrectal or transperineal ultrasound (biopsy usually done)
- *Management*
    - If > 10 year survival expected, multiple management options:
        - Surveillance (some choose to do nothing)
        - Robotic partial prostatectomy with cryotherapy (most common now)
        - Radiation (brachytherapy) – well tolerated
        - Radical prostatectomy (not often used, many complications = ED, incontinence)
    - If < 10 year expected survival due to comorbidities:
        - Surveillance
        - Leuprolide (GnRH agonist competes at pituitary and lowers testosterone through suppression of FSH)
- Complication = osteoporosis and hot flashes
- Health Maintenance
    - Screening guidelines vary depending on source (see below)

PEARL: *Screening for Prostate Cancer Debate*

There are multiple screening guidelines (WHO, ACS, AUS, USPTSF) and all disagree with each other. This makes it impossible to tell you what screening should be done. If we combine all the concerns, and the recommendations from each, we are left with:

- Screening all men with PSA is not cost effective and causes harm (too many procedures done with complications for what turns out not to be cancer)
- Screening with PSA has many false positives, and multiple pitfalls
    - Ejaculation increases PSA temporarily
    - Long term lack of ejaculation increases PSA
    - BPH increases PSA levels
    - Infection of the prostate increases PSA levels
- All of the guidelines comment on there being no need for screening in any patient whose life expectancy is less than 10 years.
- All of the guidelines comment on ethnicity and family history as being risk factors that warrant screening.
- If you combine all guidelines, all say to start screening on men > 50 years old with 10-year life expectancy with DRE plus PSA.
- Even the USPTSF (which the most stringent guidelines) states screening may be offered at age 40 to "all men who desire it".
- Hope this helps --- it is an ongoing debate --- that may be what you actually need to know most!!

Bladder Carcinoma -*#2 Cause of GU Cancer*

- *Risk Factors*
  - Smoking #1
  - M>F
  - Risk increases with age
  - Cyclophosphamide (Cytoxan)
  - Industrial exposures
- *H & P*
  - Painless hematuria
  - Frequent UTI's
  - Remember to repeat u/a after treatment of cystitis to ensure that any hematuria has resolved.
  - If still hematuria on repeat with no evidence of infection, referral is warranted
- *Labs & Diagnostics*
  - Urine cytology (3 samples)
  - Cystoscopy
  - Cysto is both diagnostic and therapeutic (with removal of tumor).
- *Clinical intervention*
  - Refer to urology (for cysto)

Renal Cell Carcinoma – *Distant #3 Cause of GU Cancer*

- *Risk Factors*
  - Smoking
  - Increases with age
- *H & P*
  - Painless hematuria
  - Rarely symptoms; that's why it is caught so late
- *Labs & Diagnostics*
  - CT with contrast
    - Usually an incidental discovery on CT for another reason
- *Clinical Intervention*
  - Nephrectomy / partial nephrectomy
  - Radiation (chemo not helpful)
- *Scientific Concept*
  - If caught before penetration of capsule or invasion of renal artery, 90% 5-yr survival;
  - If capsule or renal artery involvement, prognosis drops to 1-5% 5-yr survival;
  - Unfortunately, there are almost no symptoms; and no screening available

YOUNGER PATIENTS

Testicular Carcinoma

- *Risk Factors*
  - Cryptorchidism (undescended testicles)
- *H & P*
  - Painless mass
- *Labs & Diagnostics*
  - Ultrasound of testicle
  - If solid mass, it is cancer
- *Clinical intervention*
  - Referral to urology
  - Orchiectomy

PEARL: Testicular cancer spreads to retroperitoneal nodes (not pelvic nodes as prostate) – in embryologic growth, the testicles were up by the kidneys, and descend at 28 weeks gestation into scrotal sac. This is a germ cell tumor; metastatic spread (if present) will be to those retroperitoneal nodes: CT or PET for staging, radiation or chemo, or radical lymph nodes dissection

---

Abnormalities of Development

Cryptorchidism

- Failure of descent of the testes (descends at 28 wk gestation)
- Increased risk of testicular cancer – even if corrected
- Main reason for correction is to reduce temp of the testicle to improve spermatogenesis

Varicocele

- Varicose veins, fill the scrotum, "bag of worms"
- Clinical issue is that the testicle is warmed by blood and is almost 3 degrees warmer than it should be
- Can cause abnormal spermatogenesis (but not cancer)

Phimosis

- Foreskin tight over the glans penis
- May cause pressure during voiding
- Over time can cause renal dysfunction due to chronic increased pressure gradient during voiding
- Surgical referral if needed

Paraphimosis

- Foreskin able to be retracted

- Gets "trapped" above the glans, can strangulate
- Surgical referral for circumcision
- Most common occurrence is during Foley placement, or when cleaning

Epispadias/Hypospadias

- (Epi) Developmental anomaly where urethral opening is on the dorsal surface of the glans
- (Hypo) Developmental anomaly where urethral opening is on the ventral surface of the glans (underneath)
- If near the urethral meatus, no intervention needed
- If very proximal (near the scrotum) should be referred electively for evaluation and revision
- Urology referral most often to r/o other anomalies

Duplication of the Collecting System
"Horseshoe kidneys"

- Both are due to urogenital congenital anomalies
- As suggested there are two collecting systems for each kidney
- Predisposes the infant, child, adult to frequent UTI's due to reflux from one ureter "back-wards" to the other and back to the pelvis.
- Both are identified on IVP (intravenous pyelogram) or on CT

Vascular Problems

Testicular Torsion

- *Etiology*
    - Bell-Clapper deformity (congenital lack of posterior anchor, causing testicle to "swing" within the scrotum)
- *H & P*
    - Sudden onset of testicular pain in adolescent
    - Painful testicle in a horizontal lie
    - Loss of cremasteric reflex (tickle inside of thigh and testicle retracts)
- *Labs & diagnostics*
    - Ultrasound STAT with color (flow/Doppler) to document flow (or no flow in the case of a torsion)
- *Clinical Intervention*
    - Surgical emergency – 6 hours to get flow re-established before loss of testicle
    - Orchipexy to fix the bell clapper deformity will be done on the other side

Erectile Dysfunction

- *Etiology*
    - Mechanical problems
        - *Peyronie's disease*
    - Surgery (post-op complication)
    - Diabetes (poor perfusion)
    - Trauma
    - Drugs (many drugs)
        - Alcohol

        - Diuretics
        - Psychogenic
        - Depression
- *Loss of orgasm is most often psychogenic and not organic!*

PEARL: *Erectile dysfunction* is a general term that encompasses any reason that a man cannot have intercourse due to a problem with erection. This was formerly believed to be commonly due to psychogenic causes; but now it is well known that it is more often an organic cause (due to a drug, disorder, disease). I have included Peyronie's disease because, while the patient can achieve an erection, if there is a severe curvature due to a scar, this may prevent him from being able to have intercourse (hence, ED); and I have included priapism which is not a problem with achieving erection, but it does not stop, causing a dysfunction. Finally, there are psychogenic reasons that a man cannot maintain or achieve an erection. Keep in mind that decreased libido is not erectile dysfunction; if the question is discussing a loss of libido, think endocrine dysfunction and check testosterone and FSH levels.

Infections

Urethritis

- *Epidemiology*
    - Common infection
    - Can occur in both men and women
- *H & P*
    - Dysuria
    - Penile discharge, urethral discharge
    - No fever, no flank pain, no perineal or pelvic pain
- *Labs & Diagnostics*
    - Urethral swab for GC/Chlamydia
    - Urinalysis with culture
- *Formulating Most Likely Diagnosis*
    - Dysuria without fever, flank pain, perineal/pelvic pain
- *Therapeutics*
    - <u>To cover Chlamydia</u>
        - Azithromycin 1 gm PO
    - <u>To cover GC</u>
        - ceftriaxone 125 mg IM or Cefixime 400 mg PO
        - *Cipro 500 mg. no longer recommended by CDC due to resistance*
    - <u>To cover Trichomonas</u>
        - Metronidazole 2 gm. PO

Cystitis

- *Epidemiology*
    - Most common of urogenital infections
    - Still E. Coli most common pathogen
- *H & P*

- "Irritative voiding symptoms"
- Dysuria, urgency, frequency
- +/- hematuria
- Low grade temp < 100 F
- Low back pain (*no flank pain*)

- *Labs & Diagnostics*
  - <u>Urinalysis</u>
    - *WBC's, RBC's, + LE (leukocyte esterase), +nitrite, +bacteria*
- *Formulating Most Likely Diagnosis*
  - Irritative voiding symptoms without flank pain, or high fevers
- *Clinical Intervention*
  - Antibiotics and analgesics
    - Short three day course *only* for sexually active young women

- *Therapeutics*
  - Empirically for most common pathogen
  - Bactrim (SMX/TMP); Ciprofloxacin; nitrofurantoin
- *Health Maintenance*
  - For women = void after intercourse or prophylaxis

Pyelonephritis

- *Epidemiology*
  - Common
- *H & P*
  - +/- irritative voiding symptoms
  - Flank pain
  - Fever
- *Labs & Diagnostics*
  - WBC casts (come only from renal tubules, therefore, pyelo!)
  - Otherwise the same as cystitis
  - Leukocytosis on CBC may be present
- *Clinical Intervention*
  - If stable with no vomiting; not septic – treat as outpatient
  - If high fevers, vomiting; septic – treat as inpatient
- *Therapeutics*
  - Most antibiotics will work but,
  - Nitrofurantoin does not cover pyelonephritis
  - <u>Must do 10-14 day course; no short course therapy!</u>

Epididymitis

- *Epidemiology*
  - <40 y.o. – Chlamydia/GC
  - >40 y.o. – E. Coli
- *H & P*
  - Fever, scrotal pain
  - Irritative voiding symptoms
  - Swelling and pain of epididymis (soft tissue on the superior posterior testicle – not the testicle itself)

- *Labs & Diagnostics*
    - U/A, culture, CBC, urethral swab
- *Formulating Most Likely Diagnosis*
    - Specific description of where the pain is nails the diagnosis
- *Clinical Intervention*
    - Antibiotics!
    - Scrotal elevation, ice packs
- *Therapeutics*
    - <u>In men < 35 years (presumptive GC/Chlamydia)</u>
        - Ceftriaxone 250 mg IM in a single dose
        - PLUS
        - Doxycycline 100 mg orally twice a day for 10 days

    - <u>In men > 35 years (presumptive enteric organisms)</u>
        - Levofloxacin 500 mg orally once daily for 10 days
          OR
        - Ofloxacin 300 mg orally twice a day for 10 days
- *Formulating the Most Likely Diagnosis*
    - <u>Prehn's Sign</u> --- Relief of discomfort with scrotal elevation (just like putting your infected infected finger up pain improves, put it down, throbbing pain increases)
        - <u>Distinguishing epididymitis from torsion</u>
            - No Prehn's sign
                - No better whether it is up or down, ischemic pain no matter what!
            - No fever in torsion
            - Normal lie with epididymitis (horizontal in torsion)

Acute Bacterial Prostatitis

- *Epidemiology*
    - Fairly common infection
- *H & P*
    - Perineal pain
    - +/- irritative voiding symptoms
    - Fever, chills, nausea
- *Labs & Diagnostics*
    - CBC
    - Urinalysis & culture
    - Swab if penile discharge (usually not present)
- *Clinical Intervention*
    - *Long course antibiotic treatment (30 days)*
- *Therapeutics*
    - Bactrim DS is still recommended for 30 day treatmetn
    - Urinary fluoroquinolones (but resistance is high)
        - Levofloxacin x 30 days (very expensive)
        - Ofloxacin x 30 days (ditto)
- *Scientific Concepts*
    - Acute prostatitis increases PSA (prostatic specific antigen)

- *DO NOT* perform prostatic massage to obtain prostatic secretions
    - Can cause disseminated infection
- *Avoid instrumentation (passing a Foley can cause dissemination)*
- Consider sepsis in elderly with tachycardia, hypotension

Orchitis

- *Epidemiology*
    - Inflammation of the testicle
    - Used to be due to "mumps"
    - But now due to bacterial spread from epididymitis
- *H & P*
    - Pain with palpation of testicle
    - Fever, malaise
- *Clinical Intervention*
    - Rule out torsion
    - Ultrasound with doppler

The Prostate

Benign Prostatic Hyperplasia (BPH)

- *Epidemiology*
    - Most common benign tumor in men
- *H & P*
    - Obstructive voiding symptoms (hesitancy, splitting of stream, need to valsalva, nocturia)
    - DRE = enlarged prostate, rubbery, nontender
    - Preserved "shape" with normal sulcus
    - If one lobe enlarged = cancer
- *Labs & Diagnostics*
    - U/A, culture
    - Serum creatinine (make sure not obstructive uropathy)
    - Urodynamic studies (urology PA would do this)
- *Formulating Most Likely Diagnosis*
    - Nontender; no fever; normal shape just large
- *Clinical Intervention*
    - medications to relieve symptoms
    - surgery only if obstructing and causing renal dysfunction
- *Therapeutics*
    - <u>Alpha blockers (doxazosin, tamsulosin, terazosin, ****osin)</u>
        - Does not "shrink" prostate; smooth muscle relaxation
        - No reduction in PSA (just symptomatic relief)
        - Lowers BP (usually not a problem, but be careful in elderly)
    - <u>5-alpha reductase inhibitors (finasteride)</u>
        - Reduces size of prostate
        - Reduces PSA by 50%
- *Scientific Concepts*

  - BPH causes elevation in PSA

Other Urologic Disorders

Autosomal Dominant Polycystic Kidney Disease

- *Epidemiology*
  - Autosomal Dominant (75% will have family history)
- *H&P*
  - Hypertension
  - Enlarged or palpable kidneys (eventually)
  - Lithiasis/hematuria
- *Labs & Diagnostics*
  - Ultrasound will make the diagnosis
  - Incidentally found sometimes on CT for other reasons
- *Clinical Intervention*
  - Tight control of hypertension
  - Nephrology referral
- *Health Maintenance*
  - With good control of BP, may not need transplant
  - Most common time for transplant 50-60's

Nephrolithiasis/Urolithiasis

- *Epidemiology*
  - Calcium oxalate stones (85%)
- *H & P*
  - Ureteral colic, sudden and severe in the flank
  - Can be referred to anterior abdomen and into groin
- *Labs & Diagnostics*
  - Gross or microscopic hematuria on U/A
  - Make sure you rule out infection on urinalysis!
  - KUB will diagnose most stones
  - CT can measure stone size (if > 6mm may not pass readily)
  - Check creatinine to make sure no obstructive uropathy (not likely if normal "other" kidney)
    - KUB will not show hydronephrosis
    - US and CT will both identify hydronephrosis
- *Formulating Most Likely Diagnosis*
  - In the "wrong" patient, consider aortic dissection (uncommon to have it in the retroperitoneal space, but can happen).
    - If question wants you to choose dissection, there should be abnormal peripheral pulse or some obvious risk factor
- *Clinical Intervention*
  - Fluids
  - Pain management
  - <u>If infection, will need antibiotics and close surveillance</u>

        - Tamsulosin (Flomax) an alpha blocker is used to relax smooth muscle of urethra
            - Decreases BP, so careful
    - If large stone (8-10 mm) and infection, will need urgent urology consult to retrieve stone and place stent
- *Health Maintenance*
    - Increase fluids

Stress Incontinence

- *Epidemiology*
    - Common in women (particularly after childbirth)
    - Due to pubococcygeal muscle atrophy
    - Common in older woman (#2 after urge incontinence in geriatrics)
    - Common in men after prostatectomy
- *H & P*
    - Leakage of urine with cough/sneeze/laugh/exercise
    - Cystocele may be evident on pelvic exam with valsalva
- *Labs & Diagnostics*
    - Urinalysis to rule out cystitis as cause of incontinence
- *Formulating Most Likely Diagnosis*
    - Mechanical/structural problem
- *Clinical Intervention*
    - Kegel exercises (to strengthen P-C muscles)
    - Bladder "sling" to lift bladder and return sphincter to normal function
    - Drugs not effective

Urge Incontinence

- *Epidemiology*
    - Detrusor muscle hyperreflexia
    - Uninhibited bladder contraction causes leakage
    - Most common cause of geriatric incontinence
- *H & P*
    - History for urge to void; and then voiding before "ready"
    - No pain; no irritative symptoms
- *Labs & Diagnostics*
    - Urologic evaluation to rule out infection, tumor
- *Therapeutics*
    - Tolterodine; oxybutynin
        - Anticholinergic agents (dry mouth; urinary retention)

Male Infertility

- *Epidemiology*
    - 50% of the time, it is a male problem (what d'ya know?)
- *H & P*
    - History for toxins, alcohol, marijuana, cigarette smoking
    - Focused scrotal exam likely normal
    - May be varicocele ("bag of worms") which may keep testes too warm

- *Labs & Diagnostics*
    - Semen Analysis
        - Oligospermia (too few sperm)
        - Abnormal forms/motility
- *Clinical Intervention*
    - Urology referral if varicocele
    - Endocrine if low testosterone; or if hypogonadism

Peyronie's Disease

- Able to have erection, but scar causes a "pulling" curvature in the erect penis
    - This does not allow comfortable intercourse (hence, ED).

Priapism

- ***Definition***
    - Painful erection lasting > 4 hours
    - Think "compartment syndrome" of the penis, blood engorges penis, but no flow out – penis-threatening emergency!
- *Etiologies*
    - Sickle cell anemia
    - Desyrel (Trazodone) in high doses (per a psych PA at a review course, confirmed in Epocrates)

Erectile Dysfunction

- *Epidemiology/Etiology*
- *H & P*
    - Inability to achieve or maintain erection in order to have intercourse
    - If decreased libido, this is not ED (think endocrine problem)
    - Normal physical exam
- *Labs & Diagnostics*
    - Nocturnal penile tumescence test
        - A tension meter is placed around the flaccid penis
        - Then as the patient sleeps, it records pressures frequency and rigidity of erections
    - If no erections occur, this suggests erectile dysfunction due to organic problem.
    - If erections occur, this would suggest that everything works just fine.
        - Psychological cause most common
- *Clinical Intervention*
    - May need urologic referral if unclear etiology.
- *Therapeutics*
    - ED drugs
        - Sildenafil, tadalafil, vardenafil
        - ED drugs do not affect libido
        - Priapism has not been an issue
            - *No nitrates* with this drug
    - Prostaglandin injections
    - Devices

Renal Diseases (Nephrology)

Acid-Base abnormalities (both respiratory and metabolic) are covered in Physiology and Pathyophysiology Review, Chapter 10.

Kidney Function

The kidney's function is important to understand (but impossible to understand completely)

A few basics will help you decide if the renal problem presented to you is an acute renal problem (a problem of decreased perfusion to the kidney or obstruction to urine flow) or a chronic renal problem (which is typically autoimmune or a result of lack of perfusion that caused ischemia, or obstruction that was not "fixed" in time). Once you figure out whether the question is asking you about acute renal failure or chronic renal failure, you have a very good chance of getting the question correct!

What is the Kidney's Function?

- Synthesize erythropoietin (EPO)
- Synthesize renin
- Metabolize Vitamin D to active metabolic form (D3)
- Maintain pH of the body

Therefore, in an acute renal problem, most of the function of the kidney was fine until just a day or two ago. However, if the patient has a chronic renal problem, these functions have been lacking for months and years.

A 54 year old man presents with multiple complaints. You perform labs and find that:

Serum creatinine is 6.8 (nl 0.6-1.2)
BUN 46 (nl 0.8 – 12)
CBC shows H&H of 14/42 (normal)
CMP: Electrolytes are normal

Do these labs most likely represent an acute or a chronic cause of renal failure?

Answer/Discussion: This is an example of acute renal failure. While the patient has azotemia (elevation of BUN and creatinine), the function of the kidney has been good (no anemia, normal electrolytes). The BUN is very high and this is because the gut has not had time to help clear it yet. Look for an acute reason for renal failure in your options on the exam.

A 54 year old man presents with multiple complaints. You perform labs and find that:

Serum creatinine is 6.8 (nl 0.6-1.2)
BUN 26
CBC shows H&H of 7.4/21 (nl 14/52)
CMP: Electrolytes show marked hyperkalemia

Do these labs most likely represent an acute or a chronic cause of renal failure?

Answer/Discussion*:* This is an example of chronic renal failure with loss of renal function (anemia due to no erythropoietin; hyperkalemia and metabolic acidosis are expected due to lack of tubular function). The BUN is not as high relative to the creatinine because the gut has had some time to help get rid of nitrogenous waste products.

Osmolarity/Osmolality

The concept of osmolarity/osmolality has to do with electrolyte/water balance within the body. The two measure slightly different things, but the differences are negligible in actual clinical practice, and very confusing to explain and understand. This, I think, is beyond the scope of most exam questions, so once again, I will use simple explanations to help understanding.

Osmolarity has to do with the number of particles per liter of plasma but does not take into account the weight of the particles. Osmolality considers weight, but this is not important for the purposes of this very basic discussion.

Bedside calculations are actually in units of osmolarity, whereas laboratory measurements will provide readings in units of osmolality. In practice, there is almost negligible difference between the absolute values of the different measurements. For this reason, both terms are often used interchangeably, even though they refer to different units of measurement.

Cell membranes, generally, are freely permeable to water; therefore, the osmolality of the extracellular fluid (ECF) is approximately equal to that of the intracellular fluid (ICF) when everything is normal. Therefore, plasma osmolality is a guide to intracellular osmolality.

This is important, as it shows that changes in ECF osmolality have a great effect on ICF osmolality which can cause problems with normal cell functioning and volume. If the ECF becomes too hypotonic, water fills cells, increasing their volume and potentially lysing them. The brain tends to swell in response to hypo-osmolality (and hypo-osmolarity).

The osmolality of blood increases with dehydration, and decreases with over-hydration.

Increased osmolality will stimulate secretion of antidiuretic hormone (ADH). Recall from the physiology chapter that ADH from the posterior pituitary will cause the kidney to hold water for the body.

Decreased serum osmolality will suppress the release of ADH, resulting in decreased water reabsorption and concentrated plasma.

The two topics in the NCCPA blueprint in this section are volume excess and volume depletion:

Fluid Disorders

Volume Excess

- **Syndrome of Inappropriate (Increased) ADH <SIADH>**
    - ADH is secreted by pituitary
    - Water retained by the kidney (sodium stays the same)
- **Primary hyperaldosteronism**
    - Retention of sodium (water stays the same); therefore: increased osmolality
    - Water goes where sodium goes

Which of these will cause a hyperosmolar problem?

Answer: Primary hyperaldosteronism

Which of these will cause a hypo-osmolar hyponatremia?

Answer: SIADH --- the most common cause of hyponatremia in hospitalized and outpatients

Volume Depletion

- An obvious cause of volume depletion would be vomiting & diarrhea; dehydration
- Less obvious causes:
    - DI (diabetes insipidus)
    - Loss of water by the kidney because no ADH secretion
    - Aldosterone deficiency (Addison's, adrenal failure)
    - Loss of sodium by the kidney, because no aldosterone

Which will be hyperosmolar?

Answer: Diabetes insipidus (loss of water would cause a hyperosmolar problem, too much sodium per liter of blood volume)

Which will be hypo-osmolar?

Answer: Addison's disease. Aldosterone deficiency (loss of solute (Na) causes too little sodium per liter of blood volume, i.e. hypoosmolarity)

Nephritic Syndrome vs. Nephrotic Syndrome

These two "syndromes" are distinguished from each other by the findings on urine analysis

- Each has its own differential
- Each has different etiologies
- Look at the urine findings given to you to pick the "most likely diagnosis" based on whether the description is that of a
    - Nephritic-type problem
      OR
    - Nephrotic-type problem

In all instances, the diagnosis is made by renal biopsy (referral to nephrology). Your evaluation as the primary PA is to recognize the renal problem (the patient's presentation of painless hematuria, or painless proteinuria, and abnormal creatinine) and order the 24 hour urine to check for amount of protein loss. *Remember that 4+ proteinuria is not an amount – it is "to infinity and beyond" so you really only know the patient is losing > 3000 mg/d of protein. The definition of nephrotic-type proteinuria is > 3500 mg/d of protein loss.

Nephritic = Painless *Hematuria*

- RBC's, dysmorphic RBC's and RBC casts on urine microscopic
- Mild proteinuria/mild hypertension/mild edema

Examples:

- Post-strep glomerulonephritis
- Interstitial nephritis

Note that nephritic syndromes will have "itis" or "itic" in the name of the syndrome unless named after a physician, i.e. Berger's syndrome and Goodpasture syndrome

Nephrotic = Painless *Proteinuria*

- Few cells on urine microscopic "bland" microscopic
- Significant proteinuria (>3.5 mg/day on 24 hour urine analysis), hypertension, significant edema
- Hypoalbuminemia (causing movement of water out of the vasculature and into the patient's tissues)
- Loss of proteins needed for anti-clotting, immune function, cholesterol metabolism (i.e. thrombotic, immune, and atherosclerotic problems)

Examples:

- Minimal change disease (#1 cause in kids)
- Membranous nephropathy (note the "o" in the name like nephrOtic)

- DM and HTN cause nephrotic-type protein loss
- Amyloidosis and multiple myeloma result in nephrotic type syndrome

PEARL: The word "protein" is found in the word "**nephrotic**", which helps you remember that nephrotic problems are all about protein loss by the kidney.

Managing Chronic Kidney Disease

- CKD is the most costly disease covered by Medicare.
- The two most common causes being hypertension and diabetes, whose incidence is increasing rapidly worldwide.
    - More than 60% of adults will develop CKD in their lifetimes.
- Albuminuria is the most predictice factor in progression to kidney failure.
- It is the first indicator of progressing kidney disease, and is frequently ignored in family practice.
- New 2012 guidelines reflect the importance of intervening early in patients who develop albuminuria.
    - Dipstick for protein is sufficient in identifying patients with kidney disease (1+ or greater).
    - These patients need to go on to quantitiative evaluation (urine albumin to creatinine ratio)
    - Because 24 hour urine is so difficult to collect, spot urine (on first morning sample) is useful.
    - If confirmatory spot urine, then repeat in 2 months.
    - If second is also positive, then definition for persistent albuminuria is made.
    - Referral now to nephrology for evaluation for CKD is warranted.

- Hypertension and DM must be addressed and treated to goals in all patients identified with above screening.
- All patients with DM should be on ACE inhibitor (ACEI) or angiotensin receptor blocker (ARB)
- ACEI or ARB is indicated once albumin > 300 mg/dL in nondiabetics.

Electrolyte Abnormalities

Hyponatremia (Na < 135 mEq/L)

- *Epidemiology*
    - ***Most common electrolyte abnormality in hospitalized patients***
    - Can cause catastrophic cerebral osmotic demyelination
- *Etiology*

- Hypotonic (hypo-osmolar)
  - SIADH (syndrome of increased ADH)
    - *Most common cause in hospitalized patients*
  - Adrenal insufficiency
  - Hypothyroidism
  - Diuretics
  - Psychogenic polydipsia/beer potomania
- Hypervolemic Hypotonic (third spacing of fluid/fluid retention)
  - CHF
  - Nephrotic syndrome
  - Cirrhosis
- Hyperosmolar Hyponatremia
  - Hyperglycemia
    - Glucose "replaces" the sodium in plasma
    - Recall that glucose is not supposed to *be in the plasma*

- *H & P*
  - If acute
    - Seizures and altered mental status
    - Can be 128 with seizures
  - If chronic
    - Asymptomatic
    - Can be 108 without symptoms
- *Treatment*
  - Isotonic saline (0.9% NaCl)
  - Slowly increase sodium to about 125-130; no faster unless patient is dying
- Scientific Concept
  - Too aggressive replacement is more catastrophic than the hyponatremia itself
    - Central pontine myelinolysis

PEARL: *SIADH (The syndrome of increased ADH)*

Recall that ADH is in our pituitary gland in case we become hypovolemic. It will then be secreted and cause the kidney to hold water, increasing our fluid volume and cardiac output. So, what happens if you have "syndrome of increased ADH"? You hold water, but with the same amount of sodium. This would make you, not fluid overloaded but *water* overloaded; therefore, hypo-osmolar and hypervolemic, and hyponatremic.

The most common reason for SIADH in a patient who does not actually need more body water is any medical problem that causes a decrease in cardiac output. Consider how many patients have decreased cardiac output, or decreased renal perfusion, or decreased carotid perfusion, and are not, in fact, volume depleted!

Hypernatremia

- *Epidemiology*
  - Much less common than hypo-natremia

- *Etiology*
    - Dehydration
- *H & P*
    - Evidence of dehydration
- *Labs & Diagnostics*
    - Concentrated urine
    - Elevated BUN
    - Sodium > 145 mEq/L
- *Treatment*
    - Isotonic saline, slow replacement

Hyperkalemia (K > 5 mEq/L)

- *Epidemiology*
    - Common electrolyte abnormality
- *Etiology*
    - CRF is #1
    - ACEI's, ARB's
    - Potassium-sparing diuretics
    - Hemolysis of cells (traumatic blood draw)
- *H & P*
    - Arrhythmias as a consequence of hyperkalemia
- *Labs & Diagnostics*
    - ECG shows *tall, peaked T waves*
    - Can lead to widened QRS and life threatening arrhythmias
- *Treatment*
    - CaCO3 or CaCl, 1 amp
        - Neutralize electrical effects on heart
    - Insulin with D-50%
        - Drives glucose into the cell and takes K with it
    - Albuterol nebulized therapy
        - β agonist effect shifts K into cells (and out of serum)
    - Kayexelate
        - Oral or rectal
    - Peritoneal dialysis or hemodialysis
- *Clinical Intervention*
    - Hospitalize if:
        - K > 6
        - ECG changes

Hypokalemia

- *Epidemiology*
    - Common due to CHF therapies
- *Etiology*

  - Loop and thiazide diuretics
- *H & P*
  - Muscle cramps
  - Weakness, fatigue
- *Labs & Diagnostics*
  - ECG showing flat T waves
- *Treatment*
  - K supplement orally if at all possible
  - If given IV, give in 1-2 liters of fluid over several hours
- *Scientific Concept*
  - Increases the likelihood of dig toxicity
  - Loops + dig are often given together, so...
  - Consider hypokalemia in patient on dig who appears toxic
    - Yellow color vision
    - Nausea, anorexia
    - Tachyarrhythmias (SVT, VT)

Hypercalcemia and Hypocalemia are covered in Endocrine, Chapter 19.

ELECTROLYTE ABNORMALITIES			
ABNORMALITY	**ETIOLOGIES**	**SIGNS & SYMPTOMS**	**CLINICAL INTERVENTION**
HYPONATREMIA Sodium < 135 Ref Ranges: 135 -145 mmol/L	•SIADH •Psychogenic polydipsia •GI fluid loss •Sweating	•AMS •Seizures • ↓ BP • ↑ ICP	•Monitor I & O •Limit fluids/ water •0.9% NS IV •Give Hypertonic IV fluids •Increase levels gradually
HYPERNATREMIA Sodium > 145 Ref Ranges: 135 -145 mmol/L	•Fluid deprivation •Diabetes insipidus	•AMS •Edema •Thirst •Tachycardia	•Monitor I & O •Encourage fluids •Limit sodium •Lower levels gradually •Give hypotonic IV, 1/4 or 1/2 NS solution
HYPOKALEMIA Potassium < 3.4 Ref Ranges: 3.4 - 4.9 mmol/L	•Diuretics •Alcoholism •Nasogastric suctioning •Vomiting •Eating Disorders	•Dysrhythmia •Leg cramps •Anorexia	•Cardiac monitor •Give Oral K+(K-Dur) 20mEq = 0.1↑K •Give IV K+ (dilute & give slowly) •Educate about K+ rich foods •√ Magnesium
HYPERKALEMIA Potassium > 5.0 Ref Ranges: 3.4 - 4.9 mmol/L	•Renal failure •Crush injuries •Potassium sparing diuretics	• ♥ Dysrhythmia • ♥ Arrest • ♥ Irregular pulse • ♥ Elevated T waves • Paresthesias	•Cardiac monitor •Monitor labs/ EKG •Give oral Kayexalate •Calcium Gluconate by IV •D50%+ 10 u. Reg Insulin IV/SQ •1HR continuous Albuterol nebs •Oral or rectal Kayexalate • Dialysis
HYPOCALCEMIA Calcium < 8.9 Ref Ranges: 8.9 - 10.3 mg/dL	•Renal failure • ↓ Vitamin D •Alcoholism •Hypoparathyroidism •Crohn's disease	•Chvostek's sign •Trousseau's sign •Tetany •V-Tach •Seizures •Long QT	•Calcium supplements/ vitamin D •Increase dietary calcium •Weight-bearing exercises
HYPERCALCEMIA Calcium > 10.3 Ref Ranges: 8.9 - 10.3 mg/dL	•Hyperparathyroidism •Malignancy	•Depressed DTR's •Mental status: lethargy, confusion, weakness • ♥ Dysrhythmia •Constipation	•Oral fluids (dilute urine) •Increase fiber •Limit dietary intake •IF NO kidney disease or heart failure- give diuretics & NS *IF THERE IS kidney disease or heart failure- give CALCITONIN
HYPOMAGNESEMIA Magnesium < 1.5 Ref Ranges: 1.2 - 2.2 mg/dL	•Alcoholism •Burns •Pancreatitis	• ↑ DTR's • ↑ HR, BP •Dysrhythmia •Vertigo •Seizures	•Provide safety for seizure risk •Increase dietary intake of Magnesium: whole grains, nuts, chocolate, seafood •MgSO4 4gm P.O or give IV •Monitor DTR's
HYPERMAGNESEMIA Magnesium > 2.5 Ref Ranges: 1.2 - 2.2 mg/dL	•Renal failure •Adrenal insufficiency	• ↓HR, BP •Coma •Lethargy •Muscle weakness	•Monitor vital signs •Monitor LOC •Provide dialysis if the level is critically high

Specific Renal Diseases

Acute Tubular Necrosis

- *Epidemiology*
  - 85 % of all causes of acute kidney injury
- *Etiology*
  - Ischemia to the renal tubules causing necrosis
  - Prolonged decreased renal perfusion
  - Shock
    - Cardiogenic
    - Anaphylactic
    - Hypovolemic
    - Septic
  - Nephrotoxin damage
    - Aminoglycosides
      - Gentamycin, torbramycin
    - NSAIDs
    - Amphotericin B
    - Iodinated contrast dye
    - Myoglobin
    - Uric acid
    - Bence-Jones protein (multiple myeloma)
- *H & P*
  - Asymptomatic until later in course
- *Labs & Diagnostics*
  - Elevated creatinine
  - BUN : creatinine ratio < 20:1
  - FENA > 1 (fractional excretion of sodium)
- *Clinical Intervention*
  - Nephrology consult

Post-Strep Glomerulonephritis

- *Epidemiology*
  - Strep Group A
  - Anti-GBM associated (Goodpasture syndrome)
- *Etiology*
  - Immune-mediated
  - Not prevented with treatment of strep throat
- *H & P*
  - *Hematuria*
  - Edema/hypertension

- *Labs & Diagnostics*
  - Elevated creatinine
  - Urine microscopic with RBC's, *RBC casts*
  - *Mild proteinuria (< 3 g/d)*
- *Clinical Intervention*
  - Nephrology consult

Interstitial Nephritis

- *Epidemiology*
  - 10-15% of cases of acute kidney injury
- *Etiology*
  - Interstitial inflammatory response
  - Immune mediated
  - 70% caused by medications (almost any drug can cause it)
- *H & P*
  - *Fever & rash*
  - Arthralgias
- *Labs & Diagnostics*
  - *Eosinophia in blood*
  - Proteinuria
- *Clinical Intervention*
  - Nephrology consult

Renal Vascular Disease

- *Etiology*
  - Renal artery stenosis (RAS)
    - 90% due to atherosclerotic disease of the artery
    - 10% due to fibromuscular dysplasia of the artery
- *H & P*
  - Hypertension unresponsive to treatment
- *Labs & Diagnostics*
  - Elevated BUN & creatinine
  - Doppler US of renal arteries (cheap and no radiation)
  - CT angiography (most radiation)
  - MRA (most expensive)
- *Clinical Intervention*
  - Controversial
- *Scientific Concepts*
  - *Hallmark is marked elevation in creatinine when begun on ACEI to treat hypertension – investigate for renal artery stenosis!*

"We are all strangers to our hidden potential until we confront problems that reveal our capabilities."

-Apoorve Dubey

CHAPTER 22

Infectious Disease – 3%

Covered in Peds

Acute rheumatic fever
Erythema Infectiosum
Mumps
Pinworms
Rocky Mountain spotted fever
Roseola
Rubella
Rubeola (Measles)
Varicella zoster infection

Covered in GI

Amebiasis
Cholera
Pinworms
Salmonellosis
Shigellosis

Covered in Pulmonology

Influenza
Tuberculosis

Covered in GYN

Chlamydia
Gonococcal infections
Herpes simplex
Human papilloma virus

Covered in ENT

Epstein-Barr Virus (infectious mono)
Herpes simplex
Human papilloma virus

Introduction to the Infectious Disease Chapter

This chapter is organized by characterizing the diseases by organism (most important therapeutics will be given as well).

The problem with this section is that it covers many diseases for only 3% of the total possible questions on the test and there is so much overlap with other content areas, i.e. measles, mumps and rubella will be covered here, and in pediatrics.

I cover the diseases in detail in the content areas that most pertain (as in the example above, most of the info will be in the pediatric chapter as these diseases really do not occur in adults, and then mention them again in OB, as they pertain to a fetus). In some instances, you will note that I simply supply the same information here as I do in the content area, i.e. TB is copied and pasted in both the Pulmonary Chapter and in the ID chapter to make sure you do not miss it.

I struggled with this section, because the overlap and redundancy is puzzling to me, as are some of the topics here, and some of the topics that are conspicuously not here. Nevertheless, as I say on numerous occasions," it is what it is", so all will be covered, including some notable diseases not in the Blueprint.

This chapter is at the end of the Blueprint, and if you have reviewed the prior chapters, you should be able to "skim" most of this chapter and just focus on the most important ID topics for your 6-9 questions, HIV, syphilis, TB, etc.

Should you get a random question about babesiosis or ehrlichiosis (not in the blueprint, but possibly may show up on your exam), smile, pick your favorite letter and move on!

By Organism

Viral Infections

Human Immunodeficiency Virus (HIV)

- *Epidemiology/Etiology*
  - Blood borne virus:
    - Sexual intercourse
    - IV drug use
    - Vertical transmission (mother to child)/ delivery, placental, nursing
  - Retroviruses = HIV-1, HIV-2
- *H & P*
  - Acute infection has flulike symptoms:
    - Fever, malaise, generalized and nonspecific rash
    - Patient then becomes asymptomatic.
    - Eventually generalized lymphadenopathy develops (often the presenting symptom).
  - Differential includes: lymphoma, leukemia, other viral infections

  - Other opportunistic infections (Kaposi's, crypto, histo, PCP) suggest AIDs.
- *Blood product infusion prior to 1985*
- *Needle-stick injuries in healthcare professionals*
- *Maternal HIV infection*
- *Sexual History*
  - Unprotected receptive anal intercourse
  - Large number of partners
  - H/o STI's
  - IV drug use
- *Labs & Diagnostics*
  - <u>USPTSF</u>
    - Screen for HIV in all adolescents and adults at risk
    - Screen all pregnant women
  - <u>CDC</u>
    - Screen all high risk patients annually
    - Opt-out screening for patients
  - <u>ACP</u>
    - Encourage all patients to be screened
- *How to screen?*
  - ELISA (enzyme-linked immunoabsorbent assay), a serum test
    - Confirmation with Western Blot (HIV-1)
  - Test for HIV-2 if in an endemic area or if indeterminate HIV-1 result
  - <u>If Blot is positive</u>
    - CD4 count (normal range 500-2000 cells/uL)
    - < 200 = AIDs -defining
  - Viral load (rate of progression to AIDs and death is related to viral load)
    - Viral loads > 30,000 are 20 times more likely to die of AIDs than if undetectable
  - In successful treatment (< 400 copies/mL), better prognosis
- *Clinical Intervention*
  - PPD
  - CMV testing
  - RPR/VDRL/FTA-ABS for syphilis
  - GC/Chlamydia
  - Hepatitis A, B, C serology
  - Anti-Toxoplasma antibody
  - Dilated oththalmologic exam
- *Therapeutics*
  - Retroviral drugs in all patients with CD4 count < 350
  - <u>Antiretroviral drugs in:</u>
    - All pregnant women
    - HIV-associated nephropathy
    - Concomitant Hepatitis B
  - <u>HAART (highly active antiretroviral therapy):</u>
    - NRTIs – nucleoside revere transcriptase inhibitors
    - PIs – protease inhibitors
    - NNRTIs – nonnucleoside revere transcriptase inhibitors
    - Fusion inhibitors

        - CCR5 co-receptor antagonists
        - HIV integrase strand transfer inhibitors
    - Regimen selection is individualized based on multiple factors:
        - Virology efficacy
    - Toxicity
        - Pill burden/dosage frequency
        - Drug-drug interaction potential
        - Drug resistance
        - Comorbid conditions
    - Prophylactic therapies
        - CD4 count < 200 = Bactrim for PCP prophylaxis
- *Health Maintenance*
    - Safe sex practices
- *For those who are HIV positive:*
    - Limit exposure to toxo (cooked meat, no kitty litter, wash veggies)
    - Limit exposure to endemic areas for other funguses
- *Scientific Concept – Three categories for classifying HIV*:
    - Category A: asymptomatic HIV infection
    - Category B: HIV with symptoms or defect in T-Cell mediated immunity
    - Category C: AIDs defining opportunistic infections

Kaposi's Sarcoma: HHV – 8

- *Epidemiology*
    - Before the HIV epidemic, this was mostly a cancer of elderly Italian and Ashkenazi Jewish men
    - Now primarily seen in HIV/AIDs patients.
- *H & P*
    - Purple macules; papules, and nodules throughout body
- *Scientific concept*
    - Slow growing cancer
    - May be first clue that the patient has HIV/AIDs

Herpes Simplex (HSV 1 & 2)

- *Epidemiology*
    - HSV 1 – typically orofacial
    - HSV 2 – genital lesions
        - much overlap
        - 80% asymptomatic infection
    - In immunocompromised, minor infection can be life-threatening
        - Neonates
        - AIDs
        - Elderly, steroids, TNF-α inhibitors, azathioprine, transplant patients, etc.
- *H & P*
    - Painful ulcers on erythematous base
        - HSV 1 – gingivostomatitis/ cold sores
        - HSV 2 – genital lesions
- *Labs & Diagnostics*
    - Tissue culture is best – distinguishes HSV 1 from HSV 2

- Immunofluorescent staining of tissue from scraping of lesion
- Tzanck smear
    - Swab, on wet prep, showing multinucleated giant cells with inclusion bodies
    - Does not distinguish HSV 1 from HSV 2
- PCR-DNA
    - Especially useful in CSF
- Antibody testing
    - Not for acute infection
    - Not for recurrences

- *Most Likely Diagnosis (differential)*
    - HSV 1
    - Hand-foot-mouth disease (coxsackie virus)
    - Candidiasis (with erosions)
    - HSV 2 (painful)
    - Chancroid (painless)
    - Chancre (painless)
- *Clinical Intervention*
    - symptomatic treatment (remember, it resolves without meds due to intrinsic immune system of the patient)
    - If no resolution in 10-14 days, consider immune deficiency!
- *Therapeutics*
    - ***cyclovir
        - Acyclovir
        - Valacyclovir
        - Famciclovir
- *Health Maintenance*
    - Condom use
    - Daily dose of valacyclovir to prevent "shedding"
    - Single dose for cold sores at first tingling sensation

Herpes Zoster (Shingles)

- *Epidemiology*
    - Direct contact from lesion
    - Reactivation of latent chickenpox virus
    - Remains dormant in spinal root ganglia of nerves
    - Most common in very young, very old and immunosuppressed
- *H & P*
    - Burning in dermatome distribution of skin (often prior to eruption of vesicles)
    - Always only to midline
    - May be disseminated lesions in the elderly or very very sick
- *Labs & Diagnostics*
    - Tzank smear
- *Most Likely Diagnosis*
    - Typical dermatomal pattern to pain and vesicles
- *Clinical Intervention*
    - *Accelerate cutaneous healing*
    - *Resolve acute or chronic pain*
    - *Prevent complications*

- *Therapeutics*
    - ----cyclovir does all three above better than placebo
    - Acyclovir 800 mg. five times daily for 7 days
    - Valacyclovir 1000 gm TID for 7 days
    - Famiciclovir 750 mg. TID for 7 days
    - The ....cyclovirs are renally excreted so decrease dose in decreased GFR.
    - No med has been found to decrease incidence or intensity of postherpetic neuralgia (PHN).
- *Health Maintenance*
    - Not contagious to immune competent person who has had chicken pox.
    - Main contagion is to very young (not vaccinated) or very old, especially undergoing cancer treatment
    - VACCINATION is key to prevention
        - Now recommended by CDC for all persons ≥ 60 years.
        - Also approved for all patients ≥ 50 years.
        - Contraindicated in immunosuppression and PREGNANCY
    - PHN can be treated with gabapentin, tramadol, pregabalin, SSRI's
- *Scientific Concept*
    - If opthalmic branch of trigeminal nerve – check cornea for dendritic lesion.
    - Hutchinson's sign – vesicle on tip of nose = dendritic lesion on cornea

Cytomegalovirus infections

- *Epidemiology*
    - Transmitted sexually, congenitally, transfusion, transplanation, respiratory secretions
- *H & P*
    - Like infectious mono (sore throat, swollen glands; fairly benign in immune competent patient)
- *Labs & Diagnostics*
    - Serology
- *Therapeutics*
    - Gangciclovir
- *ScientifiG Concept*
    - Part of the TORCH screen for still births (i.e. C = CMV)
    - In AIDS (CD4<50) causes severe disease
    - Retinitis (blindness)
    - GI ulcers – esophageal CMV infection (dysphagia)
    - Pulmonary CMV

Epstein-Barr virus infections

- *Etiology/Epidemiology*
    - Infectious mono
- *H & P*
    - Sore throat with tonsillar exudates (nasty looking!)
    - Posterior cervical lymph nodes
    - Splenomegaly
    - Hepatomegaly (uncommon) with anorexia (common)

- *Labs & Diagnostics*
    - CBC shows leukopenia with relative lymphocytosis and atypical lymphocytes
    - Monospot (heterophile agglutination) --- may not be positive for 24-48 hours)
    - If LFT's are checked, will usually be elevated within two weeks of infection and remain elevated for up to six weeks
- *Clinical Intervention*
    - Check rapid strep (strep frequently accompanies mono)
- *Therapeutics*
    - None, self-limited
    - May need steroids for short course if tonsils prevent swallowing
- *Health Maintenance*
    - No contact sports x 4-6 weeks (or recheck)

- *Scientific Concept*
    - Rash all over if treated with Amoxicillin (frequently given because tonsils looks so bad)

Human Papillomavirus Infections

- *Etiology/Epidemiology*
    - HPV 6, etc. = benign warts
    - HPV 16, etc = cervical/squamous cell dysplasia; cancer
- *H & P*
    - Can be wart; flat; just irritation
- *Labs & Diagnostics*
    - HPV typing (serology, or on Thin Prep pap smear)
- *Most Likely Diagnosis*
    - Most common cause of squamous cell carcinoma (HPV 16, etc)
- *Clinical Intervention*
    - Cervical dysplasia - in women's health
    - If on vocal cords – ENT referral for biopsy
    - If skin -- biopsy
- *Therapeutics*
    - Immunosuppressants (imiquimod, topical 5-FU)
    - Cryocautery
- *Health Maintenance*
    - Gardasil vaccine available for HPV prevention
    - Available for boys since 2010
    - *See Women's Health Chapter 15 for more information.*

Influenza

- *Etiology/Epidemiology*
    - Virus
    - Common, highly contagious, genetically labile (changes every year)
- *H & P*
    - Abrupt onset
    - Fever & myalgias
    - Rhinorrhea

  - Sore throat
  - Cough
- *Labs & Diagnostics*
  - Nasopharyngeal swab
- *Most Likely Diagnosis*
  - During flu season, high index of suspicion
- *Clinical Intervention*
  - Oxygen
  - Fluids
  - Fever management
- *Secondary infections (in high risk patients) – hospitalization*
  - Most low risk patients can be followed closely OP
- *Therapeutics*
  - Oseltamivir
  - Zanamivir
  - Amantadine
- *Health Maintenance*
  - Influenza vaccine!
- *Scientific Concept*
  - Treatment must be started within 48 hours of symptom onset; the sooner the better!

Rabies

- *Etiology/Epidemiology*
  - Virus
  - Most common: #1 bats, dogs, cats, raccoons, skunks
- *H & P*
  - Patient is asymptomatic until develops disease
  - Once disease state
    - Hydrophobia
    - Thick tenacious saliva
    - Fever
    - Episodic rage alternating with calm
    - Paresthesias, paralysis
- *Labs & Diagnostics – clinical diagnosis*
- *Clinical Intervention*
  - Clean wound with soap and water – this alone reduces risk of infection!
  - Capture animal if possible – quarantined by health department
  - Rabies immunoglobulin is given directly into wound (if finger or small body part, as much as tolerated in wound, then in proximal muscles)
  - Rabies vaccine today (day 0) then day 3, 7, 14
    - This is just an IM shot in deltoid (not in abdomen like most still think)
- *Therapeutics*
  - Immunoglobulin
  - Injected into the wound itself; based on patient weight
  - Vaccine
    - Given at same time as immunoglobulin
    - Then again at day 3, 7 and 14

        - This injection is given intramuscularly just like any other injection in the deltoid
- *Health Maintenance*
    - Veterinarians
        - Prophylaxis = vaccine, then rabies antibody titer every 2 years and booters
    - Do not forget tetanus shot too!
- *Scientific Concept*
    - Rabies may not manifest for weeks after exposure
    - Even if touched by a bat, rabies is indicated!

Poliomyelitis *(not in the blueprint, but I think it is still important to comment on)*
- *Epidemiology*
    - Enterovirus
    - Fecal-oral route of infection
    - No reports since 1999 (except one in 2011 in immunocompromised patient)
- *H & P*
    - Paralysis
- *Labs & Diagnostics*
    - LP is needed
- *Clinical Intervention*
    - Strict bedrest
- *Health Maintenance*
    - Trivalent oral live poliovirus no longer in use – can cause disease
    - Inactivated parenteral vaccine is used (Salk vaccine) now

---

Fungal Infections

For these diseases look for clues to patient being immunocompromised

Candidiasis
- *Etiology*
    - Candida albicans/ glabrata/ tropicalis
- *Epidemiology*
    - Immunocompromised and diabetics
    - Inhaled steroids can cause thrush or esophageal candidiasis
- *H & P*
    - Curdy white discharge clinging to mucous walls
    - Scrapes off with Q-tip of tongue depressor
- *Labs & Diagnostics*
    - KOH scraping from skin/mucous membranes, including vagina
    - EGD with biopsy for esophageal
    - If retinal/other body parts, biopsy/culture needed
- *Most Likely Diagnosis*
    - KOH shows "pseudohyphae"

- *Therapeutics*
    - For candida albicans – fluconazole (PO) <Diflucan> or any –azole topically or vaginally
    - For non-albicans – tercanazole may work better, many resistances to fluconazole/miconazole
- *Health Maintenance*
    - Good control of AIC
    - Rinse mouth after using inhaled steroids
- *Scientific Concept*
    - If esophageal , needs EGD scoping; fluconazole
    - If vaginal needs cream or tablet

Cryptococcosis

- *Etiology*
    - Cryptococcus neoformans
- *Epidemiology*
    - AIDS/immunocompromised
    - Not contagious
- *H & P*
    - Altered mental status; HA
- *Labs & Diagnostics*
    - LP for CSF culture
    - Serum cryptococcal antigen
    - India ink positive
- *Therapeutics*
    - Amphotericin
- *Scientific Concept*
    - Most common cause of fungal meningitis in immunocompromised

HIV-RELATED PNEUMONIAS

Histoplasmosis

- Pathogen – Histoplasma capsulatum
- *Etiology/Epidemiology*
    - Bird droppings
    - Guano (bat dropping) exposure
- *H & P*
    - Pulmonary infection (asymptomatic in health people)
    - Disseminated in AIDs/immunosuppressed
- *Labs & Diagnostics*
    - Pulmonary biopsy
    - Urine antigen test
- *Therapeutics*
    - Itraconazole in mild or asymptomatic disease
    - Amphotericin (ampho"terrible") in severe disease (AIDS)

Pneumocystis – HIV Positive Patient with CD4 < 200
At this level prophylax with Bactrim (also for Tx)

- Pathogen –Pneumocystis jiroveci
- *Epidemiology*
  - AIDS with CD4<200
  - Asymptomatic in healthy individuals
- *H & P*
  - Fever, nonproductive cough
- *Labs & Diagnostics*
  - CSR (fluffy interstitial infiltrates throughout in AIDS patient)
- *Most Likely Diagnosis*
  - Any patient with HIV/AIDs, this is most likely diagnosis (if not prophylaxed)
- *Clinical Intervention*
  - Begin prophylactic antibiotics when CD4 count < 200
- *Therapeutics*
  - Bactrim DS (trimethoprim/sulfamethoxazole)
- *Health Maintenance*
  - *Start Bactrim DS when CD4<200 prophylactically
- *Scientific Concept*
  - Most common opportunistic infection in AIDs

OTHER FUNGAL DISEASES NOT IN THE BLUEPRINT:

Blastomycosis

- *Etiology*
  - Blastomyces dermatitides
- *Epidemiology*
  - Soil (dust) exposure in Ohio River Valley
- *H & P*
  - Pulmonary infection
  - Asymptomatic
- *Labs & Diagnostics*
  - Incidental finding on CXR
  - Biopsy/culture
- *Therapeutics*
  - Itraconazole, mild disease
- *Amphotericin, severe disease*

Coccidioidomycosis

- *Etiology*
  - Coccidioides immitis
- *Epidemiology*

- Entire southwest U.S. and Mexico (San Joaquin Valley Fever)
- *H & P*
    - Influenza-like illness
    - Erythema nodosum is common (purple painful nodules on anterior shins)
- *Labs & Diagnostics*
    - Blood test - serology
- *Clinical Intervention*
    - Self-limited --- no treatment needed
    - If disseminated (in HIV/AIDs patients):
        - Ketaconazle, itraconazole
    - Amphotericin
    - None of them work all that well though

Aspergillosis

- *Etiology*
    - Aspergillus fumigatus
- *Epidemiology*
    - Commonly inhaled fungus
- *H & P*
    - Bronchospasm = allergic bronchopulmonary aspergillosis
    - Mass in lung (looks like lung cancer) = aspergilloma (fungal "ball")
    - Neutropenia; very ill appearing= invasive aspergillosis

---

Bacterial Infections

Botulism

- *Etiology/Epidemiology*
    - Neurotoxin (Clostridium botulinum)
    - Home canning/ honey in infants
- *H & P*
    - Sudden onset of symptoms
    - Dipolpia; muscle weakness; dysphagia; respiratory paralysis
- *Clinical Intervention*
    - Ventilation support
- *Therapeutics*
    - Botulinum immune globulin
- *Health Maintenance*
    - No honey to kids < 1 year old
- *Scientific Concept*
    - Used in aesthetics and plastic surgery to "paralyze" muscles temporarily to decrease wrinkling
    - Paralyzes muscles in scalp to treat migraine
    - Paralyzes spasms in cerebral palsy and other neurologic diseases

Chlamydia – *(Pulmonary, Cervical, Urethral, Ophthalmologic)*

- *Etiology/Epidemiology*
  - Intracellular organism
  - Not seen on wet prep
  - Not seen on urine microscopic
- *C. trachomatis*
  - Cervix, urethra, uterus, nasopharyns, epididymis
  - Conjunctivitis (trachoma) and pneumonia in neonates
  - Most common reported bacterial STI
- *C. pneumoniae*
  - Pharyngitis, bronchitis, pneumonia
- *H & P*
  - Asymptomatic
  - Yellow discharge from cervix, penis, eye, etc.
  - Dysuria, urgency, frequency with pyuria (wbc's in urine) but no bacteria
- *Labs & Diagnostics*
  - Swab of cervix or penis
  - Culture
    - PCR-DNA
    - Voided urine sample can now be done for nucleic acid amplification testing (NAAT)
- *Clinical Intervention*
  - If urethritis without epididymitis/orchitis, or PID in women:
    - Single dose Azithromycin 1 gm. PO
    - Pending culture results, you should also cover GC (see below)
  - If epidiymitis/orchitis or PID:
    - Doxycycline 100 mg. BID x 14 days & Ceftriaxone 250 mg. IM (for GC)
- *Therapeutics*
  - Macrolides
  - Azithromycin (ok in pg)
  - Erythromycin (ointment in neonate eyes)
  - Tetracyclines
  - Doxacycline (not in pg)
  - Ampicillin
- *Health Maintenance*
  - Routine screening of sexually active young women is recommended by USPTSF as disease of the urethra and cervix is asymptomatic often
  - Barrier methods for sex
- *Scientific Concept*
  - Trachoma is the leading cause of acquired blindness world-wide
  - Remember, if there is one STI, look for others, i.e. if patient has herpes, get GC/Chlamydia cultures too!

Gonococcal infections – *(Cervical, PID, Urethral, Ophthalmologic)*

- *Etiology/Epidemiology*
  - Neisseria gonorrhoeae
  - Sexual contact/vertical transmission (mother to baby)

- *H & P*
  - Vaginal discharge is much more common in GC than in chlamydia
  - Dysuria, frequency
  - PID more common with GC than chlamydia
  - Urethral d/c in men
  - Acute epididymitis
  - Rectal infection with pain and pruritis or tenesmus
- *Labs & Diagnostics*
  - Culture is best (but not quickest)
  - DNA probe (next best)
  - PCR (assay)
  - Always get a pregnancy test if you suspect GC
  - Always check for chlamydia
- *Therapeutics*
  - Ceftriaxone 250 mg. IM plus azithromycin 1 gm or doxycycline 200 BID x 7 days(preferred)
- *Only if ceftriaxone is unavailable:*
  - Cefixime 400 mg.; plus the azithro or doxy (do test of cure in 1 week)
- *If true cephalosporin allergy:*
  - Azithromycin 2 gm PO (but do test of cure in 1 week to ensure eradication)
- *Health Maintenance*
  - Condoms/safe sex practices
- *Scientific Concept*
  - Dissemination to knee joint is common!
  - Culture should be taken from endocervix if bleeding (PCR or DNA not reliable then)
  - GI Infectious Diseases

Cholera

- *Etiology*
  - Vibrio cholerae
- *Epidemiology*
  - Contaminated food & water
  - Occurs most commonly after disaster flooding sanitation systems
- *H & P*
  - "Rice water" stools
  - Huge loss of total body water – can kill an infant quickly
- *Labs & Diagnostics*
  - Stool culture
- *Clinical Intervention*
  - Fluid resuscitation (always oral, if possible!!!)
- *Therapeutics*
  - No real treatment except for oral fluid resuscitation
    - Doxycycline is drug of choice (only if severely ill) in adults
    - Azithromycin should be used in children and pregnant women

Salmonellosis

- *Etiology*
  - Salmonella typhi

- *Epidemiology*
  - Think undercooked eggs (mayonnaise), raw cookie dough
  - Turtles
  - Travel to area endemic for salmonella
- *H & P*
  - Diarrhea
  - "Rose spots" on trunk (rose colored small papules)
  - Fever, HA plus GI symptoms above = "typhoid fever"
- *Labs & Diagnostics*
  - Stool culture (fecal leukocytes)
- *Most Likely Diagnosis*
  - Travel to an endemic area
  - Fever, symptoms within 60 days
- *Clinical Intervention*
  - Oral hydration

- *Therapeutics – only if severe symptoms*
  - Fluoroquinolones are first-line
- *Health Maintenance*
  - Vaccine is available

Shigellosis

- *Etiology*
  - Shigella *sonnei/dysenteriae*
- *Epidemiology*
  - Oral-fecal, especially in day cares among staff as well as infants
- *H & P*
  - Abrupt onset of bloody diarrhea with abdominal cramping
- *Labs & Diagnostics*
  - Stool culture, fecal leukocytes
- *Clinical Intervention*
  - Oral fluid rehydration
- *Therapeutics*
  - **Children** = TMP/SMX (Bactrim suspension)
  - **Adults** = fluoroquinolones (Cipro)
- *Health Maintenance*
  - Hand washing

Campylobacter

- *Etiology*
  - Campylobacter *jejuni*
- *Epidemiology*
  - Undercooked chicken
- *H & P*
  - Abdominal cramping
  - Fever
  - Watery/bloody diarrhea
- *Labs & Diagnostics*

  - Stool culture
- *Clinical Intervention*
  - Fluid support
- *Therapeutics (macrolides)*
  - Erythromycin
  - Azithromycin
- *Health Maintenance*
  - Hand washing
  - Cook chicken
  - Clean kitchen utensils/platters, etc
- *Scientific Concept*
  - Most common cause of infectious diarrhea in U.S.
  - Implicated in Guillain-Barre syndrome
  - Implicated in Reactive arthritis (Reiter's syndrome) along with Chlamydia

Clostridium Dificile (C. dif)

- *Etiology*
  - C. dificile
- *Epidemiology*
  - Antibiotic use (any) ; clindamycin implicated, but cephalosporins given more commonly so causes more in terms of incidence!
- *H & P*
  - High WBC count is a hallmark (30,000-50,000 is not uncommon!)
  - Frequent stools, 20-40 times per day; usually watery with distinctive odor
  - Patient can be toxic and die
- *Labs & Diagnostics*
  - Stool culture will not find it!!! need to order C. dif toxin assay
- *Most Likely Diagnosis*
  - Anyone recently on antibiotics!!!
- *Therapeutics*
  - Metronidazole - first line
  - Vancomycin (PO) – works better in the gut than if given IV
  - Stop other antibiotics
- *Health Maintenance*
  - Limit unnecessary antibiotic use, i.e. URI's
- *Scientific Concept*
  - Important iatrogenic infection – patient needs isolation precautions

Tetanus

- *Etiology*
  - Clostridium tetani neurotoxin
- *Epidemiology – break in skin*
  - Remember, not just puncture (although punctures are most susceptible)
  - Corneal abrasions, decubitus ulcers, abrasions of skin, elbows
- *H & P*
  - Tetany of jaw (trismus), neck; dysphagia
- *Labs & Diagnostics*

- None, really. Based on Physical Exam findings
- *Therapeutics*
  - If tetany, give vaccine PLUS TIG (tetanus immune globulin) PLUS Penicillin G
- *Health Maintenance*
  - Prevent with vaccination (tetanus series, then booster q 10 years
- *Scientific Concept*
  - If "clean wound" – scissors in house cutting a box, etc; needs last booster within 10 years
- *If dirty wound, (outdoor nail in foot) give tetanus booster if > 5 years from last one*

PEARL: *Reminder about Td, immunoglobulin:*

- if the person has all their childhood shots (primary immunity) --- then Td every 10 years as update whether injured or not. Td within 10 years for "clean wound" if not updated already (i.e., if the patient has had it 8 years ago, no need for booster).

- If dirty (particularly puncture wound) then within 5 years --- again even if he steps on a feces encrusted nail, but had Td 3 years ago, no need for booster.

- If the patient has not had childhood vaccines, then TIG (to fight acute tetanus_ and vaccine to start the series.

- If the patient actually has TETANUS -- then TIG is indicated as well as antibiotics.

Corynebacerium Diptheriae

- *Illness is due to a toxin (produced by the bacteria)*
- *Very uncommon now due to vaccination (DPT)*
- *Only two cases so far since 2000*
- *H & P*
  - Sore throat
  - Low grade fever
  - Adherent gray membrane on tonsils, pharynx and oropharyngeal cavity
  - Can cause severe swelling of anterior neck
- *Labs & Diagnostics*
  - Gram stain
  - Throat culture (not rapid strep!)
- *Most Likely Diagnosis*
  - "Gray membrane"
- *Clinical Intervention*
- *Therapeutics*
  - Antitoxin is the real "cure", but must be given very early in course; does not do anything for toxin already in tissue
- *Health Maintenance*
  - Vaccination!!!

Mycobacterial Infections

Tuberculosis

- Etiology/epidemiology
  - multisystem disease
  - *Most common cause of infectious disease-related mortality worldwide.*
  - Decreasing in incidence in U.S.
  - Increasing in incidence in some part of the world.
  - Prevalence of drug-resistant TB is increasing worldwide (and in the U.S.).
- H & P
  - Pulmonary TB
    - cough
    - weight loss/anorexia
    - fever & night sweats
    - hemoptysis
  - CNS TB
    - tTubercular meningitis
    - HA x 2-3 weeks with mental status changes
      - May, or may not have fever
    - chorioretinitis
  - Ortho TB
    - skeletal TB
    - back pain
    - lower extremity paralysis
    - 50% of patients with Pott disease
    - arthritis
    - monoarticular (hip or knee)
  - Genitourinary TB
    - flank pain
    - dysuria and frequency
    - painful scrotal mass, prostatitis, orchitis, epididymitis
    - PID
  - GI TB
    - nonhealing ulcers of mouth or anus
    - dysphagia
    - upper abdominal pain mimicking PUD
    - malabsorption
    - diarrhea with hematochezia
- Labs & Diagnostics
  - screening
    - Mantoux TB skin test with purified protein derivative (PPD)
- Diagnosis (if you suspect TB)
  - Acid-fast bacilli (AFB) smear and culture of sputum
  - HIV serology in all patients with positive AFB
- If positive cultures:
  - drug susceptibility testing (to identify multidrug-resistant TB (MDR-TB)
  - Direct DNA sequencing analysis, or variety of other testing

    - CXR
        - Cavitations
            - In primary TB in middle or lower lung regions
        - Noncaseating granulomas
        - Miliary TB: numerous tiny nodules in all lung fields
        - Pleural TB
- Most Likely Diagnosis
    - clues are cough/ fever/ weight loss
- Therapeutics for active TB:
    - empiric therapy until MDR testing comes back:
        - Isoniazid
        - Rifampin
        - Pyrazinamide
        - Ethambutol
- If MDR-TB is suspected (4-5 of the following):
    - Aminoglycoside (streptomycin, amikacin, kanamycin)
    - Fluoroquinolone (cipro, ofloxacin)
    - Thioamide (ethionamide)
    - Pyrazinamide
    - Ethambutol
    - Cycloserine
    - Terizodone
    - Para-aminosalicylic acid
- Therapeutics for latent TB:
    - Isoniazid
    - Rifampin
- Health Maintenance
    - Health care workers should be regularly screened.
    - You should have PPD applied after contact with known TB patient.
    - Isolate patients with possible TB (in hospital use negative pressure room).
    - high-efficiency masks (filter bacillus)
    - Isolation continues with ID precautions until sputum smear negative x 3 (2-4 weeks after beginning treatment).
- Scientific Concept – the TB testing information:
    - must be read within 72 hours of applied; if not, will need to be repeated
    - Induration and not just redness is measured (diameter of the circle), if blistered, that counts.
    - More the general population with no risk, just being screened for no reason at all:
        - 15 mm of induration or more is a POS
        - 10 mm or more is POS in:
            - recent immigrants from endemic countries
            - IV drug users
            - prisoners, institutionalized, homeless, nursing homes
            - lab personnel who work in microbiology who do mycobacteria testing
            - increased susceptibility (DM, steroids, leukemias, ESRF, anorexics)
            - children < 4 yrs

      - patients who have received BCG (if in contact with TB pt, or from TB prevalent country)
    - 5 mm or more would be a POS in:
      - HIV positive patients
      - known contact with active TB patient
      - CXR findings of nodules
      - transplant or severely immunocompromised patients
  - Remember that if severely immunocompromised patient, should also apply candida to make sure the patient is not anergic
    - In anergy, the patient has no immune response, i.e. a false negative.
    - Since we all react to yeast on our skin, if the candida is negative too, the patient is anergic and you cannot call it a negative PPD.

Atypical Mycobacterial Disease

- Etiology/epidemiology
  - There are 30 known entities that are acid fast bacilli but do not cause TB or leprosy.
    - occur in patients with underlying other diseases
      - emphysema, DM, leukemia, SLE, lung cancer, ESRF, TB, bronchiectasis
      - patients on TNF-α inhibitors
- Mycobacterium avium-intracellulare (most common in humans)
  - pulmonary
  - soft tissue
  - lymphadenitis
  - disseminated (in AIDs)
  - Mycobacterium marinum (fish tank granuloma)
- H & P
  - almost anything depending on the system infected
- Labs & Diagnostics
  - culture of tissue (biopsy, bronchoscopy)
- Clinical Intervention
  - ID is always involved
- Therapeutics
  - clarithromycin is a good start
  - sensitivities from culture is most useful
- Health Maintenance
  - manage comorbid conditions
- Scientific Concept
  - Leprosy is due to a mycobacterium too! (M. leprae)
    - Major reservoir in the U.S. is the armadillo!
    - I never knew this (but I live in WI), I'll bet those TX PA's knew this!

Parasitic Infections

Amebiasis

- Etiology – Entamoeba *histolytica*

- Epidemiology
  - fresh water; rivers;
  - fecal-oral; poor sanitation
- H & P
  - diarrhea and abdominal cramping
  - Liver abscess is most common complication
- Labs & Diagnostics
  - stool ova & parasites (not found on culture), must order separately
  - antigen PCR from serum is better
  - abdominal CT to r/o liver abscess
- Therapeutics
  - metronidazole
  - drainage of abscess

Malaria

- Etiology – Plasmodium *vivax*; *malaraie*; ovale; *falciparum* (nastiest one!)
- Epidemiology
  - mosquito vector in endemic areas (hot, humid climates)
- H & P
  - sudden onset of shaking rigors, fevers, and sweats in paroxysms (every couple of days)
  - HA, myalgias; splenomegaly
- Labs & Diagnostics
  - blood smear – look for RBC's containing malaria organisms
- Therapeutics
  - quinine
  - chloroquine
  - if G6PD deficient = do not use antimalarials --- use Doxycycline
- Scientific Concept
  - sickle cell anemia and G6PD deficiency are both genetic mutations that cause abnormalities of the RBC cell membrane; when these mutations occurred in areas endemic to malaria, it conferred a protective effect on those individuals who got the mutation
  - (see youtube video (http://www.youtube.com/watch?v=1fN7rOwDyMQ)
- Therefore, this Hgb S gene propagated as it is protective to these humans
  - the same happens with G6PD deficiency
- For this reason, these two diseases are most prevalent in areas also endemic to malaria
  - drug treatments for malaria are contraindicated in these patients

Nematodes

- Hookworms & Roundworms
- Etiology
  - Ascaris (most common – large roundworm)
  - Hookworms, (second most common)
- Epidemiology - 600-700 million infected worldwide
  - Used to be very common in US; now not so much due to good sanitation
- Hookworms

  - person defectates outside; person steps on soil infected with eggs; eggs hatch into larvae which penetrate skin of feet; transmitted to gut
- Roundworms
  - ingested from infected food products (trichinosis from undercooked pork is an example)
- H & P
  - asymptomatic usually at onset
  - causes profound anemia and nutritional deficiencies
- Labs & Diagnostics
  - eosinophilia on Wright strain of blood smear
- Therapeutics
  - antihelminthic drugs
    - mebendazole (vermox)
- Health Maintenance
  - sanitation
- Scientific Concept
  - most common still in third world countries

Pinworms

- Etiology – Enterobius *vermicularis*
- Epidemiology
  - very common – even now--- mainly in children preshool and early childhood
- H & P
  - intense perianal itching – especially at night
- Labs & Diagnostics
  - pinworm tape (scotch tape works too --- put on rectum before bed, take off in morning, and look under microscope – easy to see worms and eggs stuck to tape
- Most Likely Diagnosis
  - anal irritation from poor cleansing but tape has worms and eggs on it!
- Therapeutics
  - mebendazole (Vermox)
- Scientific Concept
  - most common nematode in U.S.

Not In Blueprint

Toxoplasmosis

- Etiology – Toxoplasma *gondii*
- Epidemiology
  - handling cat litter
  - one of five "neglected parasitic illnesses" targeted by CDC for intervention
  - no severe illness in nonpregnant and immunocompetent patients
  - high risk of vertical transmission to fetus of woman infected
  - high risk of serious illness in immunocompromised patients
- H & P
  - asymptomatic in normal patient
  - Headache, altered mental status, new onset seizure in AIDS patients with CD4 <100
- Labs & Diagnostics

  - serology
  - imaging of brain (in AIDS)
- Therapeutics
  - pyrimethamine
  - sufadiazine
- Scientific Concept
  - ring enhancing mass lesion in brain is hallmark on brain CT in AIDS
  - in vertical transmission to fetus (only if mom contracts it while pregnant)
  - stillbirth/miscarriage
  - microcephaly
  - cognitive impairment
  - vision loss
  - seizures

Rickettsial Diseases

Lyme disease

- Etiology/epidemiology – Borrelia burgdorferi (deer tick)
  - Most common vector-borne illness in the U.S.
  - Increasing in incidence and geographic spread
- H & P
  - Stage 1 (early localized disease)
    - 3-30 days after exposure
    - erythema migrans (widening circular ringed rash with central clearing)
  - Stage 2 (early disseminated disease)
    - days to weeks after initial tick exposure
    - dissemination to blood
    - fever, chills, myalgias, arthralgias
    - cardiac symptoms – AV block
    - neuro symptoms – Bell's Palsy; encephalitis
  - Stage 3 (late disseminated disease)
    - weeks to months after initial tick exposure
    - persistent/chronic
    - arthritis – 60 %
    - neuro – polyneuropathy; encephalopathy
- Labs & Diagnostics
  - **Clinical diagnosis if erythema migrans is seen – no need for labs**
  - ELISA with confirmatory western blot
  - Serologic testing has huge false positive – not for screening!
  - Serologic testing is not done for vague nonspecific symptoms without known tick exposure in endemic area!
- Therapeutics
  - Prophylactic treatment recommended ONLY IF:
    - The tick is identified as a deer tick attached for more than 36 hours
    - Prophylaxis must be within 72 hours of time tick removed
    - Doxycycline is not contraindicated
    - If not all three criteria met, benefit does not outweigh risk

- Doxycycline (>8 years of age) – not in pregnant women!
- Amoxicillin (< 8 years of age)
  - Should not be used in adults for prophylaxis (not very effective)
  - But, pregnancy warrants treatment!
    - Causes abortion, stillbirth and preterm birth
- Treatment of early disseminated infection
  - Ceftriaxone
- Treatment of late disseminated
  - With arthritis – Doxycycline
  - With CNS symptoms - ceftriaxone

- Health Maintenance
  - Prevention in endemic areas (long sleeves, long pant legs, socks)
  - Inspect for ticks after being out in the woods
- Scientific Concepts
  - Early local and early disseminated infection is eradicated in 90% with treatment
  - Must be attached for 24-48 hours in order to transmit infection
    - Removing the tick within 24 hours is sufficient
    - <5% incidence of infection from single tick bite (even if > 48 hr)
  - Ticks in the nymphal stage are most infectious (June through August)
  - Most cases of erythema migrans occur in summer

Rocky Mountain Spotted Fever

- Etiology/epidemiology – Rickettsia rickettsii (tick bite)
- H & P
  - influenza-like prodrome
  - fever; chills; ha; myalgias
  - red macular (petechial) rash 2nd through 6th day – wrists/ankles, spreads to trunk (90%)
  - myalgias
  - conjunctivitis/uveitis
- Labs & Diagnostics
  - No current test to identify acute infection
- Clinical diagnosis
  - Antibody tests are negative for the first 7-10 days of infection
- Clues:
  - Hyponatremia; thrombocytopenia, elevated LFT's
- Clinical Intervention
  - Therapeutics
    - Doxycycline (even in children!!)
    - If you avoid doxy, you risk death of the child
- Health Maintenance
  - Avoid tick bites (clothing), inspect and remove any ticks
- Scientific Concept
  - R. ricketsii infects the endothelial cells of arterioles (but is not in bloodstream), making it difficult to detect in first week of infection (85% neg in first week)
  - Immune reaction causes antibodies, detectable after 7-10 days
  - Endothelial damage causes the petechiae

Rickettsial diseases not in Blueprint

Erlichiosis (like Lyme disease, but different ☺)

- Etiology/epidemiology
    - tick vector
    - "Lone Star Lyme's " (Texas and high desert plains)
- H & P
    - fever
    - headache
    - arthralgias
- Labs & Diagnostics
    - blood smear (lab reports it to you)
- Therapeutics
    - Doxycycline
- Health Maintenance
    - mosquito repellant; aviud mosquito infested areas

Babesiosis

- Etiology - tick vector (but more like malaria)
- Epidemiology
    - Long Island, Martha's Vineyard
- H & P
    - fevers, drenching sweats
- Labs & Diagnostics
    - lab smear – has to be a manual evaluation of peripheral smear
- Therapeutics
    - None if asymptomatic disease
    - If symptomatic
        - Atovaquone plus azithromycin
    - If severe symptoms
        - Clindamycin plus quinine
    - If a child
        - azithromycin
- Health Maintenance
    - mosquito spray

Syphilis

Jarisch-Hertheimer Reaction

Primary syphilis

- Etiology/epidemiology
    - Spirochete – Treponema pallidum
    - Transmitted by sexual contact with a lesion
    - Transmitted vertically from mom to baby
    - Transmitted by blood products
    - PCN has lowered incidence, but still not eradicated
- H & P

  - Afebrile
  - Chancre occurs within 3 weeks of contact.
  - Solitary, painless, raised, firm
  - Regional lymphadenopathy
  - Heals in 4-8 weeks without treatment
- Labs & Diagnostics
  - Painless ulcer = get dark-field microscopy
  - Screening in asymptomatic = VDRL (positive 1-2 weeks after chancre appears)
  - If VDRL is positive = get FTA-ABS (fluorescent treponemal antibody screen)
- Therapeutics
  - Penicillin (changed everything!) Benzathine PCN G, 2.4 million units IM once.
- Health Maintenance
  - Chancre is highly contagious
- Scientific Concept
  - Four stages:
    - Primary
    - Secondary
    - Tertiary
- Famous people with syphilis : Bram Stoker (dracula guy), Vincent Van Gogh, Henry VIII (all those women)

Secondary Syphilis

- Etiology/epidemiology
  - After healing of chancre, the spirochete enters the blood stream
- H & P
  - Rash appears 2-10 weeks after healing chancre
  - Rash over back that resembles pityriasis rosea
  - Condylomata lata (loooks like warts) – very infectious
  - General and mild malaise, HA, fatigue
- Labs & Diagnostics
  - VDRL (100% sensitivity in secondary syphilis)
- Therapeutics
  - Benzathine penicillin G 2.4 million units IM once
- Scientific Concept
  - If you are given a significant sexual history in a patient with a scaley rash in a "christmas tree distribution", make sure to check a VDRL!

Tertiary syphilis

  - usually manifests within 3-10 years of acute infection
  - H&P
    - Skin
      - Gumma (skin lump, bone mass)
    - Cardiac
      - Aorta (saccular aneurysm of the thoracic aorta)
    - CNS
      - Altered mental status/dementia
      - Focal neurologic findings

            - CNS meningitis (neurosyphilis)
            - Vision and hearing loss
            - Argyll-Robertson pupil
                - "prostitute analogy" – pupil accomodates but does not re-act
    - Labs & Diagnostics
        - Lumbar puncture
            - Cell count, protein, VDRL-CSF
        - Therapeutics
        - Benzathine penicillin G 7.2 million units total, in 3 doses of 2.4 million units each, once per week x 3 weeks.

PEARL about syphilis treatment:

No matter what, Penicillin is the treatment of choice. Because so many people who think they are Pen allergic are not actually pen allergic, a patient with syphilis should be skin tested and undergo desensitization if necessary so that they can be given penicillin. (True of pregnant women too!)

CHAPTER 23

Hematology/Oncology/Coagulopathy – 3%

Introduction to Hematology Chapter

This section is only 3% of the total questions on the exam (so, about 7 or 8 questions), although there are many topics in this section in the Blueprint. Because there are so few total possible number of questions, do not spend an inordinate amount of time here. Focus mainly on the laboratory evaluation of the disorders.

Pearls about anemias:

- Anemias are easy to distinguish based on the MCV, i.e., how big or how small the cell is:
    - If the cells are small, the MCV will be < 80, and it is likely iron deficiency or Thalassemia anemia.
    - If the cells are large (MCV > 100), then a B-12 or Folic acid deficiency likely exists.
    - If the MCV is normal, there is likely an *acute* bleed.
        - It takes a while (120 days or more, to be precise) for a change in the "size" of the cell to occur, so if the MCV is normal, it signifies an acute change.
        - Although, anemia of chronic disease can cause either a microcytic (low MCV) or normocytic (normal MCV).
- All of these disorders are either inherited or acquired.
    - Acquired means that the patient was born "normal", and then developed an antibody that is damaging his cells, or has malnutrition that has altered the size of his cells, i.e., B-12 deficiency.
    - Inherited anemias are present at birth and will not be "cured", i.e. sickle cell.
- Leukemia arises in the bone marrow and is distinguished by the white cell count and differential
    - large numbers of otherwise *normal* WBC's suggest a *chronic* leukemia
    - look for *"blasts"* to identify *acute* leukemia
        - lymphoblast identifies an acute lymphocytic leukemia
        - myeloblasts suggest an acute myelogenous leukemia
        - monoblasts suggest an acute monoblastic leukemia
- Lymphomas arise in the lymph nodes themselves, identified by lymph node biopsy

Anemias

Aplastic anemia

- The word "aplasia" means "no cell development"
    - Therefore, decrease in *all* cell lines, and
    - hypoplastic marrow on bone marrow biopsy
- Most common cause
    - chemotherapy or radiation therapy
    - sulfa, seizure meds
- Labs & Diagnostics
    - Low RBC, low Hgb &Hct
    - Low WBC
    - Low Platelet count

    Everything low
- Clinical Intervention: refer to heme/onc

Microcytic Anemias (MCV < 80)

Iron deficiency anemia

- Most common hematologic abnormality worldwide
- Most common cause
    - due to malnutrition in children (even in US)
    - due to GI bleed until proven otherwise in adults
- H & P:
    - Skin changes (cheilitis; esophageal webs, etc) are chronic.
    - Tachycardia suggests acute development.
    - Pallor can happen in anyone – but if significant pallor, probably suggests a very low blood count
- Labs & Diagnostics:
    - Low RBC, low Hgb, low Hct
    - MCV < 80
    - *Serum Ferritin is the best and earliest indicator of iron deficiency*
    - Serum Fe is a later finding
        - It will not decrease until after ferritin stores are exhausted.
- Clinical Intervention:
    - Iron! Give oral TID; enteric coated is better tolerated
- Scientific Concept:
    - Where is iron absorbed? In the duodenum

Thalassemia

- Hemoglobinopathy inherited mainly by patients of Mediterranean descent
    - Turk, African, Greek, Italian, Moroccan, etc.
- Common in these ethnicities
- two types α & β – not important to distinguish them, electrophoresis will do that for you
    - Alpha-Thal – SE Asian and Chinese ethnicity
    - Beta – Thal – Mediterranean ethnicity

- Heterozygous forms (less severe) and homozygous forms (more severe)
- H & P
  - More the most part, asymptomatic
  - May have more symptoms when pregnant (shortness of breath, tachycardia)
- Labs & Diagnostics
  - Low RBC, low Hgb, low Hct
  - MCV < 80 – usually very low (lower than most Fe deficiency anemias)
  - *Iron studies will be normal*!
  - If severe (homozygous)
    - may have splenomegaly
    - reticulocytes from premature destruction of these "abnormal" cells
  - Hemoglobin electrophoresis is the key
- Clinical Intervention: none (for the most part)
  - *Do not give iron* (if ferritin is normal, patient does not need iron.
    - will overload the patient
  - If severe disease, refer to hematologist

Macrocytic Anemias (MCV > 100)

Vitamin B12 deficiency

- H & P
  - proprioception and vibratory sensation abnormal
  - gait ataxia
  - altered mental status
- Most common cause
  - malabsorption (vegans, bariatric patients, crohn's patients)
- Less common : Autoimmune cause
  - pernicious anemia – due to Intrinsic factor (IF) antibodies or parietal cell antibodies
- Labs & Diagnostics
  - MCV>100
  - serum B12 levels low,
  - serum Intrinsic factor (IF) antibodies , if present = pernicious anemia
- Clinical Intervention:
  - as below --- supplement with B12 (if not absorbed, give it IM)

PEARLS about B-12 deficiency:

- Vitamin B-12 is present in red meat and dairy and is stored in the body for as long as 3 years.
- For good absorption, it must combine with intrinsic factor, which is produced in the parietal cells of the gastric mucosa.
- The IF-B12 complex then is transported to the terminal ileum where it is absorbed.

Therefore, B-12 deficiency will occur in:

- Patients who do not eat red meat
  - vegans, the elderly
- those who do not make IF
  - bariatric surgery, atrophic gastritis (elderly)

- those who do not have good functional bowel
    - Crohn's, sprue patients
- those who have autoimmune destruction of their stomach lining
    - pernicious anemia
- *B-12 deficiency causes a preventable but incurable dementia if not treated.*
    - Treatment is < \$10.00/year.
    - Cobalamin is given IM monthly, for the rest of life.
    - Cobalamin may also be given as super high doses PO, or nasal spray daily --- compliance decreases with daily administration and is much more costly.

Folate deficiency

- Etiologies
    - Alcohol
    - Methotrexate
- Other causes
    - rapid turnover of cells
    - SS, spherocytosis, hemolytic anemias, etc.
- H & P
    - vague symptoms
    - but no neurologic symptoms as in B12 deficiency
- Labs & Diagnostics
    - Macrocytic anemia (MCV >100)
    - RBC folate levels
- Clinical Intervention
    - supplement with Folic Acid
- Scientific Concept
    - Why is folic acid and B12 needed? DNA synthesis

Why does folic acid and B12 deficiency cause a "megaloblastic" anemia with a "hypersegmented" nucleus?

ANSWER: Because there is decreased DNA synthesis (no mitosis), but RNA synthesis continues causing increased nuclear material.

Normocytic Anemias (MCV 80-100)

Most common causes in order:

- Acute Blood Loss
    - Not due to bone marrow or inherited problems, RBC's are made normally
    - They are "lost"
        - due to GI bleed, menorrhagia, hematoma, splenomegaly, chronic disease states, etc.
- Acute vs. chronic works very well here
    - If acute,
        - patient is tachycardic, pale, clammy extremities, and eventually hypotensive
        - RBC low, MCV normal (because the cells lost are all < 120 days old, yes?
        - Reticulocytes should be present (RDW wide)
    - If chronic

        - relatively asymptomatic presentation
        - RBC low, MCV low (cells are small)
        - no reticulocytes (RDW normal)
- Labs
    - if there is an acute loss of RBC's, there should be a BRISK reticulocytosis
        - bone marrow is responding appropriately to the blood loss by sending out reticulocytes which function, but not as efficiently as mature RBC's.
        - They are larger in size, so will cause an increase in the RDW.
        - This bone marrow response (retic count > 10% or more) is your biggest clue to an acute bleed!
- Acute reasons are obvious
    - trauma, bleed, menorrhagia, sickle cell crisis
- Chronic reasons are less obvious but *important*
    - In adults, chronic blood loss will always be assumed from the gut
        - Colorectal cancer is #2 cancer killer of humans, so rule it out first
        - Then, rule out loss from peptic ulcer disease, esophagitis, gastritis, etc.
            - These very chronic losses end up in the iron (Fe) deficiency anemia section above
- Scientific Concept
    - I am *not* talking about malnutrition here, remember, the bone marrow is doing its thing appropriately, but cells are being "lost"

Hemolytic anemias – inherited and acquired

Sickle Cell Anemia

- Epidemiology
    - Autosomal recessive – effecting B-globin gene on Chromosome 11
    - Homozygous = HbSS; heterozygous = HbAS
    - Mediterranean ethnicity: Turk, Italian, African, Greek
    - males & females – (recall that "autosomal" applies to all of us humans)
    - hemoglobinopathy which causes cells to lyse easily, damaged by the spleen
    - HbSS = chronic hemolytic anemia, chronic hyposia and splenomegaly
- **Acute**
    - massive "sickling" in response to illness, hypoxia and dehydration
    - causes "sequestration" of RBC's in the spllen
    - abdominal pain; bone pain; priapism; acute occlusions (stroke, ischemic problems in peripheral areas)
    - Labs
        - reticulocytosis (huge numbers, 10-25% (nl < 2%)
    - Therapeutics:
        - oxygen, fluids, pain management
    - Clinical Intervention
    - Hematology referral

- **Chronic**
    - Chronic hemolytic anemia
    - Ischemic necrosis changes of bone; kidney disease, cardiac disease, retinopathy

- splenomegaly
- Labs
  - low Hgb & Hct
  - no reticulocytosis
  - indirect bilirubinemia (as in all hemolytic anemias)
- Therapeutics
  - Urea
  - avoid infection, dehydration and hypoxia

- Clinical Intervention
  - all should have a hematologist following
- Health Maintenance
  - Pneumococcal vaccine (effective asplenism)
  - Influenza vaccine
  - Folic acid supplementation
  - Increased risk of pneumonia, meningitis, osteomyelitis and sepsis (essentially asplenic)
- Scientific Concept
  - First "clue" in neonate is dactylitis

G6PD deficiency

- Epidemiology
  - X-linked Recessive (so occurs most frequently in those who only get one X (men!)
  - Mediterranean and Ashkenazi Jewish ethnicities primarily effected
- H & P
  - Asymptomatic unless we cause hemolysis by giving the patient the wrong drug
- DRUGS TO AVOID:
  - All antimalarial drugs: quinidine, hydroxychloroquine, primaquine
  - Nitrofurantoin
  - Sulfa +/-
- Scientific Concepts:
  - Heinz bodies are produced due to oxidative stress (patient lacks enzyme to prevent this)
    - These Heinz bodies form precipitants on the red cell membrane, which the spleen does not like; and it destroys the cells, hence causing a hemolytic anemia (and eventually, effective asplenism)

Hereditary Spherocytosis

- Epidemiology
  - Autosomal dominant inheritance
- H & P
  - asymptomatic; to mild symptoms; to severe (rare)
  - Splenomegaly
    - Due to the abnormal shape of the cell, the spleen doesn't like it and destroys them
  - Jaundice
    - Indirect bilirubin will be elevated, as in hemolytic anemias (which this actually is, isn't it?)

- Labs & Diagnostics:
  - Mild anemia (usually), can even be normal sometimes
  - MCV low
  - *MCHC high – most important clue*
    - is the only anemia that will have an increase in the mean corpuscular hemoglobin concentration
    - it lacks central pallor so is "dark" in the middle and increases the MCHC
- Clinical Intervention:
  - daily folic acid (needed for DNA synthesis as there is rapid turnover of cells)

Autoimmune Hemolytic Anemia

- Etiology
  - Autoimmune (F>M)
  - Acquired IgG that attaches to RBC, and the complex is then destroyed by the spleen
- H&P
  - chronic anemia symptoms
- Labs & Diagnostics
  - Positive Coombs test
- Treatment
  - Prednisone
  - PRBC's if severe
- Clinical Intervention
  - heme/onc referral
- Scientific Concept
  - The clue is, this patient has autoimmune disease history, i.e. Hashimoto's or SLE, or RA

INHERITED ANEMIAS

G6PD deficiency and SS anemias were a mutation that occurred in humans. Those who lived in malaria endemic areas were "protected" from malaria due to the mutation, and so it propagated among the people who lived in the areas around the Mediterranean Sea. These are common inherited anemias.

Chronic "sicklers" present differently than patients in acute sickle cell "crisis". Chronic patients have chronic problems related to the spleen having to work overtime to get rid of abnormal cells, the bone marrow needing tons of nutrition to make all those new cells, and the chronic problem of sickled cells "clumping" in small capillaries

In addition to SS and G6PD, the other hereditary anemias also cause splenomegaly: Thalassemias and spherocytocis being the most important

All patients who have significant hemolytic anemias like these are "essentially asplenic". Their spleens are so damaged in the process of turning over cells that it does not function as it should (so like a true asplenic patient, this patient needs Pneumovax protection against encapsulated bacteria, i.e. strep pneumonia)

Anemia Review Questions

(?) A 19 y.o. female of Turkish ethnicity presents with her first pregnancy at 28 weeks gestation. As part of her menstrual history, she reports menarche at age 12 with frequently irregular periods since age 17. Her routine prenatal blood work reveals the following:

HGB 9.1 (nl 12-15)
HCT 30% (nl 36-45)
MCV 74 (nl 80-100)

What would be the next diagnostic test to order to help you distinguish iron deficiency anemia from Thalassemia?

A. **Reticulocyte count**
B. **Peripheral smear**
C. **HGB electrophoresis**
D. **Serum Ferritin**
E. **RDW**

Answer: D.

Discussion: Serum Ferritin; many of you probably chose Hgb Electrophoresis based on her ethnicity; but remember, iron deficiency anemia is the *most common medical disorder worldwide*, and while she MAY have Thalassemia, she may just need iron. Now, if her Ferritin is normal or high, she needs electrophoresis; the other tests are just not that helpful.

(?) A 32 y.o. African-American female presents to the clinic for her annual physical examination with c/o mild "fatigue" that she has noticed gradually worsening over the past 6 months. She has had no sleep or appetite issues, no changes in mood, no difficulty concentrating or recent major upheavals in her life. She has noted a gradual decrease in her exercise tolerance and feels very tired at the end of the day.

This patient's exam is entirely unremarkable including a normal resting pulse, no thyromegaly, no murmur, no peripheral edema; abdominal exam and stool guaiac are negative.

WBC 9,400 with normal diff
Hgb 9.9
HCT 28%
MCH 32 (nl 27-34)
MCV 68 (nl 80-100)
MCHC 34 (nl 31-36)

Serum Ferritin 7 (nl 13-100)

What is the most likely diagnosis?

A. **Fe deficiency anemia**
B. **Hereditary spherocytosis**
C. **Sickle Cell Anemia**
D. **G6PD Deficiency**
E. **Thalassemia**

Answer: A. Iron deficiency anemia

Discussion: A low *serum ferritin* is your earliest and best indicator of iron deficiency.

Please note, in the first question in this section, I only gave you the MCV in the stem of the question; but that was just to make you take notice. In a "real" CBC, all the other indices will be given as well. For the most part, you can ignore the other indices, *unless* the MCHC is high. I want you to get used to seeing all the indices but paying attention to the MCV primarily.

An 18 y.o. African-American female presents to the clinical annual PE c/o mild "fatigue" that she has noticed is gradually worsening over the past 6 months. She has had no sleep or appetite issues, no changes in mood, difficulty concentrating or recent major upheavals in her life. She has noted a gradual decrease in her exercise tolerance and feels very tired at the end of the day.

This patient's PE is entirely unremarkable including a normal resting pulse, no thyromegaly, no murmur, no peripheral edema; abdominal exam is normal except that spleen tip is palpable ; stool guaiac is negative.

WBC 9,400 with normal diff
Hgb 9.9
HCT 28%
MCH 32 (nl 27-34)
MCV 68 (nl 80-100)
MCHC 47 (nl 31-36)
Serum Ferritin 112 (nl 13-180)

What is the most likely diagnosis?

A. Fe deficiency anemia
B. Hereditary spherocytosis
C. Sickle Cell Anemia
D. G6PD Deficiency
E. Thalassemia

Answer: B. Hereditary spherocytosis

Discussion: Recall, hereditary spherocytosis is the *only* anemia that will have a *high* hemoglobin concentration (increased MCHC) Recall that anemia is normally due to low hemoglobin levels, but in this case that little round ball has hemoglobin concentrated in the center, unlike a normal RBC which has central *pallor*.

A 70-year-old white woman has noted a recent decrease in her energy. She lives alone and finds it increasingly difficult to keep up her one-story home. Past illnesses include mild DJD for which she takes Naprosyn 375 mg. BID and essential HTN for which she takes propranolol 40 mg. QD.

She had a hysterectomy 25 years ago for fibroids. She had a "silent" inferior wall MI, noted on her ECG about 10 years ago. She carries SL nitro, but has never had to use it. She is on estrogen replacement for osteoporosis and has hemorrhoids from time to time. She has no prior h/o PUD; has not ever had a screening colonoscopy.

ROS: denies melena, but states that she never looks at her stool

Her PE is normal; rectal exam reveals no masses, fissures, or hemorrhoids. Stool testing is positive for occult blood.

WBC 9,400 with normal diff
Hgb 9.9
HCT 28%
MCH 32 (nl 27-34)
MCV 68 (nl 80-100)
MCHC 34 (nl 31-36)

What is your clinical intervention for this little lady?

A. Have her start taking iron supplements three times a day
B. Type and screen and order 2 u. pRBC's to be transfused
C. Have her stop the Naprosyn as you suspect a peptic ulcer
D. Add PPI to her medical regimen to heal her peptic ulcer
E. Consult GI for upper/lower endoscopy

Answer: E. Consult GI

Discussion: She needs a colonoscopy as this represents a likely GI bleed; it could be PUD, it could be colorectal cancer; at any rate, she needs GI referral

An 86 y.o. WM presents with a cc: dyspnea on exertion. He has enjoyed good health and "has not needed medical attention" in 8-10 years. He has been very active, but two weeks ago began to notice shortness of breath while cleaning the gutters of his house. He takes no medications, has never been a smoker, and denies any history of cardiac or pulmonary disease.

ROS reveals no organ specific complaints.

PE is remarkable for a resting tachycardia of 104 bpm, regular rhythm.

He has pallor, normal abdominal exam with DRE negative for occult blood; he has absent vibratory sensation and proprioception at his toes bilaterally. He has no stigmata of alcoholism or chronic liver disease.

WBC 5,400 normal differential
HGB 8.6
HCT 24.4
MCV 102
Plt 154k
Peripheral smear --- hypersegmented PMN's

Based on his physical exam findings; what presumptive diagnosis do you make?

A. Fe deficiency anemia
B. Hereditary spherocytosis
C. Folic Acid deficiency
D. B-12 deficiency
E. Autoimmune hemolytic anemia

Answer: D. B-12 Deficiency

Discussion: Well, this one is easy because you have already seen A & B, but it illustrates a *macrocytic* anemia; with the neurologic abnormalities; B-12 is your most likely diagnosis. Get a serum B-12 level and go from there.

Coagulation Disorders

See coagulation physiology discussion in Chapter 10 for detailed information about hemostasis/thrombotic pathophysiology

Hemophilia A

- Factor VIII deficiency
    - severity depends on amount of Factor VIII available
- X-linked recessive (occurring primarily in males (mother is the carrier)
- H & P
    - vascular bleeding
        - spontaneous hemarthroses (bleed into a joint without trauma)
        - GI bleeds

        - intracranial bleeds
- Therapeutics/clinical intervention
    - Factor VIII
    - It takes 140 humans to make one unit of Factor VIII
        - prior to 1986 caused patients to acquire HIV, HepB, HepC

Hemophilia B
- Factor IX disorders (X-linked recessive)
- Very similar to Hem-A (but very rare)
- Treatment
    - Factor IX

Hemophilia C (Rosenthal Syndrome)
- Factor XI disorders
- Occurs in patient of Ashkenazi Jewish descent
    - Behaves more like a platelet problem (bleeding of gums, menorrhagia, epistaxis, bleeding after tonsillectomy)
- Treatment – Factor XI

Platelet Disorders

Idiopathic thrombocytopenic purpura (ITP)
- Etiology
    - idiopathic
    - most common of the *acquired* coagulopathies
    - acquired after viral infection
        - patient produces IgG to platelets (antiplatelet antibodies)
        - IgG-platelet complex gets to spleen where it is destroyed (because it's not perfectly "normal")
- H & P
    - Normal exam except for purpura (usually on lower extremities)
    - At time of diagnosis, there should be *no* splenomegaly
        - otherwise, you would be thinking leukemia, right?
- Labs & Diagnostics
    - CBC = normal
    - Platelet count = low
    - INR = normal
    - PTT = normal
    - Bleeding Time (not done because platelet count is low)
    - Antiplatelet antibodies = positive
- Clinical Intervention
    - Mild – self-limited (no reason to treat – observe and do frequent platelet counts)
    - Moderate – if < 50,000, give short course of steroid, then frequent platelet counts
    - Severe –if prednisone has little or no effect – ultimate "cure" is splenectomy

Looks like Scurvy.

Von Willebrand's disease

- Etiology
  - inherited (most common of the *inherited* coagulopathies)
- Scientific Concept
  - vWF is needed for two reasons:
    - released in response to injury, causes platelets to aggregate (stick)
    - slows the otherwise rapid degradation of Factor VIII
  - So, if you have less vWF than normal, you will have:
    - Platelets that don't stick
    - Less Factor VIII than normal (in the intrinsic/heparin/PTT pathway)
- H & P
  - bleeding of mucous membranes
    - epistaxis/bleeding gums
    - menorrhagia
    - petechiae/purpura
    - after tonsillectomy/tooth extraction)
- Labs & diagnostics – CBC with differential & platelet count, coag panel
  - CBC = normal
  - Platelet count = normal
  - Bleeding Time = prolonged
  - INR = normal
  - PTT = normal or mildly prolonged
- Clinical Intervention
  - avoid ASA and NSAID's
- Therapeutics
  - Desmopressin (DDAVP) – IV or intranasal
    - Causes secretion of vWF (for some weird reason)

Thrombotic thrombocytopenic purpura

- Etiology – unknown, but acquired
- Risk Factors
  - Shiga toxin-producing E. Coli 0157:H7
    - In children causes hemolytic uremic syndrome (thought to be very similar to TTP)
  - Platelet aggregation inhibitor drugs
  - Cocaine
- H & P
  - hallmark is altered mental status, also mucosal bleeding
- Labs & diagnostics
  - CBC = normal
  - Platelet count = low
  - Bleeding Time = prolonged
  - INR = normal
  - PTT = normal
  - D-Dimer = normal
- Clinical Intervention
  - Life-threatening emergency

    - Plasmapheresis is only known moderately effective treatment
- Scientific Concept
    - This looks just like DIC, but is distinguished from it because the coagulation factors are normal
        - The "clotting" that occurs is a result of micro-platelet clots, not fibrin clots therefore, INR is normal, PTT is normal, and D-Dimer would not be elevated (unlike DIC)

DIC (Disseminated Intravascular Coagulopathy)

- Etiology
    - catastrophic trauma/illness/stillbirth or retained products of conception
- Scientific Concept
    - All coagulation pathways and anti-clotting pathways are activated.
- H & P
    - platelet-type bleeding (Bleeding Time) *plus*
    - factor-type bleeding (INR, aPTT) *plus*
    - clotting (D-Dimer)
- Labs & diagnostics
    - CBC = anemia
    - Platelet count = low
    - Bleeding time = prolonged
    - INR =prolonged
    - aPTT = prolonged
    - D-Dimer = elevated

Thrombotic Disorders

- All are inherited
- all increase risk of clotting
- usually a positive family history for deep vein thrombosis (DVT) or pulmonary embolism (PE)
    - DVT can happen without a thrombotic disorder, however.

Antithrombin III deficiency

- Clinical intervention
    - LMWH
    - Vena caval filter

Protein C deficiency

- Clinical intervention
    - Surveillance
    - LMWH

Protein S deficiency

- Clinical intervention
    - Surveillance
    - LMWH

Factor V Leiden

- Epidemiology
    - Most common of the inherited thrombophilias
- Most common in patients of European descent
    - less common in African-Americans and Hispanic Americans
    - very uncommon in Native Americans, SE Asian Americans
- Scientific concept
    - just think in these terms:
        - if the patient has the Factor V Leiden (mutation)
        - then this will inactivate Protein C
        - and cause increased risk of clotting
- Clinical intervention
    - Surveillance
    - no screening recommended at this time
    - usually discovered after DVT
    - LMWH

Coagulation Review Questions

Normal Lab Values for the Cases:

- PLT count (140k – 400k)
- Bleeding time (3-10- minutes)
- aPTT (21-35 sec)
- INR (1.0) therapeutic (2.0-3.0)
- Fibrinogen level (200-400 mg/dL)
- D-Dimer - depends on the assay – normal ranges will always be reported --- along with an explanation –
- Normal D-Dimer (for these cases) will be reported as NEGATIVE

A 7 y.o. child presents 3 weeks after URI with purpuric lesions on his lower extremities. He otherwise appears well. PMH is unremarkable. PE is normal except for nonpalpable purpuric lesions scattered on lower extremities, a few on the skin of the trunk. --- no hepatosplenomegaly, no lymphadenopthy

CBC and differential – wnl
Plt ct 52k
Bleeding time not done
aPTT 25 sec
INR 1.1
Fibrinogen 250 mg/dL

What is the most likely diagnosis?

A. ITP – idiopathic thrombocytopenic purpura
B. TTP – thrombotic thrombocytopenic purpura
C. HUS – hemolytic uremic syndrome
D. DIC – disseminated intravascular coagulopathy
E. vWD – von Willebrand's disease

Answer: A.

Discussion: ITP is most likely in this well-appearing child; it is most common; PE is normal except the purpura (could have epistaxis and gingival bleeding too); and he is thrombocytopenic (let the words in the disease name help you too!)

A 34 y.o. female, 3 days post-partum in the ED with fever, altered mental status (AMS), and purpuric lesions on trunk and extremities.

WBC 14,000 with 5% bands and 90% seg
RBC 2.4
Hgb 10
HCT 30%
Peripheral smear --- schistocytes
Platelet count 24k

INR 1.1
aPTT 28 sec

BUN 45
Creatinine 2.3

What is the most likely diagnosis?

A. ITP – idiopathic thrombocytopenic purpura
B. TTP – thrombotic thrombocytopenic purpura
C. HUS – hemolytic uremic syndrome
D. DIC – disseminated intravascular coagulopathy
E. vWD – von Willebrand's disease

Answer: B.

Discussion: TTP – why is it not DIC (the next most likely diagnosis in this list)? because the INR and PTT are normal. This is a microangiopathic disorder (think microclots); it is difficult to treat, and prognosis is not good, but is getting better.

An 8 y.o. female presents with recent GI illness and is now markedly worse. Mother believes she is dehydrated since she is so lethargic. PE reveals mildly enlarged spleen, multiple petechiae and purpura on the lower extremities. The patient is lethargic and somnolent but A & O x 3.

WBC	10,800 with normal differential
Platelet ct	22k
aPTT	22 sec
INR	1.0
Fibrinogen	120 mg/dL
D-Dimer elevated	
BUN	65
Creatinine	3.0
U/A	4+ protein

What is the most likely diagnosis?

A. ITP – idiopathic thrombocytopenic purpura
B. TTP – thrombotic thrombocytopenic purpura
C. HUS – hemolytic uremic syndrome
D. DIC – disseminated intravascular coagulopathy
E. vWD – von Willebrand's disease

Answer: C.

Discussion: HUS; from eating undercooked chopped meat; E Coli 0157H7; let the words help you (BUN and creatinine are high, and this is called hemolytic uremic syndrome). That is called "educated" guessing if you hadn't known the answer!

A 23 y.o healthy male college student presents two weeks after wisdom tooth extraction to Student Health c/o gums still bleeding. His only other history is that of an ACL tear requiring surgery, and he describes significant bleeding into that joint with that injury.

WBC 8,000 with normal differential

HGB	15
HCT	45%
Plt ct	350k

Platelet aggregation studies show decreased platelet aggregation

aPTT	35 seconds
INR	1.0
Fibrinogen	280 mg/dL

What is the most likely diagnosis?

A. ITP – idiopathic thrombocytopenic purpura
B. TTP – thrombotic thrombocytopenic purpura

C. HUS – hemolytic uremic syndrome
D. DIC – disseminated intravascular coagulopathy
E. vWD – von Willebrand's disease

Answer: E. vWD (OK we are running out of choices here, but keep working on these – don't just guess because I have left the detractors the same

Note two things: the platelet count is *normal* and PTT is *mildly elevated*; the problem with vWD is platelets are normal but do not stick because there is not enough vWF around; and because of that, Factor VIII is degraded quickly so PTT (INtrinsic; INpatient; heparin) level goes up.

A 2 y.o. male infant is brought to the ED with swollen L knee and L wrist. The infant appears irritable but is not febrile. Careful history reveals no suspicion of abuse. PE is within normal limits except for hemarthrosis in knee and wrist and abdominal distention.

HGB	11
HCT	33%
Plt ct	150K
aPTT	55 sec
INR	1.0
Fibrinogen	250 mg/dL

What is the most likely diagnosis?

A. ITP – idiopathic thrombocytopenic purpura
B. TTP – thrombotic thrombocytopenic purpura
C. Hemophilia-A
D. DIC – disseminated intravascular coagulopathy
E. vWD – von Willebrand's disease

Answer: C.

Discussion: Hemophilia A – OK this is too easy because I just changed the one detractor; but make sure you work through those labs (quickly!). This baby is sick; child abuse is in your differential, unfortunately. However, he has normal platelets; normal INR, just the PTT is markedly high – and that is the clue. What is your biggest historical clue? He is a boy (x-linked recessive) and he has a spontaneous hemarthrosis!

A 40 y.o. WM presents to the ED c/o hematemesis and a 4 day h/o abdominal pain and melena. He gives a history of PUD linked to heavy ETOH use. He denies current medications, including OTC and denies a family history of bleeding abnormalities.

ROS – easy bruising for the past 3-4 months

PE – sclera icterus; moderate abdominal pain; smells of ETOH

Scattered ecchymosis; spider angiomas over the anterior trunk

Liver span 15 cm; RUQ tenderness; palpable spleen tip

WBC	4,500 with normal differential
Hgb	6.0
HCT	18%
Platelets	87k

AST	95 (0-30)
ALT	40 (0-38)
T Bili	3.5 (<1.1)
ALP	450 (0-125)

What is the most likely diagnosis?

A. ITP – idiopathic thrombocytopenic purpura
B. TTP – thrombotic thrombocytopenic purpura
C. Vitamin K deficiency
D. Chronic alcoholic cirrhosis
E. DIC

Answer: D.

Discussion: This patient has chronic liver disease; therefore is not making albumin, coag factors (except VIII), and is having a bleeding diathesis; thrombocytopenia accompanies liver disease frequently. This could be Vitamin K deficiency, as alcoholic do not typically eat lots of dark green leafy veggies; and in clinical practice, you might give some Vit. K and see what happens; but I think his liver is gone.

Bone Marrow Cancers

PEARL: Leukemias all have in common too many white blood cells (hence the Latin word leuk (white) emia (too many). What distinguishes acute leukemia from chronic leukemia?

The markedly abnormal blasts that are present in the acute (and more severe) leukemias. These blasts do not function, and therefore should not be released by the bone marrow. If the CBC shows leukemia with lymphoblasts, it is an acute lymphocytic leukemia. If it shows leukemia with monoblasts, it is an acute monocytic/monoblastic leukemia, etc. When there is leukemia, but most of the cells are normal mature lymphocytes, the patient has a chronic lymphocytic leukemia. And so on; (this was covered in the Labs & Diagnostics Chapter 6)

Acute lymphocytic leukemia

- Etiology
    - bone marrow cancer
- Epidemiology
    - children 3-7 years old = peak incidence
- H & P
    - So, how many children present with:
        - Fever?
        - Lymphadenopathy?
        - Pretty much all of them, right?
    - BUT hepatosplenomegaly makes you investigate further
        - Therefore, the abdominal exam should be performed on all children who present with fever and lymphadenopathy to r/o hepatosplenomegaly!
- Labs
    - high WBC (thus, leukemia)
    - mostly blasts (thus, acute)
    - 20% or more lymphoblasts (thus, acute lymphocytic leukemia)
- Clinical intervention
    - bone marrow biopsy
    - referral to peds heme/onc
- Prognosis
    - excellent if caught early
    - 80% cure rate

Chronic lymphocytic leukemia

- Etiology
    - bone marrow cancer
- Epidemiology
    - older men (> 70 yrs)
- H & P
    - asymptomatic (maybe sweats and fevers)
    - painless lymphadenopathy
    - hepatosplenomegaly

- Labs
  - high WBC (thus, leukemia)
  - mostly mature/normal WBC's (thus, chronic)
  - 90% normal lymphs (thus, lymphocytic)
- Clinical intervention
  - bone marrow biopsy
  - referral to heme onc
- Prognosis
  - Good
  - 25% live more than 10 years (and they start out at 70!)

Acute myelogenous leukemia

- Etiology
  - bone marrow cancer
- H & P
  - SICK
  - bleeding (platelet type bleeding)
  - AMS, fevers
  - +/- hepatosplenomegaly
- Labs
  - high WBC (thus, leukemia)
  - mostly blasts (thus, acute)
  - mostly myeloblasts (thus acute myelogenous leukemia)
- Clinical intervention
  - no drug therapy - only bone marrow transplant
- Prognosis - poor

Chronic myelogenous leukemia

- Etiology
  - bone marrow cancer
- H & P
  - may be asymptomatic
  - may have fevers/night sweats
  - lymphadenopathy and hepatosplenomegaly
- Labs
  - high WBC (thus, leukemia)
  - mostly mature/normal WBC's (thus, chronic)
  - mostly segs (thus, chronic myelogenous leukemia)
- Clinical intervention
  - bone marrow biopsy
  - GLEEVAC (genetically engineered drug, 98% control of acute phase)
- Prognosis
  - fairly good, unless transformation to blast crisis
- Complication
  - blast crisis --- turns into an "acute" leukemia, and death usually follows unless bone marrow transplant is successful

Multiple myeloma

- Etiology
    - bone marrow starts to produce excessive plasma protein (Bence-Jones)
    - this plasma protein damages kidneys; causes bone resorption
- Epidemiology
    - older adults >65 yrs
- H & P
    - signs/symptoms of renal failure
    - bone pain
    - "punched out lytic lesions of the skull"
- Labs
    - Urine dip is negative! (because it "dips" for albumin) this is NOT albumin –
    - Found on 24 hour urine --- it's a plasma protein
    - Order urine electrophoresis on the 24 hour urine collection
- Clinical intervention
    - treat renal failure
    - no real treatment

White Blood Cell Review Questions

To do this section adequately, make sure you review normal WBC and differential; and left shift and right shift in Labs & Diagnostics, Chapter 6.

I am not even going to give you any clinical hints here: I want you to give it your best shot just based on these WBC differentials:

WBC 18,000
Differential:

SEGS	**92**
BANDS	**5**
LYMPHS	**8**
EOS	**0**
BASO	**0**

What is the most likely diagnosis?

A. Bacterial infection
B. Viral infection
C. AML
D. CML
E. ALL

Answer: A. Bacterial infection; the classic "left shift" --- too many WBC's (nl 4,000 to 10,000), too many SEGS (normal ~ 70%); too few LYMPHS (nl ~20%); bands are not really normal (maybe 1 or 2, but no more)

WBC 3,500
Differential:

SEGS	48%
BANDS	0
LYMPHS	52% (22% reactive)
MONOS	2
EOS	1
BASO	0

What is the most likely diagnosis?

A. CLL
B. ALL
C. AML
D. CML
E. Viral infection

Answer: E. Viral infection; the classic *right shift*; this is typical for infectious mononucleosis; low to normal WBC; with low SEGS and high LYMPHS with reactive lymphocytes; not high enough for leukemia; and no blasts

WBC 54,000
Differential:
SEGS 91
BANDS 5
LYMPHS 4
EOS 0
BASO 0
COMMENT: toxic granulation and dohle bodies

What is the most likely diagnosis?

A. CLL
B. ALL
C. Leukemoid reaction
D. CML
E. AML

Answer: C. Leukemoid reaction; now hopefully, the item writer would describe a pretty sick patient to you; this patient has a severe bacterial infection; the only way to know for sure though is to treat the infection and see if this all resolves. If not, then he deserves to see Heme/Onc. In some overwhelming infections, the patient's WBC may actually go down and BANDS go high; this is because the WBC are dying faster than the bone marrow can make more; that's why it sends out those immature bands.

WBC 52,000
Differential:

SEGS	88
BANDS	5
LYMPHS	3
EOS	0
BASO	0
META MYELOCYTES	4
MYELOBLASTS	5

What is the most likely diagnosis?

A. CLL
B. ALL
C. Leukemoid reaction
D. CML
E. AML

Answer: D. CML, and why? Because there is a leukemia (word means "excess whites") and the BLASTS are never OK; but there are not many of them; and most of the cells are "normal" segmented neutrophils; making this: a CHRONIC myelocytic leukemia. Compare this to the leukemoid reaction; the reason CML is the better answer here is because of the immature forms; although I have seen a few of these in bad infections too!

WBC 145,000
Differential:

SEGS	2
LYMPHS	96
EOS	0
BASO	0
LYMPHOBLASTS	2

What is the most likely diagnosis?

A. CLL
B. ALL
C. Leukemoid reaction
D. CML
E. AML

Answer: A. CLL, and why? Because there is a leukemia and the BLASTS are never OK; but there are not many of them; and most of the cells are "normal" lymphocytes; making this: a CHRONIC lymphocytic leukemia

WBC 180,000
Differential:

SEGS	2
LYMPHS	10
EOS	0
BASO	0
LYMPHOBLASTS	88

What is the most likely diagnosis?

A. CLL
B. ALL
C. Leukemoid reaction
D. CML
E. AML

Answer: B. ALL, and why? Because there is a leukemia; and the BLASTS are never OK and the high numbers of them means this is acute and not chronic; and it is the lymphoblasts that are elevated; so if you put that all together you get: acute lymphocytic leukemia (ALL)

WBC 167,000
Differential:
SEGS 30
LYMPHS 4
META 12
PROMYELOCYTES 4
MYELOBLASTS 42

What is the most likely diagnosis?

A. CLL
B. ALL
C. Leukemoid reaction
D. CML
E. AML

Answer: E. AML; and why? Because there is a leukemia and the BLASTS are never OK; what kind of blasts ARE they? Myeloblasts, i.e. Acute Myeloblastic Leukemia (let the words help you!)

WBC 9,500
Differential:
SEGS 62
BANDS 0
LYMPHS 22
EOS 16
BASO 0

What is the most likely diagnosis?

A. Left shift
B. Right shift
C. Leukemoid reaction
D. Allergic reaction
E. Normal differential

Answer: D. Allergic response or worms; that are what increased eosinophils mean; in US it is likely allergic; in third world country; most likely a worm burden in the gut.

Lymph Node Cancers

Hodgkin's Lymphoma

- Etiology
  - lymph node cancer
- Epidemiology
  - most common cancer of young adults
- H & P
  - *painless* lymph node enlargement without cause (no skin infection, etc)
  - usually *supraclavicular* or in neck – painless >1 cm
  - may or may not have systemic symptoms
    - weight loss, night sweats
- Clinical intervention
  - lymph node biopsy
  - pathology shows Reed Sternberg Cells – refer to heme onc

Non-Hodgkin's Lymphoma

- Etiology
  - lymph node cancer
- Epidemiology
  - all ages, but more likely older adults
- H & P
  - painless diffuse lymphadenopathy
  - often with systemic symptoms of weight loss, sweats
- Clinical intervention
  - lymph node biopsy – referral to heme onc

PEARL: If you are asked to distinguish lymphoma from leukemia, order a CBC. If the CBC is normal, the patient does not have bone marrow cancer, so biopsy one of those nodes!

Oncological Emergencies

All of these topics have been covered elsewhere in the review of content.

I am creating a list here of the more common of the oncologic emergencies, and when appropriate, the particular cancer with which each emergency is most commonly associated

Endocrinologic/Metabolic emergencies – see Endocrine, Chapter XXX for info on each

- adrenal insufficiency – treat with hydrocortisone 100 mg. IV
  - mets (lung, breast, melanoma)
  - chronic steroid administration (brain cancers, etc)
- SIADH – treat with furosemide, or Demeclocycline (to induce diabetes insipidus)
  - most common cause of hyponatremia in clinical medicine

  - lung cancer most common, but can occur in any cancer
- Tumor Lysis Syndrome (acute destruction of cancer cells, releasing intracellular substances)
  - hyperkalemia – see chapter 6 --- briefly, Dextrose 50%, insulin, albuterol, dialysis
  - phosphotemia (combines with calcium and deposits in tissues) - dialysis
  - hyperuricemia – IV hydration, prophylactic allopurinol prior to chemotherapy
- Hypercalcemia (breast, lung, renal, ovarian)
  - poor prognostic indicator when present

Hematologic Emergencies

- hyperviscosity syndrome – keep patient well hydrated
- neutropenia (WBC < 500 cells/mL) normal is 4,000 to 10,000 cells/mL
  - a byproduct of both chemotherapy and radiation therapy
  - 30% increased risk of death from sepsis
  - fever is most common presenting sign

Renal/Urologic Syndromes

- Bladder cancer – hemorrhage, obstruction, infection

Dermatologic Emergencies

- hypersensitivity reactions
- drug extravasation during chemotherapy

Gastrointestinal Emergencies

- nausea and vomiting
  - watch electrolytes and replace fluids
  - prevention with antiemetics

Pain

- aggressive treatment
  - avoid "oligoanalgesia" or underuse of pain medications
- first line = opiates
- NSAID's are adjunctive – watch renal function, stomach ulcers
- Steroids – very useful to reduce inflammation

CHAPTER 24

Pediatrics – Unknown Percentage of the Exam

Introduction to Pediatrics Chapter

This is an unknown % of the test – we have never been told how many pediatrics questions will be present on the exam. The most important topics to consider, therefore, are the most common, the most life threatening, and the ones that change frequently (immunization schedules).

Also worth reviewing, are the drugs that should not be used in kids (at the end of this chapter).

Cardiovascular

Cyanotic congenital heart problems

Transposition of the Great Vessels

- Epidemiology
  - Most common of the cyanotic congenital heart defects
  - 60-70% male
  - Presentation severity depends on other co-anomalies
- H & P
  - Cyanosis and failure immediately after birth
- Labs & Diagnostics
  - Echocardiogram
  - Catheterization
- Clinical Intervention
  - Keep ductus arteriosis open
  - Allows fetal circulation to help with oxygenation of peripheral tissues
- Therapeutics
  - IV prostaglandin E (keeps ductus open)
- Scientific Concept
  - If concomitant large VSD or PDA, may not be as cyanotic as expected
  - If untreated, 90% mortality in first year
  - With surgery, > 90% survival

Tetralogy of Fallot

- Definition
    - VSD
    - RVH
    - RV outflow obstruction
    - Overriding aorta
        - Right sided aortic arch
- H & P
    - Cyanosis
- Labs & Diagnostics
    - Echocardiogram
    - Holter monitor (arrhythmias are common)
- Clinical Intervention
    - Cardiology and CT surgical referral
    - Primary surgical repair at about one year
- Health Maintenance
    - Need endocarditis prophylaxis
- Scientific Concept
    - Sudden onset of severe symptoms occur and are treated by bringing infants knees up to chest and calming the infant (decreases venous return)

Hypoplastic left heart syndrome

- Epidemiology
    - Uncommon
    - Abnormal development of left ventricle
    - Usually associated with coarctation of aorta, patent foramen ovale
    - Universally lethal if not surgically transplanted; or surgical intervention
- H & P
    - Profound cyanosis
- Labs & Diagnostics
    - Often discovered on fetal ultrasound
- Clinical Intervention
    - Surgery

Acyanotic congenital heart problems

Ventricular septal defect

- Epidemiology
    - **Most common** of congenital heart defects (2/1000 live births)
    - Left sided blood (oxygenated) flows through defect to right side
    - *No* cyanosis
- H & P
    - Small defect = loud murmur (more turbulence through smaller opening)
    - Large defect = may not even hear murmur
    - Will result in pulmonary hypertension (too much right sided blood flow and pressure from all that blood going from left to right)

- Labs & Diagnostics
    - Echocardiogram
- Clinical Intervention
    - Surgical closure
- Health Maintenance
    - Dental prophylaxis no longer needed after repair

Atrial septal defect

- Epidemiology
    - Second most common acyanotic congenital heart defect
- H & P
    - Usually asymptomatic
    - **Widely split and fixed S2**
- Labs & Diagnostics
    - Echocardiogram
- Clinical Intervention
    - Should be closed surgically
    - Patent foramen ovale can cause embolism and stroke
- Health Maintenance
    - Dental prophylaxis is no longer needed after repair

Patent ductus arteriosus (PDA)

- Epidemiology
    - Should close shortly after birth to allow two ventricle circulation
    - Circulating prostaglandins may cause ductus to remain open
- H & P
    - **Machine-gun continuous murmur**
- Labs & Diagnostics
    - Echocardiogram
- Clinical Intervention
    - Prostaglandin inhibitors
- Therapeutics
    - Indomethacin is most common NSAID used
- Scientific Concept
    - the other continuous murmur in childhood is the venous hum
    - the venous hum disappears if you lie the child supine or turn his head
    - in contrast, PDA murmur does not go away
    - also, the PDA murmur is louder and "machine-gun" like

Coarctation of the aorta

- Epidemiology
    - Relatively common anomaly – 5-10% of children
    - commonly associated other anomalies:
        - bicuspid aortic valve (2/3 of patients with CoA)
        - VSD
- H & P
    - Signs and symptoms of CHF

        - JVD/fluid retention
        - pulmonary edema/hypertension
    - BP high in arms
    - BP low in legs; absent or weak femoral pulses
    - May have muscle wasting of lower extremities
    - Murmur from bicuspid aortic valve
- Labs & Diagnostics
    - EKG showing LVH (high voltage)
    - CXR showing "rib notching"
        - notches in the ribs where the enlarge arterioles of the chest wall cause erosions of bone
    - Echocardiogram
- Clinical Intervention
    - PGE-1 to keep the PDA open
    - Surgical correction
- Scientific Concept
    - Increased incidence of coarct in Turner syndrome

Benign Murmurs in Children

Still's murmur

- Most common benign murmur in childhood
    - Present age 2 to adolescence
- Heard along left lower and midsternal border
- Musical (?), short systolic ejection murmur
- Grad I-II, diminishes with standing, sitting, Valsalva
- No work up needed unless other concerns (failure to thrive, etc)

Venous Hum

- Common murmur of childhood
    - Usually after age 3
- Heard in upper right and left sternal borders
- Can radiate to neck bilaterally
- Continuous musical hum, Grade I-II
- Disappears when child is supine, or if you compress the jugular vein
- No work up needed unless other concerns (failure to thrive, etc)

Infectious diseases

Group B Strep

- Epidemiology
    - 30% of all mothers are colonized
    - Leading cause of morbidity and mortality in neonates
    - Highest risk in preterm

- H & P
  - Onset < 7 days
  - Apnea is first sign
  - Sepsis, pneumonia, meningitis
- Clinical Intervention
  - Prophylactic antibiotics in any mother not screened
  - Prophylactic antibiotics in any mother with positive culture
  - Prophylactic antibiotics in any mother with GBS infection at any time during pregnancy
- Therapeutics
  - IV Penicillin G
  - IV ampicillin
  - IV Clindamycine for PCN allergy
- Health maintenance
  - Screening in pregnancy (see OB)

Acute rheumatic fever (uncommon in US, common in other countries)

- Epidemiology/etiology
  - Systemic immune response to rheumatogenic strain of β-hemolytic strep Group A
  - Produces stiffness, deformity of valve cusps; shortening of chordae tendinae; fusion of the commissures of the valves
  - Mitral valve involved 50-60% of cases
  - Aortic valve + mitral = 20% of cases
  - Tricuspid and pulmonic involved much less often
- H & P
  - Major criteria (Jones) – need two of the following
    - Carditis
    - Pericarditis, or
    - Cardiomegaly, or
    - CHF, or
    - Mitral or aortic regurgitant murmurs
    - Erythema marginatum or subcutaneous nodules
    - Sydenham chorea
      - choreiform (involuntary slithering movements of the extremities, sometimes tongue) which is permanent
    - Polyarthritis (large joints, redness, swelling, no destruction)
  - Minor criteria (Jones)
    - Polyarthralgias (pain without physical findings)
    - Prolongation of PR interval (first degree AV block)
    - Elevation of ESR (sed rate) or CRP (C-reactive protein)
- Labs & Diagnostics
  - Echocardiogram
- Clinical Intervention
  - Complete bedrest till all inflammatory markers and fever are resolved
- Therapeutics
  - Primary prophylaxis

  - Acute treatment with PCN for strep throat *plus*
  - Secondary prevention
  - Prevention of recurrent episodes
    - Benzathine penicillin G, 1.2 million units IM one time, or
    - Procaine penicillin 600,000 units IM once daily for 10 days
- Health Maintenance
  - Prevention of recurrence is the most critical step in management!
  - RF with carditis & significant residual heart disease
    - Benzathine penicillin G, 1.2 million units IM every 3-4 weeks *for minimum of 10 years after latest episode, usually for life*
  - RF with carditis but no residual heart disease (except mild MR)
    - Benzathine penicillin G, 1.2 million units IM every 3-4 weeks *for minimum of 10 years or until age 25 (whichever is longer)*
  - RF with no carditis
    - Benzathine penicillin G, 1.2 million units IM every 3-4 weeks *for minimum of 5 years or until age 18-21 (whichever is longer)*
- Scientific Concept
  - Recurrence is most common in those with carditis
    - 20% recurrence in the next five years

Kawasaki's disease (mucocutaneous lymph node syndrome (see also CV peds)

- Epidemiology
  - Uncommon
  - Idiopathic (viral??) probably autoimmune
  - Occurs in children < 5 y.o.
  - Usually self-limited and mild course, but major complications rarely
  - Major complication is coronary artery vasculitis
  - Can cause a heart attack (in a 3 year old!)
  - Can destroy the vessels in the heart
- H & P
  - High fever for one to two weeks or longer
  - (does not respond to treatment with Tylenol or ibuprofen)
  - Rash on trunk
  - Swollen Lips And Throat ("strawberry tongue")
  - Swollen Lymph Nodes
  - Peeling Hands And Feet
- Labs & Diagnostics
  - Clinical diagnosis – no specific lab test
- Clinical Intervention
  - Hospitalize
  - Cardiology consult/ Rheumatology consult/ ID consult
- Therapeutics
  - IV immunoglobulin
  - Aspirin
- Scientific concept:
  - To make the diagnosis clinically you need:
    - Five days of high fever PLUS four of the following:
    - Red lips, strawberry tongue

        - Conjunctivitis
        - Adenopathy
        - Rash on trunk
        - Desquamation of hand

Pulmonary

Hyaline membrane disease (infant respiratory distress syndrome)

- Epidemiology
    - Common cause of pulmonary complications in premature infants
    - Occurs in > 50% of infants born < 28 weeks
    - Occurs in 33% born 32-38 weeks
    - More common in preterm males than females
    - Due to lack of surfactant
- H & P
    - Respiratory Difficulty At Birth That Gets Progressively Worse
    - Cyanosis
    - Flaring Of The Nostrils
    - Tachypnea
    - Grunting Sounds With Breathing
    - Chest retractions
- Labs & Diagnostics
    - CXR shows "ground glass" appearance (reticulogranular pattern)
    - Echocardiogram may be done to r/o cardiac cause of respiratory symptoms
- Clinical Intervention
    - Therapeutics
        - Oxygen
        - CPAP
        - Artificial surfactant
        - Mechanical ventilation
- Health Maintenance
    - Lecithin/sphingomyelin ratio (L/S ratio) done on amniotic fluid
    - Dexamethasone given to mom may hasten lung maturity if threatened preterm delivery

Croup

- Epidemiology
    - Common in children
    - Smallest airways have greatest distress
    - Adults will get laryngitis
- H & P
    - Barking cough
    - Inspiratory stridor
    - No drooling (that would be epiglottitis)
    - Lung fields are clear
- Labs & Diagnostics

    - Plain film may show steeple sign
- Clinical Intervention
    - If no inspiratory stridor, no treatment except symptomatic (see below)
        - Some give a single dose of dexamethasone (fairly good data)
    - If inspiratory stridor
        - Give racemic epinephrine (nebulized) & dexamethasone
- Therapeutics
    - Epinephrine
    - Dexamethasone (as above)
- Health Maintenance
    - Prevention is just hand washing (no vaccine available)
    - Humidified air usually improves stridor and difficulty breathing
- Scientific Concept
    - Viral, no treatment
    - Clinical judgement --- no lab testing to prove it

Respiratory syncytial virus (RSV) /Acute bronchiolitis

- Epidemiology
    - Paramyxovirus
    - Leading cause of hospitalization in infants < 6 months
    - Major cause of morbidity and mortality in infants
    - Risk factors for severe disease
        - Prematurity/low birth weight
        - Age < 6 months
        - Congenital heart disease
    - Is thought to be a major contributing factor in bronchospasm later in life
- H & P
    - Low grade fever
    - Tachypnea (apnea can also occur)
    - Wheezing
    - Increased work of breathing
    - Hyperinflated lungs
- Labs & Diagnostics
    - Rapid RSV available (culture is standard of care)
- Clinical Intervention
    - Supportive treatment (only very very ill get therapy)
    - Humidified air
    - Albuterol found not very effective (75% hospitalized anyway)
    - Racemic epinephrine is better (30% are hospitalized)
    - Ribavirin is the only drug found to help at all
    - Ventilator support if needed
- Therapeutics
- Health Maintenance
    - No vaccine!
    - RSV-IG IV (for infants with pulmonary disease or prematurity)
    - Palivizumab --- monoclonal antibody against RSV for at-risk patients with underlying cardiopulmonary disease - extremely expensive
    - Handwashing/ isolating ill children

- Scientific Concept
    - Bronchodilators do not work!!!!
    - Steroids do not work!!!!

Foreign body aspiration

- Epidemiology
    - Most commonly, objects are swallowed and not aspirated
    - Have high index of suspicion in child who develops sudden onset of cough and is not ill
- H & P
    - Focal wheeze; may not have any abnormality
- Labs & Diagnostics
    - Inspiratory film may show no abnormality
    - Expiratory film may show "air trapping"
        - focal area aerated and rest of lobe is collapsed
- Clinical Intervention
    - Referral to pulmonary medicine
    - Anesthesia and bronchoscopy
- Scientific Concept
    - When you inhale, bronchioles dilate (air can move past FB)
    - When you exhale, bronchioles "collapse" to move air out (air trapping behind the FB)

Cystic fibrosis

- Epidemiology
    - Autosomal recessive disease of eccrine and exocrine glands
        - Lungs
        - Pancreas
        - Liver
        - All mucous production (cervix, urethra)
- H & P
    - Meconium ileus in neonate is big clue
    - Nasal polyps in children is big clue
- Labs & Diagnostics
    - Sweat chloride test
- Clinical Intervention
    - pulmonary medicine referral
- Therapeutics
    - medications for infections, no cure
- Health Maintenance
    - All possible vaccinations/immunizations
- Scientific concepts
    - If pneumonia, cover pseudomonas besides other pathogens

Acute epiglottitis

See Chapter 12, Pulmonary Medicine.

- This disease used to be common, life-threatening in children, but now with the usage of HIB vaccine, almost never occurs in children.

Pertussis

See Chapter 12, Pulmonary Medicine.

- This disease used to be most common in unvaccinated children; but now older children and adults are developing pertussis apparently because vaccines thought to be lifelong, have "worn off". Children are now given DTaP; adults are now given Tdap booster instead of just tetanus toxoid – revaccinate at 10 years and with booster every ten years to age 65.

Gastroenterology/Nutrition

Reye's syndrome (not in blueprint)

- Definition
    - Fatty liver with encephalopathy
- Epidemiology
    - Rare and severe complication of influenza (usually B)
    - Can occur after other viral infections
    - Associated with aspirin use in viral infections
- H & P
    - Change in mental status
- Labs & Diagnostics
    - Hypoglycemia
    - Increased LFT's
    - *Increased blood ammonia*
- Clinical Intervention
    - supportive
- Therapeutics - none
- Health Maintenance
    - *No aspirin during viral infections*
- Scientific Concept
    - 30% mortality
    - Rapidly advancing liver failure
    - Cerebral edema

Pyloric stenosis

- Epidemiology
    - Most common cause of intestinal obstruction in infancy
    - Due to hyperplasia and hypertrophy of the muscles of the pyloris causing a "mechanical" obstruction from the stomach to the duodenum
- H & P
    - Non-bilious vomiting, usually with each meal (70%)
    - Failure to thrive, poor weight gain, lethargy
    - "palpable olive" sign
- Labs & Diagnostics

- Electrolytes
- US is imaging study of choice

- Clinical Intervention
  - Replace fluid loss (20 cc/kg NS IV)
  - NPO
  - Surgical consult

Intussusception

- Epidemiology
  - occurs mainly in infants (but also in the very elderly)
  - <1% mortality if caught early
  - death in 2-5 days if not recognized
- H & P
  - colicky, severe and intermittent abdominal pain
  - vomiting
  - **currant jelly mucous stools*
  - *R hypochondrial sausage shaped mass with empty RLQ*
    - called the Dance sign
- Labs & Diagnostics
  - plain films positive 60%
  - barium enema is main diagnostic tool
    - corrects the problem sometimes too!
- Clinical Intervention
  - *air enema* is treatment of choice
  - of not successful:
  - laparoscopic repair (sometimes needs to be done open)
- Therapeutics
  - fluids, bowel rest

Volvulus

- Description
  - twisting of a portion of bowel around the mesenteric attachment
  - if involving artery, can lead to ischemia and necrosis
- Epidemiology
  - children usually get a midgut volvulus involving the SMA (superior mesenteric artery)
  - the elderly more often get a sigmoid volvulus
- H & P
  - vague and nonspecific symptoms
  - abdominal pain; constipation; failure to thrive
  - intermittent bilious vomiting
- Labs & Diagnostics
  - no specific labs
  - Upper GI with contrast and Barium enema
  - CT with contrast
  - US is not very useful
- Clinical Intervention
  - *emergent* surgical referral

Meckel's Diverticulum

- Description
  - Remnant of embryologic tissue – incomplete absorption of the vitelline duct (pouch)
- Epidemiology
  - Most common congenital anomaly of the small intestine
  - 2% of population
- H & P
  - *asymptomatic*
    - usually an incidental finding on imaging for another reason
    - occasionally inflammation in the diverticulum can occur and cause pain and fever
  - *rectal bleeding* is most common presentation
- Labs & Diagnostics
  - Meckel scan (radionucleotide scan)
  - other imaging no help
- Clinical Intervention
  - Surgery if bleeding is significant
- Scientific Concept
  - According to Mayo, "Meckel's Diverticulum is frequently suspected, often looked for, and seldom found."

Lactose intolerance

- Epidemiology
  - common
  - ethnic predisposition
    - Asian, African, South American ethnicity is most common
- H & P
  - loose stools
  - abdominal bloating and pain
  - flatulence
  - borborygmi
- Labs & Diagnostics
  - no abnormalities
  - lactose loading (reproduces symptoms)
  - lactose avoidance improves symptoms
- Clinical Intervention
  - Avoidance of lactose
- Therapeutics
  - Lactaid
- Scientific Concept
  - differential diagnosis includes
    - celiac disease
    - inflammatory bowel syndromes
    - irritable bowel syndrome
  - remember,
    - celiac and inflammatory bowel will produce malabsorption
    - lactose intolerance and IBS will not

Constipation

This is covered in Chapter 13, Gastrointestinal Medicine, and is similar for children and adults. This is a very common presentation for sudden and severe abdominal pain in children which occurs after eating a meal. Remember, there is no fever, and stool is usually palpable in the bowel. Do not get CT imaging on a child with constipation; this constitutes too much radiation (100-200 times the radiation of a CXR!)

Umbilical hernia

- Epidemiology
    - very common, especially in premature infants
- H & P
    - bulge of umbilicus, circumferential
    - at the insertion point of the umbilical cord
    - easily reducible
    - infant is *asymptomatic*
- Labs & Diagnostics
    - none
- Clinical Intervention
    - spontaneously resolves with time

Rotavirus

- Epidemiology
    - leading worldwide cause of dehydrating gastroenteritis in children
    - highest incidence between 6 months and 2 years
    - 500,000 deaths/yr in children < 5 years
    - fecal-oral route
- H & P
    - 2-3 day prodrome of fever and vomiting
    - 10-20 BM's/day follows
- Labs & Diagnostics
    - PCR of stool is preferred method
- Clinical Intervention
    - oral rehydration
    - replenishment of electrolytes
- Health Maintenance
    - two oral vaccines are available
    - given at 2, 4, 6 months
- Scientific Concept
    - usually mild and self-limiting
    - older vaccines had increased risk of intussusception
        - this has almost been eliminated
        - risk of intussusception is higher in rotavirus infection than with vaccine now

Gastroesophageal reflux disease (GERD)

- Epidemiology
    - used to rarely be diagnosed
    - now very common diagnosis

- H & P
  - frequent or recurrent vomiting
  - frequent or persistent cough or wheezing
  - refusing to eat or difficulty eating (choking or gagging with feeding)
  - heartburn, gas, abdominal pain, or colicky behavior (frequent crying and fussiness) associated with feeding
  - regurgitation and re-swallowing
  - complaining of a sour taste in their mouth
- Labs & Diagnostics
  - Upper GI or barium swallow
  - pH probe
  - upper endoscopy
  - gastric emptying study
- Therapeutics
  - PPI (proton pump inhibitors)
    - omeprazole, lansoprazole, etc
- Scientific Concept
  - Many other symptoms are sometimes blamed on gastroesophageal reflux, but much of the time, we really are not sure whether reflux actually causes them. Other problems seen in young children and infants that may be blamed on GERD include:
    - colic
    - poor growth
    - breathing problems or wheezing
    - recurrent pneumonia

Phenylketonuria (PKU)

- Epidemiology
  - autosomal recessive
  - screening available
- H & P
  - normal at birth
  - if untreated:
    - cognitive impairment
    - seizures, and other CNS abnormalities
- Labs & Diagnostics
  - urine for phenylketones (not supposed to be present!)
  - that's why it is called phenylketonuria!
- Clinical Intervention
  - phenylalanine (PHE) restricted diet
- Therapeutics - none
- Health Maintenance
  - in U.S. the diet is in force for lifetime
- Scientific Concept
  - liver enzyme phenylalanine hydroxylase is nonfunctional
  - normally to be used to convert phenylalanine to tyrosine
  - then phenylketones build up and cause damage

Orthopedics/Rheumatology

Congenital Hip Dysplasia

- Epidemiology
  - fairly uncommon
    - firstborn
    - female > male
  - failure to diagnose it in early infancy leads to
    - deterioration of the hip joint
    - hip arthritis
  - treatment is most effective in the newborn period
- Etiology
  - familial/genetic predisposition
  - breech presentation
  - "swaddling" in some cultures
- H & P
  - diagnosis is made on physical exam
    - Barlow maneuver
      - with hip flexed try to push the femoral head out of the acetabulum over the posterior rim
    - if Barlow is negative, do the Ortalani maneuver
      - widely abduct the hip into the socket and feel for a clunk as the hip reduces back into the socket
- Labs & Diagnostics
  - imaging is unreliable in infants < 6 weeks of age
  - Ultrasound in children 6 weeks to 4 months
- Clinical Intervention
  - Pavlik harness – keeps hips externally rotated

Legg-Calve Perthes

- Epidemiology
  - boys, 4-10 year of age
  - delayed bone age
  - short stature
  - usually unilateral
  - sometimes associated with trauma; usually not
- Etiology
  - avascular necrosis of the femoral head
- H & P
  - painless limp at first
  - can have referred knee pain
  - pain as bone is lost
  - limited range of motion
- Labs & Diagnostics
  - A/P of the hip with frog leg views

  - loss of bone of femoral head
    - takes 12-40 months through stages
  - bone scan to evaluate if suspicious
- Clinical Intervention
  - referral to ortho
  - femoral osteotomy results in better ROM later
- Scientific Concept
  - This is the pediatric hip pain in the short kid!

Slipped Capital Femoral Epiphysis
- Epidemiology
  - much less common than Perthes
  - 10-16 years old
  - often bilateral
  - in obese kids
- H & P
  - hip pain
  - often referred to knee
  - no fever or other constitutional symptoms
- Labs & Diagnostics
  - A/P with frog leg views
    - femoral head "slips off"
    - displaced inferiorly and posteriorly
- Clinical Intervention
  - ortho referral
  - operative internal fixation
    - to prevent avascular necrosis
- Scientific Concept
  - This is the hip/knee pain occurs in chubby boys!

Osgood-Schlatter's
- Epidemiology
  - one of the most common causes of knee pain in the adolescent
- Etiology
  - benign, self-limited knee condition
  - due to repetitive strain on the secondary ossification center of the tibial tubercle.
- H & P
  - pain and edema of the tibial tubercle
- Clinical Intervention
  - Initial treatment: ice for 20 minutes every 2-4 hours.
  - Analgesics and NSAIDs
  - Avoid pain-producing activities (eg, sports that involve excess amounts of jumping)
    - But ONLY avoidance if symptomatic (does not change anything otherwise)
  - Referral to ortho if not improving

Torus Fractures (Buckle fractures)
- Epidemiology
  - extremely common injuries seen in children

- Etiology
    - Because children have softer bones, one side of the bone may buckle upon itself without disrupting the other side
    - this is also known as an incomplete fracture
- Clinical Intervention
    - splint immediately
    - referral to ortho for cast
    - usually a short duration, usually about three weeks
    - these injuries tend to heal much more quickly than the similar Greenstick Fractures

Greenstick Fractures

- Etiology:
    - Because a child's bones are much more pliable than adult bone, an incomplete, or 'greenstick,' fracture may occur.
    - one side of the cortex has broken and one side is bent; therefore it is classified as an incomplete break.
- Clinical Intervention
    - closed reduction (to "bend" the bone in position)
    - casting for about six weeks

Clavicular Fracture

- Etiology/epidemiology
    - most common of pediatric fractures due to fall or being struck
- H & P
    - unable to lift arm; deformity visible and palpable
- Labs & Diagnostics
    - plain films
- Clinical Intervention
    - cradle sling or Figure of 8
- Scientific Concept
    - "If the bones are in the same room, they will heal!"

Supracondylar humeral fracture

- Mechanism of injury
    - falling on outstretched hand (FOOSH)
- Epidemiology
    - ages 6-7 is peak
    - most common elbow fracture in kids (>50%)
    - extension type 98%
- H & P
    - pain at elbow
    - pain with pronation/supination
    - make sure to check radial and median nerve function
    - check all pulses
- Imaging: "fat pad sign" is presumptive for fracture, even if fracture not seen
- Clinical intervention
    - long arm posterior molded splint
    - referral to ortho for f/u casting

- This fracture is most common cause of radial nerve injury

Salter-Harris Classification

This mnemonic requires you to imagine the bones as long bones, with the epiphyses at the base.

- I – S = **Slip (separated or straight across)**. Fracture of the cartilage of the physis (growth plate)
- II – A = **Above**. The fracture lies above the physis, or **A**way from the joint.
- III – L = **Lower**. The fracture is below the physis in the epiphysis.
- IV – T = **Through**. The fracture is through the metaphysis, physis, and epiphysis.
- V – R = **Rammed (crushed)**. The physis has been crushed.

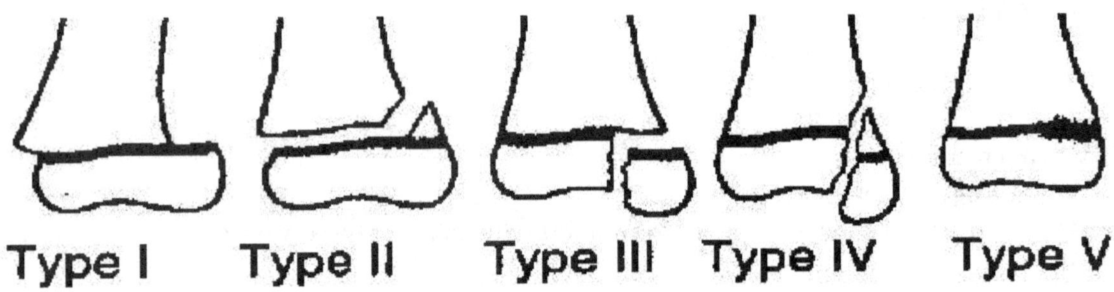

Nursemaid's elbow

- Mechanism of Injury
    - usually hand was pulled, or arm was tugged, i.e. swinging a child by the arms while playing
- Epidemiology
    - 1-4 years old is most common
- Etiology is slippage of the head of the radius under the annular ligament. The distal attachment of the annular ligament covering the radial head is weaker in children than in adults, allowing it to be more easily torn.
- H & P
    - sudden refusal to move the arm
    - no trauma, fall, nothing striking it
    - The forearm is usually flexed 15-20 degrees at the elbow, and the forearm is partially pronated.
    - Often, the weight of the affected arm is supported with the other hand.
    - *Erythema, warmth, edema, bruising or other signs of trauma are absent.*
    - Distal circulation, sensation, and motor activity are normal.
    - Tenderness at the head of the radius may be present.
    - The patient resists supination/pronation as well as flexion/extension of the forearm.

- Imaging not needed if no trauma and typical MOI
- Clinical Intervention
    - Closed reduction
        - This is accomplished by immobilizing the elbow and palpating the region of the radial head with one hand.
        - The other hand applies axial compression at the wrist while supinating the forearm and flexing the elbow.
        - As the arm is manipulated, a click or snap can be felt at the radial head.
        - A click noted by the examiner has a positive predictive value of > 90%

Scoliosis

- Epidemiology
    - This is an uncommon spinal condition in which the spine abnormally rotates and curves from side to side.
    - The incidence of scoliosis is roughly 2 in 100.
    - It usually develops later in childhood or adolescence and is more common in young girls than boys.
    - In more severe cases, the child may suffer potentially serious complications such as respiratory difficulty and physical deformities.
- H & P
    - measure the curvature of the spine with a scoliometer
        - patient flexed forward
- Clinical Intervention
    - Early diagnosis is the key in limiting the extent of the curvature.
    - Curvatures of 10 degrees or less are not considered true scoliosis.
    - Curves less than 30 degrees are usually watched and followed through serial x-rays.
    - Curvatures beyond 30 degrees are often treated by an orthopedic brace to help limit curvature.
    - If a brace fails to control the progression of the curve, surgery is considered.

Kyphosis

- Epidemiology
    - The incidence of kyphosis is approximately 1 in 1,000.
    - an exaggerated curvature of the spine that gives the back a rounded appearance due to:
        - poor posture
        - osteoporosis
        - long term use of steroids
        - spine tumors
- Clinical Intervention
    - A curve of more than 45 degrees should be referred to orthopedics.
    - If a kyphotic curve is more than 75 degrees, surgery may be an option. The doctor may choose to straighten and fuse the vertebrae of the abnormal segment together to stabilize the spine and relieve any pain associated with the instability.

Osteosarcoma

- Etiology/epidemiology
    - Boys > girls

   - 10-25 y.o.
- H & P
   - long bone pain
   - pathologic fracture of long bone
- Labs & Diagnostics
   - sunburst appearance on xray
- Clinical Intervention
   - removal of limb
   - Oncology referral

Juvenile rheumatoid arthritis

- Epidemiology
   - most common chronic rheumatologic disease in children
   - one of the most common chronic diseases of childhood
- Etiology is unknown, and the genetic component is complex
- H & P
   - arthritis present for at least 6 weeks before diagnosis (mandatory for diagnosis of JRA)
   - morning stiffness or gelling phenomenon and arthralgia during the day
   - school absences or limited ability to participate in physical education classes
   - spiking fevers occurring once or twice each day at about the same time of day
   - rash on the trunk and extremities
   - pain, warmth, or erythema of the joint
- Labs & Diagnostics
   - Inflammatory markers: Erythrocyte sedimentation rate (ESR) or CRP level
   - Complete blood count (CBC) and metabolic panel
   - Liver function tests and assessment of renal function with serum creatinine levels
   - Antinuclear antibody (ANA) testing
   - Plain film (especially if only single joint)
- Basic radiographic changes in JIA include the following:
   - Soft tissue swelling
   - Osteopenia or osteoporosis
   - Bony erosions
   - Intra-articular bony ankylosis
   - Growth disturbances
- Referral to pediatric rheumatologist

Neurology

Cerebral Palsy

- Etiology/epidemiology
   - 2-3/1000 births (increased in preterm and in small for dates term babies)
   - fetal asphyxia not proven as a cause (but still widely believed)
- H & P
   - motor and postural dysfunction(spastic – upper motor neuron stymptoms)
   - cognitive impairment (up to 60%), can have normal cognition
   - seizure disorders in 50%

- Clinical Intervention – supportive for patient and family

Febrile seizures

- Epidemiology
  - most common seizure in children 6 months to 5 years
  - 2-5% of pediatric population
  - 30% will have recurrence with febrile illness
  - if seizure < 12 months old, 50% chance of recurrence
- H & P
  - generalized seizure lasting < 15 minutes
  - fever (usually untreated)
  - normal neurologic exam
    - must not have developmental delay/issue
    - must not have congenital anomalies
    - must not have nuchal rigidity/AMS
- Labs & Diagnostics
  - no labs or diagnostics related to seizure
  - workup for cause of seizure
  - *No CT indicated*!
    - if CT indicated, then it is NOT a febrile seizure!
- Clinical Intervention
- Therapeutics
  - none
  - no evidence that anti-seizure meds are indicated
  - seizures are too intermittent and meds have side effects
- Health Maintenance
  - treat fever
  - reassurance of parents
- Scientific Concepts
  - 2% rate of epilepsy by age 25
  - 1% rate in all people by age 25
  - in child < 2 months, you need a negative LP to call it
  - consider LP in children < 12 months

Absence seizure

- Epidemiology
  - almost always begin in childhood
  - usually cease by 20 years of age
    - occasionally replaced by different type of seizure
- H & P
  - impairment of consciousness (therefore a "generalized" seizure)
  - loss of postural tone sometimes
  - sometimes enuresis
  - blank stares, sometimes in mid-sentence
  - automatisms
    - lip smacking
  - abrupt return to normal
- Labs & Diagnostics

  - EEG
- Clinical Intervention
  - neurologic referral
- Therapeutics
  - ethosuximide is drug of choice
  - valproic acid
- Scientific Concepts
  - if EEG shows normal background with bursts of activity and
  - normal to above normal intelligence
  - good prognosis for cessation of the seizures

Psychiatry

Attention Deficit Disorder (ADD/ADHD)

- Etiology/epidemiology
  - familial
  - male> female
  - onset < 7 y.o. typically
  - other psychiatric disorders are common
- H & P
  - school disruption; discipline difficulties; difficulty sitting still (hyperactivity)
  - difficulty concentrating; finishing assignments (inattentiveness)
  - in order to make diagnosis this must be in both social and academic or work setting
- Labs & Diagnostics
  - r/o hyperthyroidism; caffeine excess
- Clinical Intervention
  - behavioral management
- Therapeutics
  - psychostimulants
    - Adderall
    - Concerta
- Health Maintenance
  - meds may cause weight loss
  - failure to thrive
  - concern for decreased growth
  - potential for abuse
- Scientific Concept
  - in order to make diagnosis this must be in *both* social and academic or work setting

Autistic disorder/spectrum

- Etiology/epidemiology
  - male:female, 3:1
  - consider Fragile X
  - occurs with cognitive disorders
  - 25% have seizure disorder
- H & P
  - abnormal development noted shortly after birth

  - failure to smile
  - failure to make eye contact
  - failure to nurse/thrive
  - impaired ability to communicate both verbally and nonverbally
  - abnormal pitch and tone of speech; abnormal speech patterns
  - repetitive motor movements
  - preoccupation with items instead of people
  - hypersensitivity to tactile stimulation (averse to being touched, or touching some-one/thing)
- Labs & Diagnostics
  - NONE – may get basic labs, CT imaging or MR of brain
- Clinical Intervention
  - behavioral management
  - OT/PT
- Therapeutics
  - to treat behaviors (OCD/aggression)
- Scientific Concept
  - no conclusive proof linking autism to vaccination; encourage vaccination

---

Urology

Wilm's Tumor (nephroblastoma)

- Etiology/epidemiology
  - Most common childhood abdominal malignancy
  - Survival rates 80-90%
- H & P
  - Asymptomatic
  - Abdominal mass (80%)
  - Abdominal pain in only 25%
- Labs & Diagnostics
  - CBC
  - Chemistries (BUN/creatinine, electrolytes)
  - Urinalysis
  - Renal ultrasound
  - CT scan (when tumor identified)
  - CXR for metastasis
- Most Likely Diagnosis
  - Same presentation as neuroblastoma and polycystic kidney disease
- Scientific Concept
  - Associated with other urogenital anomalies

Abnormalities of development are covered in Urology Chapter 21:

- Cryptorchidism
- Duplication of the collecting system
- Horseshoe kidneys
- hypospadias/epispadias

NEPHROLOGY

Hemolytic Uremic Syndrome

- Etiology/epidemiology
  - Most common cause of renal failure in childhood
  - Autoimmune (angiopathic – very much like TTP, only affecting kidneys)
  - E Coli 0157:H7 but also many other bacterias (campylobacter, yersinia, strep pneumo, etc, etc, etc)
- H & P
  - Gastroenteritis (80%) with bloody diarrhea (50%)
  - Fever (50%)
  - Acute renal failure (97%)
- Labs & Diagnostics
  - CBC – anemia, hemolysis
  - Chemistries (BUN/creatinine, electrolytes)
  - Urinalysis
  - Stool cultures (shigatoxin)
- Clinical Intervention
  - Hospitalization
  - Nephrology consult
- Scientific Concept
  - Not a lot of good treatments – just like TTP, plasmapheresis (plasma exchange) has been used with some success

---

Eye/ENT

Dacryoadenitis/Nasolacrimal duct obstruction

- Epidemiology
  - plugged lacrimal duct causing inflammation/infection
- H & P
  - Mild swelling of upper or lower inner lid
  - Sometimes purulent discharge from the duct
- Labs & Diagnostics - none
- Clinical Intervention
  - Massage
  - Warm compresses
  - Referral to ophthalmologist if not resolving for lacrimal duct exploration
- Therapeutics
  - Antibacterial eye drops if purulent discharge and eyelid redness and swelling

Acute Otitis Media

- Epidemiology
  - Most common in children due to short, wide Eustachian tubes
  - Very common in Down Syndrome for the same reason
- H & P
  - Red, bulging TM
  - No vibration with insufflation

- Labs & Diagnostics: none needed
    - Clinical Intervention
    - Observation vs. treatment --- debatable lately (in U.S., we usually treat)
- Therapeutics
    - **Amoxicillin 80-90 mg/kg/day in divided doses**
- Scientific Concepts
    - Same pathogens as acute sinusitis and community acquired pneumonias (because it is all connected)
    - Amoxicillin 20-40 mg/kg/day can still be used, *but higher dose (above in therapeutics)will cover dose dependent strep pneumo resistance and is most commonly used in younger kids*

PEARL: There is a push to reduce our antibiotic use in patient's with AOM (as they have been doing in Europe for years now). These are the newest guiding principles we should follow:

- Determine the likelihood that the source is bacterial:
    - A visible middle ear effusion (bulging TM) and otalgia
    - New onset otorrhea not due to OE
    - If not, don't treat with antibiotic!
- Weigh benefits against the risks of antibiotics (I just saw a 9 mo old with C. dif!!!)
- If antibiotics are warranted, use judicious prescribing strategies
    - 10 days duration for < 24 months
    - 7 days for kids older than this (I will admit that I am not doing this clinically)

Serous Otitis Media/Otitis Media with Effusion

- Epidemiology
    - Common
    - Due to prolonged eustachian tube dysfunction
    - Viruses
    - Allergic rhinitis
- H & P
    - No fevers, nontoxic
    - Conductive hearing loss is common
    - Popping and crackling with yawning
    - Serous fluid in middle ear
    - TM is not red!
    - Sluggish or no vibration with insufflation
- Labs & Diagnostics: none, clinical diagnosis
- Clinical Intervention
    - Decongestants are no longer used in children
    - OK to try in adults (with no hypertension or heart disease)
    - Referral to audiology for testing hearing if small child (to preserve normally developing speech patterns)
    - Tympanostomy tube placement referral
- Therapeutics
    - If you use antibiotic, direct it empirically at the most common pathogens for the ears, nose and throat (S. pneumo, H. flu, M. catarrhalis)

Strep pharyngitis

- Epidemiology
    - still very common in school-aged children
    - uncommon cause of rheumatic fever in U.S.
        - due to frequent testing and antibiotic use
    - common cause of rheumatic fever worldwide
- H & P
    - fever
    - exudative tonsillitis
    - anterior cervical adenopathy
    - *without* rhinorrhea, cough
- Labs & Diagnostics
    - rapid strep is 90% sensitive
    - culture should be done if you need better sensitivity
- Therapeutics
    - PenVK is still drug of choice
- Health Maintenance
    - no school until on PCN for 24 hours
    - rapidly travels through classrooms
- Scientific Concept
    - treating strep only prevents rheumatic fever
    - does not prevent glomerulonephritis
    - always look for asymmetry = peritonsillar abscess
    - mono looks like strep, usually worse
        - amox used to treat strep in mono patient will cause rash

Oral candidiasis (thrush)

- Epidemiology
    - Common
    - Usually in neonate from acquiring yeast at time of birth
- H & P
    - White, curdy discharge on inner cheek
    - Scrapes off with tongue depressor
- Labs & Diagnostics
    - KOH shows pseudohyphae
- Therapeutics
    - Nystatin powder, reconstituted in water, swab on inside of cheeks

Nasal polyps

- Epidemiology
    - Cystic Fibrosis
- Clinical Intervention
    - consider sweat chloride test
- Scientific Concept
    - The following are clues to CF in a child:
        - nasal polyps
        - meconium ileus

        - thick tenacious secretions

Infectious diseases

Mumps

- Epidemiology
    - Last outbreak 2006 in Midwest US
    - Outbreak (minor) in Canada 2010 in unvaccinated kids at camp
- H & P
    - Parotitis (enlargement of parotid gland)
    - In adult men, orchitis can occur (testicular pain)
- Labs & Diagnostics
    - None – based on clinical parotitis
- Therapeutics -none
- Health Maintenance
    - MMR vaccine seems to give lifelong immunity to mumps
- Scientific Concept
    - Most parotitis now due to duct stone (and occurs most often in adults)
    - Orchitis (if mumps in adult man) can cause permanent infertility
    - Can cause meningitis

Roseola

- Epidemiology
    - 3 mos to 4 years
- H & P
    - Rhinorrhea, conjunctivitis
    - High fever (up to 104-105) x 4-5 days
    - Fever drops, and rash appears
- Labs & Diagnostics
    - none
- Clinical Intervention
    - None needed
    - Treat fever to prevent febrile seizures and for comfort
- Therapeutics
    - none
- Health Maintenance
    - No vaccine available
- Scientific Concept
    - No significant sequelae
    - Most important complication could be febrile seizure (which is usually quite benign)

Rubeola (Measles)

- Epidemiology
    - 10-14 days prodrome before rash
- H & P
    - fever
    - coryza (nasal congestion, sneezing, sore throat)

- cough
- bilateral conjunctivitis
- photophobia
- Koplik spots are pathognomonic (red spots with white centers on inside of cheeks)
- rash starts on face and behind the ears, papular that coalesce; then on trunk, extremities, then palms and soles

- Labs & Diagnostics
  - IgM measles antibodies
- Clinical Intervention
  - Isolation to prevent spread
- Therapeutics – none
  - Ribavirin has had some effect in people with severe disease
- Health Maintenance
  - MMR vaccination
- Complications
  - Encephalomyelitis
  - Pneumonia
  - Secondary skin infections

Rubella

- Epidemiology
  - Oral droplets
  - 14-21 day incubation period
- H & P
  - Arthralgias
  - Mild symptoms of fever and malaise
  - Posterior cervical and postauricular nodes week before rash
  - Rash is maculopapular on face, then to trunk, then extremities
- Labs & Diagnostics
  - IgM antibodies
  - Otherwise, like most viral illnesses, mild leukopenia
- Clinical Intervention
  - None needed for child
  - Main concern in pregnant woman
- Therapeutics - none
- Health Maintenance
  - Vaccination for children to prevent infection in pregnant females
- Scientific Concept
  - Congenital rubella
  - Cataracts
  - Hearing loss
  - Congenital heart defects
  - Rash

Varicella

- Epidemiology
  - 14-21 day incubation period

    - Contagious by droplets, or by contact with lesions
- H & P
    - Fever and malaise 1-2 days before vesicles erupt
    - Pruritic fluid filled droplets (dewdrops on a rose petal), crusts develop
- Labs & Diagnostics – none needed – clinical diagnosis
- Clinical Intervention
    - Limit contact (usually too late) – very contagious
- Therapeutics - none
- Health Maintenance
    - Varicella vaccine is effective
    - First dose at 12-15 months, second at 4-6 years
    - Avoid aspirin (high risk of Reye's syndrome)
- Complications
    - In kids – secondary infections (impetigo)
    - In adults, especially pregnant women, pneumonia which can be very severe and cause acute respiratory distress syndrome
    - Zoster is possible after initial varicella infection

Dermatology

Diaper dermatitis

- H & P
    - Irritant red "rash" over buttocks and thighs from contact with urine or feces
    - NOTE – redness is on convex parts of butt and thighs (not in the skin folds)
- Labs & Diagnostics
    - KOH would be negative for "pseudohyphae", therefore not yeast
- Clinical Intervention
    - Barrier (Vaseline)
    - Frequent diaper changes
- Therapeutics
    - No yeast cream for this!
- Health Maintenance
    - Biggest occurrence is during diarrhea; frequent diaper changes and some kind of barrier ointment with each diaper change
- Scientific Concept
    - Let the KOH be your friend --- if pos = candida, if neg = irritant

---

Febrile Children with Rashes

(all of these topics are covered earlier in the book, this is just a "summary" for quick reference --- use the buzz words I have here to trigger your memory, and if you still need more, look back in the corresponding chapters)

- bacteremia (i.e. purpura in meningitis, etc)
    - fever precedes rash, be suspicious if the child is very ill
- Scarlet fever (2nd disease)

  - strep throat with a sand paper-like rash
    - rash in groin and around neck
  - no better, no worse, than a strep throat but parents freak!
  - treat like strep throat
- Scalded Skin Syndrome (4th disease)
  - staph aureus
  - bullous painful lesions, red skin around area, fever
  - distinguished from a nasty diaper rash by the fever!
- Viral exanthems
  - measles (1st disease), rubella (3rd disease), varicella
- Erysipelas
  - bright red, well demarcated, painful rash, usually head
- Henoch-Schonlein purpura
  - purpuric lesions with renal failure and hematuria
  - vasculitis due to IgA, C3 (autoimmune)
- Kawasaki syndrome
  - High fever x 1-2 weeks or more (resistant to treatment)
  - Red, cracked lips and "strawberry tongue"
  - Rash on trunk
  - Potentially life-threatening coronary artery vessel disease
- Lyme disease
  - erythema migricans after tick bite
- Rocky Mountain Spotted Fever
  - rash
  - palms & soles
  - cardiac disease

The Six "Diseases" of childhood that cause rashes

1. Rubeola (measles)
2. Scarlet fever (Strep Grp A)
3. Rubella (German measles)
4. Scalded Skin (staph aureus)
5. Fifth's disease (Parvovirus B-19)
6. Roseola

Drugs Not To Be Used In Pediatric Patients

Antimicrobials

- Quinolones – cartilaginous abnormalities, bone defects
- Tetracyclines (TCN, minocycline, doxycycline) – abnormal formation/color of teeth

CV drugs

- ACEI's and ARBs (contraindicated in pregnancy)
- Anti-lipid drugs (not given in pregnancy)

Psych

- Lamictal – Black box warning – Stevens-Johnson syndrome in kids < 16 y.o.

PEDIATRIC IMMUNIZATION SCHEDULE FROM THE CDC

Recommended Immunization Schedule for Persons Aged 0 Through 6 Years—United States • 2011
For those who fall behind or start late, see the catch-up schedule

Vaccine ▼ Age ▶	Birth	1 month	2 months	4 months	6 months	12 months	15 months	18 months	19–23 months	2–3 years	4–6 years
Hepatitis B[1]	HepB	HepB			HepB						
Rotavirus[2]			RV	RV	RV[2]						
Diphtheria, Tetanus, Pertussis[3]			DTaP	DTaP	DTaP	see footnote[3]	DTaP				DTaP
Haemophilus influenzae type b[4]			Hib	Hib	Hib[4]	Hib					
Pneumococcal[5]			PCV	PCV	PCV	PCV				PPSV	
Inactivated Poliovirus[6]			IPV	IPV	IPV						IPV
Influenza[7]					Influenza (Yearly)						
Measles, Mumps, Rubella[8]						MMR		see footnote[8]			MMR
Varicella[9]						Varicella		see footnote[9]			Varicella
Hepatitis A[10]						HepA (2 doses)				HepA Series	
Meningococcal[11]										MCV4	

Legend:
- Range of recommended ages for all children
- Range of recommended ages for certain high-risk groups

Recommended Immunization Schedule for Persons Aged 7 Through 18 Years—United States • 2011
For those who fall behind or start late, see the schedule below and the catch-up schedule

Vaccine ▼ Age ▶	7–10 years	11–12 years	13–18 years
Tetanus, Diphtheria, Pertussis[1]		Tdap	Tdap
Human Papillomavirus[2]	see footnote[2]	HPV (3 doses)(females)	HPV series
Meningococcal[3]	MCV4	MCV4	MCV4
Influenza[4]	Influenza (Yearly)		
Pneumococcal[5]	Pneumococcal		
Hepatitis A[6]	HepA Series		
Hepatitis B[7]	Hep B Series		
Inactivated Poliovirus[8]	IPV Series		
Measles, Mumps, Rubella[9]	MMR Series		
Varicella[10]	Varicella Series		

Legend:
- Range of recommended ages for all children
- Range of recommended ages for catch-up immunization
- Range of recommended ages for certain high-risk groups

"Believe you can and you're halfway there."

-Theodore Roosevelt

CHAPTER 25

Miscellaneous Topics

Genetics

Genetics has been added to the curricula of all PA programs as of 2008; and has been recognized as a very important component of almost all disease entities (if not all). For this reason, I am adding a brief section to remind you of some basic genetic principles:

These are the most basic Mendelian inheritance patterns
- autosomal dominant
- autosomal recessive
- X-linked dominant
- X-linked recessive

All humans (male and female) have autosomes (so if the questions is about "autosomal whatever" then it is equally distributed between the genders
- X-linked diseases will occur most commonly in men
    - They can occur in women, but the female baby would have to get the X (affected gene) from dad who actually has that disease, and an X (affected gene) from mom who "carries" the gene but doesn't express the disease
    - A boy baby simply needs to get the carrier gene from mom to express the disease
- There are very few X-dominant and Y-dominant diseases; so few that it's not worth mentioning (so pay more attention to Autosomal dominant/recessive, and X-linked recessive)
- Pedigrees help to suggest a hereditary pattern of inheritance
    - Mendelian inheritance patterns (autosomal dominant, etc)
    - or a familial pattern (HNPCC, etc)

In trying to figure out pedigrees:
- darkened square = affected male
- darkened circle = affected female
- small dot in square or circle = "carrier" male or female, not necessarily affected

In trying to figure out a specific pedigree:
- If there are both squares and circles in every generation (the mutation occurs quite frequently) = autosomal dominant
- If there are both squares and circles but "skipping" of generations (the mutation occurs only occasionally throughout several generations = autosomal recessive
- If there are almost exclusively squares = X-linked recessive

Use the pedigree examples below toidentify most likely genetic pattern:

Autosomal Dominant:

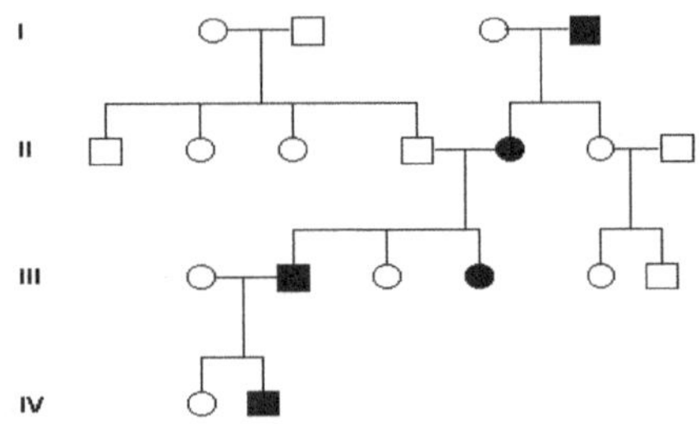

Phenotype of the following disorders:

- Von Willebrands Disease
- Marfan's syndrome
- Hypertrophic Cardiomyopathy
- Familial Adenomatous Polyposis (FAP)
- Polycystic Kidney Disease
- Huntington's Chorea

Autosomal Recessive:

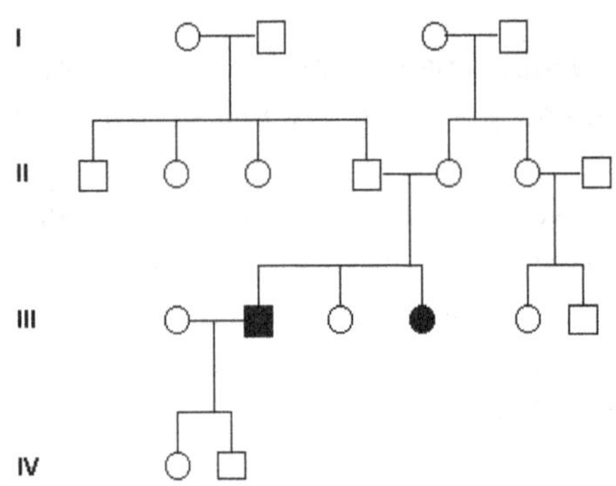

Phenotype of the following disorders:

- Cystic Fibrosis
- Sickle Cell Anemia
- Hemachromatosis
- Wilson's disease

X-Linked Recessive:

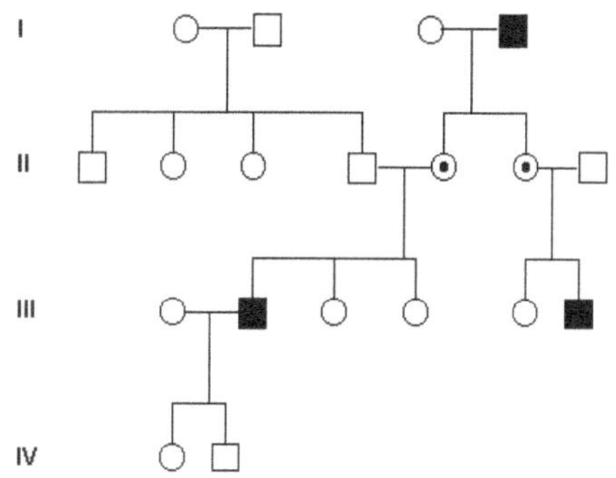

Phenotype of the following disorders:

- G6PD deficiency
- Hemophilia-A
- Color Blindness

Extra autosome = Down Syndrome (extra chromosome 21)

Extra sex chromosome = Klinefelter's syndrome (XXY)

Missing sex chromosome = Turner Syndrome (XO)

Fragile X

Many disease entities which have a genetic component are multifactorial in nature(Type 2 DM, HIV, CAD)

Basic findings of the genome project:

- Humans have far fewer genes than expected (30-35K)
- Each gene codes for more proteins than was expected (3 proteins/gene)
- The male mutation rate is 2x that of the female
- Only two amino protein substitutions per 20,000 typically occur from one individual to a next

Basic genetic laboratory testing

- Molecular genetics lab (DNA extraction and PCR – Fragilc X)
- Cytogenetics lab (FISH – karyotype interpretation - Down Syndrome)
- Biochemical genetics lab (enzyme testin g- i.e. Tay Sachs)

Impact on the prevention of disease with the current state of genetic understanding

- Changes in medical surveillance can occur with patients known at risk
- Drugs are being developed for specific genotypes of patients
- Gene therapy and development of specific drugs for specific disease entities

Ethical and legal considerations and controversies surrounding

- Screening for genetic abnormalities
- Prenatal testing
- Carrier testing
- Confidentiality
- True informed consent prior to testing
- Discrimination issues
- Paternity issues

GINA – The Genetics and Information Nondiscrimination Act of 2008

Title I – prohibits discrimination against a patient for health insurance due to genetics information. This does not protect the patient from discrimination for life insurance or longterm care.

Title II – protects patient from discrimination for employment due to genetic information discovered.

Toxidromes

Toxidrome	Mechanism	Signs and Symptoms
Opioid	opioid receptor	sedation, miosis, decreased respirations
Anticholinergic	muscarinic acetylcholine receptors	altered mental status, sedation, hallucinations, mydriasis, dry mucous membranes, decreased bowel sounds and urinary retention "mad as a hatter, dry as a bone, red as a beet"
Cholinergic	nicotinic and muscurinic acetylcholine receptors	seizures, miosis, lacrimation, diaphoresis, bronchospasm, bronchorrhea, vomiting, diarrhea, bradycardia
Sympathomimetic	alpha and beta adrenergic receptors	agitation, mydriasis, tachycardia, hypertension, hyperthermia, diaphoresis
Sedative-hypnotic	GABA receptors	sedation, miosis, decreased respirations
Serotonin Syndrome	serotonin receptors	altered mental status, tachycardia, hypertension, hyperreflexia, clonus, hyperthermia

ANTIDOTES FOR COMMON POISONINGS

Poison/overdose	Sns/Sxs of poisoning	Antidote	Mechanism of action
Acetaminophen	0-24 hr – vomiting 48 hr– elevated LFTs Days – liver failure	Mucomyst (N-acetylcysteine)	Glutathione substitute- binds toxic metabolite of acetaminophen
Benzodiazepines	Drowsiness, bradycardia, respiratory depression	Flumazenil (note: flumazenil has severe toxicity issues – much debate about its safety) Supportive care is usually best	
Beta Blocker or Calcium Channel blocker	BB: coma; bradycardia; hypotension; respiratory depression CCB: flushing hypotension, reflex tachycardaia, seizures	Glucagon	Has beta agonist effects; promotes movement of glucose (along with calcium into cell)
Digoxin	Anorexia, nausea, vomiting, vision changes, tachyarrhythmias, AV dissociation	Digibind CHECK Potassium level!	
Heavy metal poisoning (lead most common) but also copper, mercury, arsenic)	Penicillamine (also used in Wilson's disease)		
Anticholinergics (antihistamine, antidepressants)	Dry mouth; urinary retention, tachycardia and hypertension, hyperthermia	physostigmine	

ACLS Pharmacology

ACLS is not in the blueprint; and is not a requirement of being a PA; but it may appear on the exam – this is a brief review, just in case! Here is what's new in the past 10 years:

- Begin CPR as soon as possible
  - (this hasn't changed, but emphasis on *compressions*, not breathing)
- BLS is changing (was ABC's, now CAB)
- CAB = circulation, then airway, then breathing
- *nothing works as well as CPR and defibrillation!*

- Acidosis problems in a pulseless nonbreather
  - patient will be acidotic due to CO_2 retention and Lactic Acid production
  - no longer use more than an amp or two of bicarbonate
    - doesn't cross blood brain barrier--- now use HYPERVENTILATION

Key Drugs (many fewer drugs to learn now):

make it simple and just memorize the bolded drugs

Pressors

- **Epinephrine**
  - best at increasing myocardial and cerebral blood flow
  - 1mg every 3-5 minutes throughout code
- vasopressin (ADH)
  - alternative to epi (but just use epi if available, no improved outcome)
  - vasoconstriction (let the latin help you)
  - increases coronary perfusion pressure

Antiarrhythmics

  - no meaningful survival with these drugs--- CPR is still key --
- **amiodarone**
  - sustained VF/VT (defib is better)
- lidocaine
  - has never been proven to help survival

Heart rate agents

- **atropine**
  - to speed up heart
- **adenosine**
  - to slow down heart

Torsades

- **$MgSO_4$**

Other pressors (cardiogenic shock -- SBP<90 for more than 30 minutes)

- **dopamine**
  - low dose – increases right atrial perfusion

    - mid range dose – increases HR, contractility
    - high dose – vasoconstrictor – increases BP
- dobutamine

CHAPTER 26

Diagnosis by Symptoms

In this chapter, I would like you to "put it all together" and use the very brief description and minimal words in the stem to come up with the MOST LIKELY DIAGNOSIS. Recall that this knowledge & skills area is 18% of your entire exam!

As you take the exam, you will realize that there is a great deal of other information given (in the form of lab results, historical clues; imaging results, etc.)

As you will see as you do the worksheets in this chapter, only a little bit of information can give you a good head start in identifying the "most likely diagnosis", especially if you feel that you are running out of time and the questions are just too long.

Try to move through these quickly, as if you were at the end of a block, and had 10 questions left, but only 7 minutes to finish.

Practice makes perfect. Take these test-taking skills now to PanceMaster quizzes and do 30 Q quizzes on the top 6 content areas (CV, Pulm, GI, Ortho, EENT, Women's Health), and see how you do!

The BEST utilization of PanceMaster in preparing for your exam:

Do not just frantically do Q.s! Select Q's from the top 6 weighted areas.

Time yourself --- do not allow yourself more than 60 min. for 60 Q.; and do 60-minute blocks to get practice in timing!

Then, have a piece of paper numbered 1-60.

- On the ones you know for sure -- just answer them
- If you are making a COMPLETE GUESS (and you will guess often!)--- mark that one G
- If you are stuck between A & C -- and you answer A -- them mark C
- Or if you are stuck between three choices, select one and mark your other two options

Then, quickly go over all your incorrect answers (especially if it is one you THOUGHT you knew for sure)

Then, go over all the CORRECT ones with a G --- or the ones where you incorrectly guessed the "other one".

So your paper should look something like this:

1.	G 4.	C/E 7.
G 2.	5.	G 8.
3.	A 6.	9.

For the G's (the ones you guessed on)- look at them and see if they are just stupid zebras that you should just let go == then FORGET ABOUT IT -- i.e. erlichiosis --- who the heck cares about that unless you see it often -- just let it go --- you have to get SOME wrong! However, if your G is about CHF drugs – even if you got it CORRECT, go back to that section in the book.

Next, look at the ones where you were stuck between the answer you chose and (in the example of Question 6 above --- A. Let's say you chose B, and you got it correct, but you still need to review *WHY* you chose the correct answer, since you were clearly stuck between B and A.

In my example #7. You selected an answer, but also thought C or E might be correct. Review this Q, *even if you got the answer correct*, so you know *why* your answer was correct.

ANY other questions, email me, you should have a response within 24-48 hours; if not email again, I am committed to all PAs passing their exams and will help in any way I am able!!

Now work on these, and then get going on PanceMaster questions – you will learn a lot if you use the above method as you review your practice exams.

Hyperbilirubinemia

Select the most likely diagnosis given this minimal information for each vignette from the following list (you may only use each diagnosis once)

1. NASH (nonalcoholic steatohepatitis)
2. Hepatitis A
3. Hepatitis B
4. Hepatitis C
5. Gilbert's syndrome
6. Acute cholecystitis
7. Hepatoma (primary liver cancer)
8. Pancreatic cancer

A. A 17 y.o. presents with abdominal pain which turns out to be constipation. Entire workup is negative except for a mildly elevated T. bilirubin and elevation of the indirect bilirubin fraction.

B. A 17 y.o. presents with abdominal pain, jaundice on physical exam with RUQ discomfort, anorexia. He has just returned from a trip to the Midwest to assist the Red Cross after a flood.

C. A 17 y.o. presents with abdominal pain, jaundice on physical exam with RUQ discomfort, anorexia. He has had six sexual partners in the past six months.

D. A 32 year old presents for routine care; he is asymptomatic; in history-taking, he admits to IV drug use in his youth; labs show moderate elevation of LFT's and mild direct bilirubinemia.

E. A 44 year old female with BMI 38 presents for routine physical exam. A comprehensive metabolic panel is done which shows mild elevation of ALT and AST with normal bilirubin and rest of labs all within normal limits.

F. A 48 y.o. obese female presents with three month history of RUQ pain after eating, and now has 2 hours of sustained RUQ discomfort, positive Murphy's sign and jaundice with mild fever.

G. A 62 year old male presents with jaundice, and vague epigastric discomfort which has been present for the past 2-3 months. He has been previously healthy. His RUQ ultrasound shows no liver or GB abnormalities; pancreas is obscured by gas and stool in bowel.

H. A 62 y.o. smoker, with significant long term alcohol intake and diagnosis of cirrhosis presents with six month h/o RUQ discomfort and anorexia. He has icteric sclera and has lost 18 pounds unintentionally. He is afebrile and has otherwise normal PE.

DISCUSSION:

In evaluating a patient who presents with jaundice, the first thing to do is determine whether this is a chronic problem or an acute problem.

Then, are the transaminases most elevated (ALT/AST), or is it the biliary tree enzymes (Alk ptase, GGTP, 5'nucleatidase) that are most significantly elevated?

Next, is it primarily a direct bilirubin elevation, or an indirect bilirubin elevation.

Direct bilirubin is conjugated, allowing the kidneys to help the liver get rid of bilirubin. In a direct bilirubin elevation, therefore, there will be positive bilirubin on a urine dip.

Indirect bilirubin is unconjugated, so the kidney cannot help get rid of it. The urine will be yellow and negative for bilirubin on the urine dip.

Direct bilirubin is due to many many different reasons.

Indirect bilirubin is only due to two main reasons: hemolysis of RBC's (sending too much bilirubin to the liver.

Dyspnea

Select the most likely diagnosis given this minimal information for each vignette from the following list (you may only use each diagnosis once)

1. CHF
2. Community acquired pneumonia (CAP)
3. Normal pregnancy changes
4. Iron deficiency anemia
5. Mitral stenosis
6. Acute exacerbation of COPD
7. Pulmonary embolism
8. Pericardial effusion/tamponade

A. A 28 y.o. female presents with history of menorrhagia for the past six months and dyspnea, particularly with exertion.

B. A 64 y.o. male smoker who had the "stomach flu" last week presents with new onset of peripheral edema and dyspnea on exertion. Chest x-ray shows diffuse patchy infiltrates and cardiomegaly. EKG shows new Q waves in leads II, III, and avF.

C. A 64 y.o. male smoker who had the "flu" last week presents with a single shaking rigor yesterday, with fever, cough productive of thick discolored sputum and dyspnea.

D. A 38 y.o. female presents with dyspnea, tachycardia, tachypnea and mild hypoxia with pleuritic chest pain but no cough. She is 36 weeks pregnant and has just returned from an overseas flight for her mother's funeral.

E. A 38 y.o. female presents with complaint of dyspnea; peripheral edema in her ankles and fingers worsening in the past 3-4 weeks. She is 38 weeks pregnant. Her PE is normal; with normal DTR's and no clonus. CBC is normal with normal platelet count; normal LFT's and renal function.

F. A 64 y.o. male presents 3 weeks after aortic valve replacement with increasing dyspnea with exertion, but now even at rest. He has no chest pain. His BP is 92/84; his jugular vein is markedly distended. He has low voltage on an ECG with pulsus alternans. CXR shows significant cardiac silhouette enlargement which is new since last CXR just before discharge after surgery.

G. A 64 y.o. male presents with increasing dyspnea on exertion, but now also at rest. He has cough productive of yellow sputum increased compared to his "usual" daily cough. He has a 60 pk-yr history of smoking.

H. A 38 y.o. female presents with complaint of worsening dyspnea with exertion. She is 28 weeks pregnant and has bibasilar rales on exam with a grade II-III/VI diastolic rumbling murmur which radiates into her axilla and back. She had a murmur noted at her first OB visit, but this is a significant change. ECG is normal; CXR shows pulmonary revascularization and prominent pulmonary vasculature.

Chest pain

Select the most likely diagnosis given this minimal information for each vignette from the following list (you may only use each diagnosis once)

1. GERD
2. Costochondritis
3. Pleuritis
4. Panic disorder/hyperventilation syndrome
5. Rib fracture
6. STEMI
7. Pulmonary embolism
8. Unstable angina

A. A 23 y.o. male presents with chest pain that increases with deep breathing following a recent URI. He has no rales or rhonchi, but a friction rub is heard when he is supine along the lateral lung fields.

B. A 23 y.o. male presents with chest pain that increases with deep breathing following a recent URI. VS are normal; there is pain to palpation of the chest wall at the left sternal margin at ribs 2,3,4.

C. A 32 y.o. female on birth control pills and recent bunionectomy surgery presents with chest pain that increases with deep breathing. HR 124; RR 24; BP 130/98; Pulse ox 92% T99.4

D. A 42 y.o. woman who had a fall this afternoon presents with chest pain that increases with deep breathing. She splints with breathing and pulse ox is 92%. She is a smoker

E. A 52 y.o. male presents with retrosternal chest pressure that began while shoveling the snow two hours ago. He has mild diaphoresis. ECG shows ST elevation in leads II, II and avF.

F. A 52 y.o. male presents with retrosternal chest pain which occurred while laying down after Thanksgiving dinner. He has had similar symptoms before; never with exertion; usually after meals, particularly after having a cigarette and drink after his dinner. HR 64; RR 16; BP 140/70; Pulse ox 98%.

G. A 52 y.o. female presents with tingling of her hands and around her lips; numbness of her lips; diaphoresis; HR 132; RR 28; BP 190/90; T 98.9; Pulse ox 100%. She was seen by you in the ER three days ago and diagnosed with metastatic lung cancer and is being worked up to identify the primary cancer.

H. A 52 y.o. male presents with retrosternal chest pressure that began while shoveling the snow, but resolved after 20 minutes of rest. He now is asymptomatic; but did note the same discomfort while climbing up a flight of stairs, and so presents. ECG is normal; cardiac enzymes are normal x 1 set.

Abdominal pain

Select the most likely diagnosis given this minimal information for each vignette from the following list (you may only use each diagnosis once)

1. Constipation
2. Hemorrhagic ovarian cyst
3. Peptic ulcer disease
4. Diverticulitis
5. Acute pancreatitis
6. Appendicitis
7. Splenic rupture
8. Ectopic pregnancy
9. Acute cholecystitis

A. A 72 y.o. male with fever and LLQ pain for two days presents......

B. A 16 y.o. male with fever and RLQ pain for 12 hours presents.......

C. A 42 y.o. female with fever and RUQ pain for 12 hours presents.....

D. A 4 y.o. male, afebrile, with diffuse abdominal pain since eating dinner presents.....

E. A 23 y.o. pregnant female with sudden onset RLQ pain presents.......

F. A 23 y.o. nonpregnant female presents midcycle with sudden onset LLQ pain.....

G. A 32 y.o. businessman with epigastric gnawing pain for two to three weeks presents....

H. A 60 y.o. male with LUQ pain two hours after colonoscopy presents......

I. A 43 y.o. male with RUQ pain two days after ERCP presents........

DISCUSSION: In evaluating abdominal pain, let the location and quality of the pain narrow your differential. Pay careful attention to the vital signs (particularly fever, tachycardia). The age of the patient may completely change your differential. Information about the patient's alcohol intake, or association of the pain with food also points you toward the most likely diagnosis. Also, pay attention to the acute or chronic nature of the complaint; often this will help you identify the answer.

Headache

Select the most likely diagnosis /etiology given this minimal information for each vignette from the following list (you may only use each diagnosis once)

1. Migraine HA
2. Subarachnoid hemorrhage
3. Tension (myofascial HA)
4. Lead poisoning
5. Meningococcal meningitis
6. CN III palsy
7. Cluster HA
8. Epidural hematoma
9. Subdural hematoma

A. A 16 y.o. with FH of migraine presents with monthly unilateral HA with associated photo-phonophobia, nausea and normal neuro exam.

B. A 6 y.o. with neg FH presents with "clumsiness" and HA; neuro exam shows a gait ataxia. He has chronic complaints of abdominal pain; and is anemic on CBC.

C. A 62 y.o. with PMH of DM presents with 45 minute history of HA with lid ptosis and abnormal EOM's; no papilledema.

D. A 28 y.o. with neg PMH/FH presents with sudden onset of "worst HA of my life"

E. A 38 y.o. presents with HA after trauma occurring 3 hrs PTA with brief LOC; CT shows blood which crosses the parietal suture along the inside of the cranium

F. A 38 y.o. has onset of severe HA and altered mental status 20 minutes after head trauma with LOC; CT shows a lens shaped collection of blood which does not cross the parietal sutureline.

G. A 22 y.o. college student presents to Student Health during midterm week with HA that feels like a tight band around her head and neck muscle stiffness. Her PE is completely normal.

H. A 22 y.o. college student presents to Student Health during midterm week with HA, fever, stiff neck and purpuric rash on extremities.

I. A 42 y.o. male presents with unilateral pain with lacrimation of the eye, and mild conjunctival injection. This HA has been present for 8 days, and seems to occur once every year or two for a week or more for the past 6-8 years.

DISCUSSION: When trying to identify the most likely etiology of a headache, pay attention to the chronicity (or acute-ness) of the complaint. A severe HA that occurs every month is less ominous than a severe HA for the very first time in a patient. An abnormal neurologic exam ALWAYS must be investigated, and suggests a more serious etiology. The description of the HA alone may give you the clue without any additional information. Any rash at all with fever and HA increases the risk of meningitis, and is a life-threatening emergency.

Diarrhea

Select the most likely diagnosis given this minimal information for each vignette from the following list (you may only use each diagnosis once)

1. Celiac disease
2. Irritable bowel syndrome
3. Giardia
4. Clostridium dificile
5. Crohn's disease
6. Ulcerative colitis
7. Laxative abuse
8. Salmonellosis

A. A 34 y.o. patient presents with diarrhea ongoing for more than a year with negative work up. She has recently been diagnosed with anorexia and has BMI 17.

B. A 34 y.o. patient presents afebrile with diarrhea for 3 days following a camping trip to the boundary waters; the diarrhea is nonbloody; profuse and watery

C. A 34 y.o. patient presents febrile (T 101.4) with diarrhea for 3 days which is small volume and with bright red blood.

D. A 34 y.o. patient presents with diarrhea, on and off for more than a year with workup that shows iron deficiency anemia; B12 deficiency; but no significant weight loss

E. A 34 y.o. patient presents with diarrhea, on and off for about 3-4 months, with low grade fevers; weight loss of about 15 pounds. The stools are bloody; frequently with nocturnal diarrhea.

F. A 34 y.o. patient presents with alternating constipation and diarrhea ongoing for since college; no fever; no blood in her stool; no weight loss. Her workup shows no nutritional deficiencies.

G. A 34 y.o. patient presents with diarrhea, on and off for more than 4 months; with low grade fevers; weight loss of more than 10 pounds; she has RLQ cramping; and has had two perianal abscesses in the past three months.

H. A 34 y.o. patient presents with diarrhea which is severe and began after 6 week course of broad spectrum antibiotics for osteomyelitis after a dog bite with open fracture of her R hand.

Discussion: Most important is to pay careful attention to ACUTE or CHRONIC; the differential is drastically different. Inflammatory bowel diseases are chronic in nature, although pay present acutely with specific symptoms related; dysentery is acute in onset. IBS by definition is functional and so should not have any nutritional deficiencies. Celiac disease and any other inflammatory disorders will cause deficiencies of vitamins (celiac will primarily affect iron which is absorbed in the duodenum; Crohn's will have more B12 deficiency due to terminal ileus involvement where B12 is absorbed) C dif is the answer if there has been chronic antibiotic use (in the past several months); camping = giardia (although other pathogens can be seen too)

Vomiting

Select the most likely diagnosis given this minimal information for each vignette from the following list (you may only use each diagnosis once)

1. Hydatidiform molar pregnancy
2. Food poisoning
3. Increased CSF pressure (mass effect of tumor)
4. Gastroenteritis
5. Hyperemesis gravidarum
6. Mallory Weiss Tear
7. Digoxin toxicity
8. Bulimia
9. Variceal hemorrhage
10. Boerhaave's syndrome

A. A 32-year-old pregnant female presents at 10 weeks gestation with severe vomiting for the past two weeks. Her HCG is appropriate for dates; as is her uterine size.

B. A 32-year-old pregnant female presents at 10 weeks gestation with severe vomiting for the past two weeks. Her HCG is at least three times the expected HCG for her dates; and uterus is large for dates at about 14-16 week size.

C. A 32-year-old kindergarten teacher presents with 4 hours of vomiting and onset of diarrhea now that vomiting has resolved with T 100.8; abdominal cramping, rhinorrhea, and myalgias.

D. A 42-year-old male presents with severe wretching and diarrhea; six hours after eating lunch of a chicken sandwich that he kept in his truck overnight .

E. A 42-year-old male presents with vomiting mainly when laying down at night; he has progressing daily headaches; and has noted change in vision in his peripheral fields bilaterally.

F. A 42-year-old male with sudden onset of severe retrosternal tearing sensation after wretching for about three hours with marked anxiety; CXR shows air in the mediastinum.

G. A 42-year-old male presents with vomiting for three hours after heavy binge drinking during a Packer game; his last emesis had some bright red blood that he noted in the toilet.

H. A 52-year-old male with long history of alcohol abuse presents after waking from sleep with vomiting of large amounts of blood; he has no pain; but is hypotensive and tachycardic.

I. A 62-year-old male with h/o CHF due to ischemic cardiomyopathy presents with anorexia and vomiting for the past couple of days; he complains of yellow color vision; and has tachycardia; ECG shows SVT at rate of 180 bpm.

J. A 21-year-old female college student presents to Student Health with lightheadedness and near syncopal episode. She admits to vomiting "occasionally" but denies abdominal pain. Her exam is normal except for erythema of her oropharynx. Her CBC is wnl; her electrolytes show marked hypokalemia with K of only 2.8.

Vomiting (continued)

Discussion: Again, this is about acute vs. chronic. After you have figured out if it is acute or chronic, ask yourself a few more questions: Is it infectious? (fever) Is this a varsity drinker? (variceal bleed) Is it painful (Boerhaaves)? or painless (Mallory-Weiss)?

The next most common cause is the most lethal: cardiogenic syncope – pay attention to three main clues: #1 DURING exertion- remember, you should have good BP during exertion-if not, it suggests a significant obstruction; #2 murmur – this can suggest aortic stenosis; mitral stenosis, hypertrophic myopathy; myxoma, #3 arrhythmias (v fib; v tach, a fib, SVT, etc)

Hearing loss

Select the diagnosis that would have Weber test lateralizing to the "bad ear" with abnormal air : bone conduction:

A. Chronic otitis media
B. Presbycusis
C. Otosclerosis
D. Cerumen impaction
E. Meniere's disease
F. Acoustic neuroma
G. Otitis media with effusion (SOM)

Discussion: Remember, the Weber is using the tuning fork to "bypass" the conductive system from the pinna, canal, TM, ossicles, and middle ear/Eustachian tube in order to vibrate the perfectly normal Acoustic nerve. Therefore, the "bad" ear can suddenly hear again!

Similarly, since air conduction is the problem here; the Rinne will vibrate CN VIII through the mastoid bone, so bone conduction is better than air conduction

Now – just reverse this and select the diagnoses that would cause Weber to cause sound to the "good' ear and preserved air>bone conduction

Vertigo

Select the most likely diagnosis given this minimal information for each vignette from the following list (you may only use each diagnosis once):

1. Meniere's Disease
2. Acoustic Neuroma
3. Vertebrobasilar stroke
4. Acute labyrinthitis

A. A 72-year-old patient presents with one week of progressive dizziness. On exam, a vertical nystagmus does not fatigue with maneuvers. There is a cranial nerve palsy with a ptosis of the right lid.

B. A 28-year-old female presents 10 days after a "bad cold" with sudden and severe dizziness, nausea and vomiting; tinnitus and hearing loss with fullness in her left ear. The nystagmus is horizontal and fatigues with head maneuvers.

C. A 62-year-old patient presents with ongoing issues of episodic mild vertigo; worse when he has been off his CHF "diet". He has associated low-pitched blowing tinnitus and a sensorineural hearing loss in the left ear.

D. A 42-year-old patient presents with sudden unilateral hearing loss. It is sensorineural. He describes continuous disequilibrium that has been very slowly getting worse over the past couple of weeks.

Discussion: The most important thing to figure out in a questions about vertigo, is whether the vertigo is "peripheral", i.e. coming from the cochlea, labyrinth and semicircular canals; or whether it is "central" coming from a tumor, mass in the cerebellum, cerebellar stroke.

Look for clues about the sudden severe nature (peripheral); the nystagmus (horizontal & fatigable is most likely peripheral; vertical or rotatory with no fatigability is most likely central). Also always look for those RF's for stroke – that may be your only clue.

One more comment – and the most difficult thing to do clinically – is to make sure that "dizziness" is not actually lightheadedness from orthostasis. So, if orthostatic VS are abnormal, go there!

Treatment is with meclizine – an antihistamine with anticholinergic SE's like dry mouth, urinary retention.

Central vertigo needs referral – in in ER, CT of head; but most likely in clinic, then MRI with contrast would be indicated.

Syncope

Select the most likely diagnosis given this minimal information for each vignette from the following list (you may only use each diagnosis once):

1. Arrhythmia
2. Vasovagal/neurocardiogenic syncope
3. Hypertrophic cardiomyopathy

A. A 13 year old girl presents having had a syncopal episode during a blood draw. The entire history and physical exam is normal. She is feeling completely fine 15 minutes later with normal vital signs.

B. A 26 year old college student has a syncopal episode while running sprints in a football practice. He is awake and alert now but still diaphoretic; vital signs are now normal.

C. A 63 year old male is taken to the ER after having a syncopal episode during the middle of the night when up to void. He felt lightheaded prior to the episode, but remembers very little since that time. History and physical exam are normal except for the fact that the patient has had triple vessel coronary stents, and is currently being treated for hypertension and hyperlipidemia.

Discussion: Most syncopal episodes (40%) are a result of an "overactive" autonomic nervous system. A perfect example is the PA student at the OR table – anxious, terrified, has not had anything to eat or so she does not have to scrub out. After becoming interested in the case, her parasympathetic system counteracts that fight-or-flight response and drops her BP and HR. If you are not perfusing your brain, nature will put your brain on the floor and let gravity perfuse it.

The most lethal cause of syncope is cardiogenic. A missed diagnosis here has almost a 30% one-year mortality rate. So, look for the clues of the syncope occurring *during exertion* –this almost always suggests obstruction to flow from the LV to the carotids (aortic valve stenosis, no CO, etc). Likewise, pay attention to murmurs – again suggesting obstruction to flow (so most likely *stenotic* valve disorders). And pay careful attention to arrhythmias (irregular irregular pulse, palpitations), as atrial fib is both common and lethal if clots are going to the brain.

Vision loss/disturbance

Select the most likely diagnosis given this minimal information for each vignette from the following list (you may only use each diagnosis once)

1. Central retinal artery occlusion
2. Central retinal vein occlusion
3. Ocular migraine
4. Optic neuritis
5. Temporal (Giant cell) arteritis
6. Retinal detachment

A. A 64-year-old male with hypertension, diabetes, and coronary artery disease presents to the ER with sudden onset of vision loss in his L eye. He describes mild discomfort, but is not markedly uncomfortable. External inspection is normal; visual acuity is poor. Fundoscopic exam shows darkening of the retina with exudates, hemorrhages and optic disk edema in his L eye. R eye exam is normal.
B. A 72-year-old female presents with visual disturbance in her R eye vision. She has had 2-3 weeks of mild R sided unilateral headache. She has had generalized malaise and low grade fevers. Her visual acuity is decreased in the R eye; otherwise the eye looks normal.
C. An 80-year-old patient presents with sudden loss of vision in his L eye. He has longstanding h/o atrial fibrillation. His INR was subtherapeutic three days ago at 1.2, his warfarin was doubled last night. He denies any pain. Visual acuity is markedly impaired. Fundoscopic exam shows a very pale retina; there is a red "spot" in the area of the macula.
D. A 32-year-old female presents with visual disturbance in her R eye vision over the past 3-4 hours. She reports change in her color vision, with loss of bright color vision. She has mild discomfort behind her R eye. Visual acuity is decreased. External eye exam is normal. On fundoscopic exam her R optic disk is edematous; L is normal.
E. A 52-year-old female with Type I DM since age 10, presents with sudden change in vision in her R eye. She states that this morning she noticed bright flashes of light in her vision which was sporadic. She has noted many floaters in her vision since waking too. Now she feels like she is slowly losing her vision from top to bottom. Visual acuity is markedly decreased. Fundoscopic exam is markedly abnormal.
F. A 32-year-old female presents with visual disturbance in her R eye vision, which is now resolving after 20-30 minutes. She presents with R unilateral headache pain with photo-phonophobia, nausea and vomiting. Her visual acuity is normal; and complete eye evaluation is now normal.

Optic disk/cup changes

Select the most likely diagnosis given this minimal information for each vignette from the following list (you may only use each diagnosis once)

1. Chronic open angle glaucoma
2. Optic neuritis
3. Central retinal vein occlusion
4. Papilledema

A. A 32-year-old female presents with visual disturbance in her R eye vision over the past 3-4 hours. She reports change in her color vision, with loss of bright color vision. She has mild discomfort behind her R eye. Visual acuity is decreased. External eye exam is normal. On fundoscopic exam her R optic disk is edematous; L is normal.
B. A 52-year-old woman presents with complaint of headache, which has been worsening over the past month, occasional vomiting but mainly when supine, and now visual disturbance which is mild. Her neurologic exam is significant for weakness in her R grip strength. On fundoscopic exam, both optic disks are significantly edematous.
C. A 64-year-old male with hypertension, diabetes, and coronary artery disease presents to the ER with sudden onset of vision loss in his L eye. He describes mild discomfort, but is not markedly uncomfortable. External inspection is normal; visual acuity is poor. Fundoscopic exam shows darkening of the retina with exudates, hemorrhages and optic disk edema in his L eye. R eye exam is normal.
D. A 68-year-old male presents to clinic with complaint of visual changes which have been on-going for several months. He has not seen an eye doctor is more than 10 years; although he does wear glasses. On exam, his visual acuity is 20/300 OD; 20/450 OS. Slit lamp exam is normal. Fundoscopic exam shows a mildly enlarged cup:disk ratio on the R, but a markedly enlarged cup on the L. His tonopen pressures are 24 OD and 32 OS.

Discussion: I think you get the point after doing these questions that swelling of the disk accompanies many visual concerns. First, pay attention to whether or not the disk swelling is bilateral or unilateral. If bilateral, it is increased CSF pressures, so think brain! If unilateral, then you need to look at the rest of the retina. If the retina is fine, then it is an optic nerve problem (neuritis). If the retina is involved, then there is some back up of blood into the cup/disk (vein occlusion).

In chronic glaucoma, "cupping" occurs over a long period of time of untreated intra-ocular pressures. In cupping, the disk is not bulging or edematous – the cup is HUGE relative to the disk. So, as always, pay careful attention to the words you are reading.

Painful Red Eye

Select the most likely diagnosis given this minimal information for each vignette from the following list (you may only use each diagnosis once)

1. Acute angle closure glaucoma
2. Iritis/uveitis
3. Bacterial conjunctivitis
4. Corneal abrasion

A. A 22-year-old college student presents with "pink eye", with diffuse conjunctival injection of her L eye, purulent d/c; normal visual acuity; and no fluorescein stain uptake on Wood lamp exam.
B. A 22-year-old college student presents with a painful "pink" eye, with diffuse conjunctival injection of her L eye; watery tearing discharge, normal visual acuity, and positive uptake of fluorescein stain on Wood lamp exam to the lateral aspect of her cornea.
C. A 56-year-old female presents to the urgent care center with sudden onset of severe headache, L eye pain, blurring of her vision, abdominal pain and vomiting. She has no fever. She was in the movie theater when she began developing the eye pain first, and then the rest of her symptoms. Her visual acuity is decreased; her L eye is mid-dilated and fixed; has a limbic flush; cloudy cornea. On slit lamp there are cells in the anterior chamber.
D. A 56-year-old female presents to the urgent care center with sudden onset of L eye pain, blurring her vision, severe photophobia, and nausea. She denies trauma or FB. Her PMH is significant only for Rheumatoid Arthritis. On exam, she has pain in the L eye with both direct and consensual light response; and pupil is noted to be sluggish. The conjunctiva is mildly injected with a limbic flush.

Discussion: The two most important to rule out may cause permanent damage if not treated early. So, make sure to review iritis/uveitis – which is really an autoimmune phenomenon, and almost always associated with RA or SLE

Acute/Chronic kidney injury

Select the most likely diagnosis given this minimal information for each vignette from the following list (all patients have a creatinine of 3.4) You may only use each diagnosis once:

1. Post-strep glomerulonephritis
2. Minimal change disease
3. Hemolytic uremic syndrome
4. Obstructive uropathy
5. Pre-renal azotemia
6. Diabetic nephropathy

A. A 6 yo presents with petechiae on his legs and trunk, puffy eyelids and lips, hematuria. He has had diarrhea ever since being at a picnic where burgers were served. U/A shows RBC's, 1+ protein. CBC shows significant anemia, schistocytes, and thrombocytopenia.
B. A 78 yo diabetic male presents with malaise and weakness. As part of his work up, he is noted to have hyperkalemia with K 5.4, CBC with marked normocytic anemia. He has a low T Protein.
C. A 6 yo presents with puffy eyelids and lips, no hematuria. U/A shows no RBC's, 4+ protein, no WBC's and a few broad casts. CBC is normal.
D. A 78 yo diabetic male presents with severe lower abdominal pain. He has moderate dementia and lives in a nursing home. Exam shows distended abdomen. DRE shows markedly enlarged prostate. U/A is normal. 750 cc. of urine was drained and Foley was placed.
E. A 6 yo presents with brown colored urine, puffy eyelids and lips. He finished a 10 day course of antibiotics for strep throat about a week ago. U/A shows > 50 RBC's, 1+ protein, no WBC's, RBC casts are present. CBC is normal.
F. A 78 yo diabetic male was "found down" at his home by his daughter. She has no idea how long ago he had fallen. He is lethargic, confused, and is brought to ER. CBC is wnl; u/a shows specific gravity > 1.030; BUN is 58, creatinine is 3.4.

Discussion: In kids, there are three main renal failure diseases: post-strep GN which is a ***nephritic syndrome*** following strep (and not prevented by appropriate treatment of strep throat). There is minimal change disease which is a ***nephrotic syndrome***, is idiopathic, and usually has a good prognosis. There is HUS, due most often to toxin from E Coli O157:H7 which causes a microangiopathic destruction of tissue (in kids, primarily kidney – though other organs are involved) – it has a poorer prognosis than the other two. Of them post-strep GN is most common; minimal change disease is the most common of the *nephrotic syndromes* in kids – yet not too common, and HUS, fortunately, is pretty rare. We had an epidemic at our Children's hospital several years ago from undercooked hamburgers at a Ponderosa – which then closed.

Rash

1. Pityriasis rosea
2. Secondary syphilis
3. Nummular eczema
4. Tinea corporis (ringworm)
5. Lichen planus
6. Candidiasis
7. Rubeola
8. Rubella
9. Kawasaki's syndrome
10. Scarlet Fever

A. An 8 yo presents with rash. It is pruritic. There are multiple "ringed" areas on his trunk. He has no lichenification in the popliteal and antecubital fossae. KOH is positive.

B. A 21 year old presents with a rash. It is salmon-colored, scaly edges and mildly pruritic. It is found on his back primarily. He has no lesions of palms or soles. He has mild URI symptoms.

C. A 38 yo female presents for vaginal itching. On speculum exam, there are white areas on the vaginal mucosa. The mucosa is mildly red. The white patches scrape with tongue depressor.

D. An 8 yo presents with rash. She is unvaccinated. She has fever, is ill-appearing, has fairly marked cough; marked bilateral conjunctivitis, tiny white-blue patches on her buccal mucosa

E. A 3 yo presents with fever, sore throat. On exam has "strawberry tongue", red, enlarged, exudative tonsils with cervical lymphadenopathy and circumoral pallor. There is a fine rash over his anterior chest and lower abdomen.

F. A 21 year old presents with a rash. It is salmon-colored, scaly edges and mildly pruritic. It is found on his back primarily. He also has lesions of palms or soles. He has no URI symptoms.

G. A 38 yo female presents for vaginal itching. On speculum exam, there are white areas on the vaginal mucosa. The mucosa otherwise is normal. The white patches do not scrape off. Wickham's striae is noted on vaginal walls.

H. An 8 yo presents with rash. She is unvaccinated. She has no fever, is well-appearing. The rash if bumpy and red. She has posterior cervical and occipital adenopathy.

I. A 3 yo presents with fever, sore throat. On exam he has "strawberry tongue", red, enlarged tonsils with cervical lymphadenopathy and bright red, blistered, desquamating lips.

J. An 8 yo presents with rash. It is pruritic. There are multiple "ringed" areas on his trunk. He has lichenification in the popliteal and antecubital fossae. KOH is negative.

Answer Key:

Hyperbilirubinemia

Answers: 1 E; 2 B; 3 C; 4 D; 5 A; 6 F; 7 H; 8 G

Dyspnea

Answers: 1 B; 2 C; 3 E; 4 A; 5 H; 6 G; 7 D; 8 F

Chest pain

Answers: 1 F; 2 B; 3 A; 4 G; 5 D; 6 E; 7 C; 8 H

Abdominal pain

Answers: 1 D; 2 F; 3 G; 4 A; 5 I; 6 B; 7 H; 8 E; 9 C

Headache

Answers: 1 A; 2 D; 3 G; 4 B; 5 H; 6 C; 7 I; 8 F; 9 E

Diarrhea

Answers: 1 D; 2 F; 3 B; 4 H; 5 G; 6E; 7 A; 8 C

Vomiting

Answers: 1 B; 2 D; 3 E; 4 C; 5 A; 6 G; 7 I; 8 J; 9 H; 10 F

Hearing Loss

Conductive hearing loss: A, C, D, G

Sensorineural hearing loss: B, E, F

Vertigo

Answers: 1 C; 2 D; 3 A; 4 B

Syncope

Answers: 1 C; 2 A; 3 B

Vision Loss/Disturbance

Answers: 1 C; 2 A; 3F; 4 D; 5 B; 6 E

Optic Cup/Disk Changes

Answers: 1 D; 2 A; 3C; 4B

Painful Red Eye

Answers: 1 C; 2 D; 3 A; 4 B

Acute/Chronic Kidney Injury

Answers: 1 E; 2 C; 3 A; 4 D; 5 F; 6 B

Rash

Answers: 1 B; 2 F; 3 J; 4 A; 5 G; 6 C; 7 D; 8 H; 9 I; 10 E

Appendix A – Updates

NEW ACC/AHA Guidelines

Cardiovascular Risk Assessment – Nov 12, 2013
These guidelines differ from the former ATP III guidelines of the National Cholesterol Education Program (NCEP)

*The new guidelines have broadened the concept of CV risk to include both stroke and myocardial infarction. Instead of 10-year risk assessment it uses **lifetime** risk assessment as endpoint.*

There were four parts to the guidelines:

1. Risk assessment
2. Lifestyle changes
3. Treatment of blood cholesterol
4. Management of overweight and obesity

Part I synopsis: Risk assessment

In order to establish risk, at least one or more of the following assessments need to be done:

- Family history
- High sensitivity C-reactive protein (hs-CRP)
- Coronary artery calcium score
- Ankle-brachial index

The following factors were considered "uncertain at present":

- apoB
- chronic kidney disease
- albuminuria
- cardiorespiratory fitness

Part 2 synopsis: Lifestyle Changes

Dietary changes were emphasized including:

1. Interventions to decrease LDL cholesterol (nothing new here!)
    a. Increase fruits, veggies and whole grains
    b. Add low-fat dairy, poultry and fish
    c. Non tropical vegetable oil and nuts
    d. Decrease sugar, sugar-sweetened beverages and red meat

2. Interventions to decrease HTN
    a. All the same as above PLUS,
    b. Decrease Na intake to
        i. <2400 mg/day

    ii. Better would be <1500 mg/day
    iii. Best would be <1000 mg/day which has been proven to lower SBP
  c. DASH plan
    i. Increase Ca and K intake

Part 3 synopsis: Treatment of Blood Cholesterol (new and important!)

- No strong evidence to support prior LDL or non-HDL targets of < 100 mg/dL or < 70 mg/dL for either primary or secondary prevention of CVD.
- Goals no longer are aimed at cholesterol levels but at overall risk for the patient (using the "tool")This new "tool" was developed that looks at all RF for CVD, including:
    - LDL cholesterol
    - Age
    - Gender
    - SBP
    - Smoking
    - DM
- **And – they are making it easier for us by recommending STATINS over any other cholesterol meds (unless the patient cannot tolerate statin therapy)**

There are risks associated with Statin therapy --- otherwise we would all just starting taking it as kids! So there are more specific guidelines that address this risk : benefit ratio.

#3 & 4 in the list take into account the score using the "tool" for estimating risk:

1. Patients with clinically relevant ASCVD should receive high-intensity statin therapy (defined as a daily dose that lowers cholesterol level by approximately >50% on average). Examples of such agents would be rosuvastatin 20 to 40 mg or atorvastatin 80 mg. But, if adverse events occur as a result of high-intensity statin treatment, the guidelines advise trying a moderate-intensity statin (defined as a drug that lowers LDL cholesterol 30% to <50% on average).
2. Patients with primary LDL cholesterol levels of at least 190 mg/dL should also be treated with high-intensity statins.
3. Patients with type 1 or type 2 diabetes mellitus and an LDL level of at least 70 mg/dL should receive a moderate-intensity statin. But, those with a 10-year ASCVD risk exceeding 7.5% should be treated with a high-intensity statin.
4. Patients without evidence of CVD or diabetes, but whose 10-year risk of ASCVD is at least 7.5%, and whose LDL cholesterol levels are between 70 mg/DL and 189 mg/dL should receive either a moderate- or a high-intensity statin

Part 4 synopsis: Management of Overweight and Obesity

Identifying patients who need to lose weight

- Measure height and weight and calculate BMI at annual visits or more frequently. *(Evidence Grade E-Expert Opinion)*
- Use current cutpoints to identify overweight/obese adults at risk for CVD and obese adults at risk for all-cause mortality. *(Evidence Grade A-Strong)*
    - Overweight: BMI of >29.0-29.9 kg/m^2
    - Obesity: BMI of > 30 kg/m^2

- Advise overweight/obese adults that elevated BMI raises the risk of CVD, type 2 diabetes, and mortality. *(Evidence Grade A-Strong)*
- Measure waist circumference at annual visits or more frequently in overweight and obese adults; advise them of risks inherent in high waist circumference. Cutpoints continue to be those recommended by the NIH/NHLBI (> 40 inches in men and > 35 inches in women)[2] or the WHO/IDF (> 94cm for men and > 80cm for women).[3] *(Evidence Grade E-Expert Opinion)*

Matching treatment benefits with risk profiles

- Counsel overweight and obese adults with CV risk factors that even modest, sustained weight loss of 3 to 5 percent can produce meaningful health benefits, and greater weight loss produces even greater benefits. *(Evidence Grade A-Strong)*

Diets for weight loss

- Prescribe a diet for overweight and obese adults, which is part of a comprehensive lifestyle intervention. Clinicians can choose from one of three potential interventions. *(Evidence Grade A-Strong)*
- 1,200-1,500 kcal/day for women and 1,500-1,800 kcal/day for men500 kcal/day or 750 kcal/day energy deficit
- One of the evidence-based diets that restricts certain food types (such as high-carbohydrate foods, low-fiber foods, or high-fat foods) in order to create an energy deficit by reduced food intake
- Prescribe a calorie-restricted diet, based on the patient's preferences and health status, preferably under the guidance of a professional nutritionist *(Evidence Level A-Strong)*

Lifestyle intervention and counseling

- Advise overweight and obese individuals to participate for at least six months in a behaviorally based comprehensive lifestyle program that facilitates adherence to a lower calorie and increased physical activity regimen. *(Evidence Grade A-Strong)*
- Prescribe on-site high-intensity comprehensive weight loss intervention (individual or group sessions). *(Evidence Grade A-Strong)*
- Electronically or telephone-based weight loss programs that include personalized feedback can be utilized, but will yield less weight loss than face-to-face interventions. *(Evidence Grade B-Moderate)*
- Some evidence-based commercial programs that provide comprehensive lifestyle interventions can be prescribed as an option. *(Evidence Grade B-Moderate)*
- Very low calorie diets (<800 kcal/day) should be used only in limited circumstances under supervision of trained practitioners in a medical care setting. *(Evidence Grade A-Strong)*

- Advise patients to participate in their comprehensive program for at least one year. *(Evidence Grade A-Strong)*
- For weight loss maintenance, prescribe face-to-face or telephone-delivered maintenance programs that provide regular contact with a trained interventionist. *(Evidence Grade A-Strong)*

USPTSF Updated Guidelines

Three new recommendations from the USPTSF

- Screening and management of obesity in adults
    - BMI ≥30
    - Refer for behavior interventions
        - Multidisciplinary approach
        - Results in 6% weight loss/year
- Preventing falls in community-dwelling older adults
    - Physical therapy + Vit D supplement is effective in decreasing falls
- Vitamin D and calcium supplementation to prevent fractures
    - INSUFFICIENT EVIDENCE – not warranted in higher than usual doses
    - 400 IU Vit D/1000 mg. calcium is recommended

Updated pertussis guidelines

Top 10 cause of death in children globally; despite vaccines available.
Vaccine failure identified; outbreaks occur every 3-5 years.
2012 48,000 cases mostly in infants, children, and adolescents
In infants, neurologic impairment due to hypoxia – seizures and encephalopathy

Clinical manifestations – highly contagious; incubation of 7-10 days;

Three stages:

- Catarrhal – 1-2 weeks – runny nose, low grade fever, mild, occasional cough (like a "cold") lacrimation and conjunctival injection is common;
- Paroxysmal – 2-8 weeks – worsening persistent cough accompanied by post-tussive emesis; whoop most severe in the nighttime – lasts 3 months if not treated;
- Convalescence --- months – increased cough with viruses; coughing bouts

Diagnosis

- Suspect in all who have cough > 2 weeks and one of the following:
- Paroxysma of cough
- Inspiratory whoop
- Posttussive emesis
- If known exposure, presume pertussis
- PCR and culture should be done if symptoms < 2 weeks

- Nasopharyngeal swab culture is gold standard (not very sensitive, but very specific)

Prevention

- DTap (4 months to 6 years); Tdap booster ages 11-12; Tdap booster ages 19-64 one time; then boost with Td every ten years; ages 65 and older (since July 2011), approved as a one time booster

Treatment

- primary prevention is BEST
- Post-exposure prophylaxis
- Azithromycin first line and can be used in infants less than 1 month
- clarithromycin first line - can be used in infants 1 mo or older
- Bactrim – may be used in infants older than 2 months

Lab & Imaging Updates

Hgb A1c (since 9/2010)

- can now be used to *screen* for diabetes in select patients
- patients who *cannot be screened* for DM with HA1c include:
    - pregnant patients (use the usual FBS, 28 week oral GTT, and the 3 hr GTT if needed)
    - anemic patients (if not enough blood, A1C will be falsely low and miss some diabetics) or anyone with hemolytic anemia. Which diseases are these?
    - Fe deficiency, folic acid deficiency, B 12 deficiency
    - Thalassemias
    - hemolytics: spherocytosis, sickle cell, G6PD
    - donation of blood
    - hemorrhage/menorrhagia

2012 Molecular tests available

- MRSA & VRE
- GC
- c. dificile
- TB
- Mycoplasma
- Chlamydia
- Legionella

Systemic Nephrogenic Sclerosis

- Gadolinium (used as contrast in MRI study) is ***CONTRAINDICATED*** in patients with renal insufficiency
- In the past, this was the preferred method over CT with contrast to protect the kidneys – turns out that was WRONG!

Therapeutics Updates

Statins

- FDA statement that statins increase A1C levels and glucose levels (but benefit still outweighs the risk)

Fibrinolytics in AMI

- now can be given full dose and coronary angiography is still able to be performed
- in the past, full dose fibrinolytic therapy was a contraindication to performing a cath

Acute Sinusitis Treatment Guideline changes

- Amoxicillin-clavulanate (rather than amoxicillin alone) is recommended since the 2012 Infectious Disease Society guideline revision.
- "High-dose" (2 gm BID or 90 mg/kg/day BID) Amoxicillin-clavulanate (Augmentin) is recommended for :
    - regions with high penicillin-nonsusceptible S. pneumonia
    - those with severe infection (toxicity with fever > 102F)
    - recent hospitalization
    - daycare attendance
    - immunocompromised
- Doxycycline or a respiratory fluoroquinolone is recommended for patients allergic to PCN (but not in children)
- Recommended course is 5-7 days; in children 10-14 days is still recommended.
- NOT RECOMMENDED
    - Macrolides, TMP/SMX (Bactrim), 2nd and 3rd generation cephalosporins *are not recommended* due to high rates of resistance.
    - Fluoroquinolones *are not recommended* due to toxicity, cost and emerging resistance.

Asthma management

Dulera

Management of Gonorrhea (changing treatment based on resistances)

n April 2007, the CDC ceased to recommend fluoroquinolone antibiotics for treatment of gonorrhea in the United States.[1] This change was based on analysis of data from the CDC's Gonococcal Isolate Surveillance Project (GISP), which showed that the prevalence of fluoroquinolone-resistant gonorrhea cases in heterosexual men had reached 6.7%, an 11-fold increase from 0.6% in 2001. Fluoroquinolones may be a treatment option for disseminated gonococcal infection if antimicrobial susceptibility can be documented.

With fluoroquinolones no longer advocated, the drugs recommended for treatment of gonorrhea are limited to cephalosporins. However, gonococcal resistance to cephalosporins has also been increasing in the United States. GISP data showed that from 2000 to 2010, the percentage of isolates with elevated minimum inhibitory concentrations rose from 0.2% to 1.4% for cefixime and from 0.1% to 0.3% for ceftriaxone.

Consequently, the CDC no longer recommends the use of oral cephalosporins for gonococcal infections. For treatment of uncomplicated urogenital, anorectal, and pharyngeal gonorrhea, the CDC recommends a single IM dose of ceftriaxone 250 mg together with either a single oral dose of azithromycin 1 g or twice-daily oral administration of doxycycline 100 mg for 7 days.

If ceftriaxone is not readily available, cefixime 400 mg can be given orally in combination with either azithromycin or doxycycline; if ceftriaxone cannot be given because of severe allergy, azithromycin 2 g can be given orally in a single dose. However, patients treated with one of these alternative regimens should return 1 week after treatment for a test of cure.

Patient management updates

Cardiac surgical updates

- Transcatheter AVR (aortic valve repair) approved by FDA if patient is not eligible for open heart procedure
- CABG over PCI in those with DM and multivessel disease

BLS (basic life support) changes:

Used to be: ABCs = airway, then breathing, then circulation

Now: CAB = circulation (chest compressions), then airway and breathing

Evidence has shown that chest compressions are more important in the initial couple of minutes of basic life resuscitation of a pulseless nonbreather. Not sure when this would change on the exam, but watch for it!

ACLS

- In my opinion, there should not be ACLS questions on the exam since it is not an ARC-PA standard, nor is it a requirement for being a PA (unless our hospital or doc requires it).
- That said, here are the basic things to remember:
- now there is use of a capnography device (measures CO2 levels) during resuscitation – measure of proper ventilation
- Epinephrine is still the mainstay of treatment medically – give Q 5 min
- Atropine is useful in bradycardic rhythms

- Amiodarone will be one of the meds for almost any arrhythmia they may throw at you – won't get you 100% of the Q's correct, but good enough for 90%!

Infectious Disease Updates – Outbreaks 2008-2012

HIV

- Three shortterm antiretroviral therapies administered simultaneiously with a single dose of nevirapine, resulted in only a 1% rate of resistant mutations.
- test all, treat positive - the new mantra –to reduce transmission
- give retroviral drugs for high risk (prophylactically) new for 2012

Pertussis (34,000 cases 2010-2012) resulting in new guidelines to re-vaccinate all with pertussis when getting tetanus booster

- NEW - On October 27, 2010, the ACIP voted to recommend:
- use of Tdap regardless of interval since the last tetanus or diphtheria containing vaccine,
- use of Tdap in certain adults ages 65 and older, and
- use of Tdap in under-vaccinated children ages 7 through 10 years.

West Nile virus (mosquito outbreaks); increase in incidence

Salmonellosis (resurgence in incidence)

Anal Cancer (presumably due to HPV infection)

Fungal meningitis (due to contaminated steroids used in epidural injections for back pain)

Measles (222 new cases in 2011)

Mumps (minor incidence 16 in 2011, but used to be zero)

Hepatitis C (24 new drugs in use as investigative)

Appendix B

American Cancer Society Guidelines for the Early Detection of Cancer

The American Cancer Society recommends these screening guidelines for most adults. These do NOT necessarily correlate completely with the World Health Organization guidelines (WHO); or each individual "College's" guidelines, i.e. ACOG; ACG but it is the most recent set of guidelines published to date.

NOTE: these guidelines do not include those patients at *high risk;* those patients have already been covered in the individual disease topic areas above.

Breast cancer

- Yearly mammograms are recommended starting at age 40 and continuing for as long as a woman is in good health (unfortunately, this is hotly debated!) WHO says not until age 50.
- Clinical breast exam (CBE) about every 3 years for women in their 20s and 30s and every year for women 40 and over (this is even being debated as a cause of unnecessary biopsies!)
- The American Cancer Society recommends that some women -- because of their family history, a genetic tendency, or certain other factors -- be screened with MRI in addition to mammograms.
    - The number of women who fall into this category is small: less than 2% of all the women in the US.

Colorectal cancer and polyps

- Beginning at age 50, both men and women should follow one of these testing schedules:
- Tests that find polyps and cancer
    - Flexible sigmoidoscopy every 5 years*, or
    - Colonoscopy every 10 years, or
    - Double-contrast barium enema every 5 years*, or
    - CT colonography (virtual colonoscopy) every 5 years*
- Tests that primarily find cancer
    - Yearly fecal occult blood test (FOBT)**, or
    - Yearly fecal immunochemical test (FIT) every year**

If any of the tests above are positive, a colonoscopy should be done.

** The multiple (3) stool take-home test should be used. One test done by the doctor in the office is not adequate for testing. A colonoscopy should be done if the test is positive.

Cervical cancer (last update 3/2012)

Finally, the USPSTF and ACOG and ACS all agree on guidelines!

- All women should begin cervical cancer screening at age 21 years old. Women younger than 21 need not be tested regardless of age of sex initiation or other risk factors.
- From age 21-29; pap smear screening should be done every 3 years. HPV testing *need not be done* for screening. May be done for diagnosis.
- Beginning at age 30 until age 65, Pap smear plus HPV-DNA should be done every 5 years. If no HPV screening, then Pap smear every three years
- Women 65 years of age or older who have had 3 or more normal Pap tests in a row and no abnormal Pap test results in the last 10 years may choose to stop having Pap tests (even if she has new sexual partners)
- Women who have had a total hysterectomy (removal of the uterus and cervix) may also choose to stop having Pap tests, unless the surgery was done as a treatment for cervical cancer or pre-cancer.
- HPV vaccination does not change these screening guidelines.

Endometrial (uterine) cancer

The American Cancer Society recommends that at the time of menopause, all women should be told about the risks and symptoms of endometrial cancer. Women should report any unexpected bleeding or spotting to their doctors.

Some women -- because of their personal and family history -- may need to consider having a yearly endometrial biopsy. (See DUB/endometrial cancer in Women's health Ch. 15 for risk factors)

Prostate cancer

The American Cancer Society recommends that men make an informed decision with their clinician about whether to be tested for prostate cancer. Research has not yet proven that the potential benefits of testing outweigh the harms of testing and treatment. The American Cancer Society believes that men should not be tested without learning about what we know and do not know about the risks and possible benefits of testing and treatment.

African American patients or patients who have a first degree relative (father or brother) who had prostate cancer before age 65, should probably start screening at age 45. (See Urology, Ch. 21)

Cancer-related check-up

For people aged 20 or older having periodic health exams, a cancer-related check-up should include health counseling and, depending on a person's age and gender, exams for cancers of the thyroid, oral cavity, skin, lymph nodes, testes, and ovaries, as well as for some non-malignant (non-cancerous) diseases. This mainly means a good history-taking and complete physical exam!!!!

Patients should always be counseled in order to reduce their cancer risk at each yearly exam.

- Testicular self exam in adolescent school and athletic physicals
- Breast self exam in all women, starting in early adulthood
- Smoking cessation
- Maintenance of a healthy weight.
- Regular physical activity.
- Healthy nutrition.
- Limit alcohol intake to one drink/day for women and two drinks/day for men.
- Skin protection at all times when outdoors.
- Regular check-ups and cancer screening tests as indicated.

REFERENCES

American Cancer Society. Cancer Facts & Figures 2011. Atlanta, Ga: American Cancer Society; 2011.

Levin B, Lieberman DA, McFarland, et al. Screening and Surveillance for the Early Detection of Colorectal Cancer and Adenomatous Polyps, 2008: A Joint Guideline from the American Cancer Society, the US Multi-Society Task Force on Colorectal Cancer, and the American College of Radiology. CA Cancer J Clin. 2008;58.

Saslow D, Boetes C, Burke W, et al for the American Cancer Society Breast Cancer Advisory Group. American Cancer Society guidelines for breast screening with MRI as an adjunct to mammography. CA Cancer J Clin. 2007;57:75-89.

Smith RA, Cokkinides V, Eyre HJ. American Cancer Society guidelines for the early detection of cancer, 2006. CA Cancer J Clin. 2006;56:11-25.

Smith, RA, Cokkinides V, Brawley OW. Cancer screening in the United States, 2008: A review of current American Cancer Society guidelines and cancer screening issues. 2008. CA Cancer J Clin. 2008;58:161-179.

Last Medical Review: 02/25/2010
Last Revised: 06/23/2011

Appendix C

Standard Precautions

Standard precautions are infection control practices used to prevent transmission of diseases that can be acquired by contact with blood, body fluids, non-intact skin (including rashes), and mucous membranes. These measures must be used when providing care to all individuals, whether or not they appear infectious or symptomatic.

Hand Hygiene

Hand hygiene refers to both washing with plain or anti-bacterial soap and water and to the use of alcohol gel to decontaminate hands. When hands are not visibly soiled, alcohol gel is the preferred method of hand hygiene when providing health care to patients.

Hand hygiene should be performed before and after the following: contact with a patient, immediately after touching blood, body fluids, non-intact skin, mucous membranes, or contaminated items (even when gloves are worn during contact), immediately after removing gloves, when moving from contaminated body sites to clean body sites during patient care, after touching objects and medical equipment in the immediate patient-care vicinity, before eating, after using the restroom, and after coughing or sneezing into a tissue as part of respiratory hygiene.

Personal Protective Equipment (PPE)

PPE includes items such as gloves, gowns, masks, respirators, and eyewear used to create barriers that protect skin, clothing, mucous membranes, and the respiratory tract from infectious agents.

Wear gloves when touching blood, body fluids, non-intact skin, mucous membranes, and contaminated items. Gloves must always be worn during activities involving vascular access, such as performing phlebotomies.

Wear a surgical mask and goggles or face shield if there is a reasonable chance that a splash or spray of blood or body fluids may occur to the eyes, mouth, or nose.

Wear a gown if skin or clothing is likely to be exposed to blood or body fluids.

Remove PPE immediately after use and wash hands. It is important to remove PPE in the proper orer to prevent contamination of skin or clothing.

If PPE or other disposable items are saturated with blood or body fluids such that fluid may be poured, squeezed, or dripped from the item, discard into a biohazard bag. PPE that is not saturated may be placed directly in the trash. (We put too many things into the red bags!)

Needle stick and Sharps Injury Prevention

Safe handling of needles and other sharp devices are components of standard precautions that are implemented to prevent health care worker exposure to blood borne pathogens.

The Needlestick Safety and Prevention Act mandates the use of sharps with engineered safety devices when suitable devices exit.

- The safety devices on needles and other sharps should be activated immediately after use.
- Used needles should be discarded immediately after use and not recapped, bent, cut, removed from the syringe or tube holder, or otherwise manipulated.
- Any used needles, lancets, or other contaminated sharps should be placed in a leak-proof, puncture-resistant sharps container that is either red in color or labeled with a biohazard label.
- Do not overfill sharps containers. Discard after 2/3 full or when contents are at the "full" line indicated on the containers.
- Used sharps containers may be taken to a collection facility such as an area pharmacy, hospital, or clinic that provides this service.

Cleaning and Disinfection

Some pathogens such as norovirus and Clostridium difficile are not inactivated by commercial disinfectants routinely used in local public health settings. In situations where contamination with these pathogens is suspected, a bleach solution (1:10) is recommended for disinfecting contaminated surfaces and items.

Respiratory Hygiene (Cough Etiquette) <new since the SARS scare!!!>

Patients in waiting rooms or other common areas can spread infections to others in the same area or to local public health agency staff. Measures to avoid spread of respiratory secretions should be promoted to help prevent respiratory disease transmission. Elements of respiratory hygiene and cough etiquette include:

- Covering the nose/mouth with a tissue when coughing or sneezing or using the crook of the elbow to contain respiratory droplets.
- Performing hand hygiene (hand washing with non-antimicrobial soap and water, alcohol-based hand rub, or antiseptic hand wash) immediately after contact with respiratory secretions and contaminated objects/materials.

- •Asking patients with signs and symptoms of respiratory illness to wear a surgical mask while waiting common areas or placing them immediately in examination rooms or areas away from others. Provide tissues and no-touch receptacles for used tissue disposal.

Safe Injection Practices

Outbreaks of hepatitis B and hepatitis C infections in US ambulatory care facilities have prompted the need to re-emphasize safe injection practices. All health care personnel who give injections should strictly adhere to the CDC recommendations - Safe Injection Practices which include:

- •Use of a new needle and syringe every time a medication vial or IV bag is accessed

- •Use of a new needle and syringe with each injection of a client

- •Using medication vials for one client only, whenever possible

Appendix D

Immunization Guidelines

Recommended Adult Immunization Schedule—United States - 2014

VACCINE ▼ GROUP ▶ AGE	19-21 years	22-26 years	27-49 years	50-59 years	60-64 years	≥65
Influenza [2,*]	1 dose annually					
Tetanus, diphtheria, pertussis (Td/Tdap) [3,*]	Substitute 1-time dose of Tdap for Td booster; then boost with Td every 10 yrs					
Varicella [4,*]	2 doses					
Human papillomavirus (HPV) Female [5,*]	3 doses					
Human papillomavirus (HPV) Male [5,*]	3 doses					
Zoster [6]					1 dose	
Measles, mumps, rubella (MMR) [7,*]	1 or 2 doses					
Pneumococcal polysaccharide (PPSV23) [8,9]	1 or 2 doses					1 dose
Pneumococcal 13-valent conjugate (PCV13) [10,*]	1 dose					
Meningococcal [11,*]	1 or more doses					
Hepatitis A [12,*]	2 doses					
Hepatitis B [13,*]	3 doses					

Footnotes — Recommended Immunization Schedule for Adults Aged 19 Years and Older—United States, 2013

NEW FOR 2014

Pregnant adolescents should receiveTdap in every pregnancy between weeks 27 and 36 regardless of their last Td or Tdap vaccination.

TRAVEL VACCINES

Recommended Vaccinations

The U.S recommends the vaccines in the table above to protect travelers from illnesses present in other parts of the world and to prevent the importation of infectious diseases across international borders. Which vaccinations you need depends on a number of factors including your destination, whether you will be spending time in rural areas, the season of the year you are traveling, your age, health status, and previous immunizations.

New for 2014 are several new vaccinations for infants who are traveling to areas with endemic high rates of meningitis. These are not "routine" and would be advised based on CDC updated information.

Required Vaccinations

The only vaccine required by International Health Regulations is yellow fever vaccination for travel to certain countries in sub-Saharan Africa and tropical South America. Meningococcal vaccination is required by the government of Saudi Arabia for annual travel during the Hajj.

Resources

NCCPA (www.nccpa.net)

This is your best resource for ANYTHING you need to know about the test, i.e. content, tasks, scoring, administration, scheduling

Visit the NCCPA website at least quarterly for new information about changes, proposed changes, and other information pertinent to certification/recertification

Pay attention to the NCCPA networker newsletters that come to your Inbox – these are IMPORTANT to read

Review Courses

CME Resources – This is the premiere "Chicago" review course since 1996; more than 20,000 attendees. It is available now in many cities throughout the U.S. year round. I am a speaker, so I have an interest to disclose; however, based on feedback from surveys from an independent surveyor, CME Resources repeatedly comes out on top. Visit the website at: www.cmeresources.com

AAPA – Your source for a yearly "mega" conference with topics in anything you could possibly think of. In the two-year cycle where you need to test, you should once again attend lectures in topics that are in your areas of weakness in those top five or six content areas most heavily weighted. This organization also provides you with JAAPA, an online and print journal of articles in the "Certification/Recertification Series". This is an excellent resource for review (see below). Visit the website at: www.aapa.org

State and Local Chapters – your state and local chapters are a great way to review PANCE/PANRE topics, but as is typical of most humans, we tend to attend lectures in our area of knowledge. As you get to that two-year window prior to the exam, you should start attending lectures in areas of weakness, in topics that are relevant to the top five or six most heavily weighted content areas.

Online Testing Software

I feel very strongly that everyone preparing for either exam MUST do online test practice. We are all human, and most of us would prefer a paper test, but this test is online – a skill set independent of the medical information – so do yourself a favor and practice ONLINE!

Included FREE with this book:

www.pancemaster.com

A $65.00 value; you have access to the question bank *until you pass your test.*

Established in 2010, PanceMaster is designed to fill the need for an affordable and applicable study system to help PA students and practicing PAs pass their national certifying exams.

PanceMaster is a computerized testing environment that currently contains more than 1300 test questions. This study system is not a medical school question bank modified and marketed to PAs, but is designed from the ground up by a panel of practicing Physician Assistants with PA education in mind. Our user-friendly website allows users to personalize their study, tailoring to their individual strengths and weaknesses. The timed testing mode mirrors that of the PANCE/PANRE, easing test day anxiety. The questions are based on the NCCPA content blueprint and cover each topic through carefully crafted questions and detailed explanations that help increase understanding.

PanceMaster is constantly moving forward; the question bank continues to grow; routine review of each question keeps the information current, and thorough statistical analysis ensures that our customers have access to the highest quality question bank on the market. Prepare with PanceMaster and prepare for success!

Others online resources available (alphabetically):

ExamMaster

- www.exammaster.com/other-health-fields/physician-assistant

Kaplan

- www.kaptest.com/PANCE/PANCE-Prep/pance-lol.html

NCCPA

- www.nccpa.net/SelfAssessment.aspx
    - this site does not provide you with the correct answers nor explanations
    - but it allows you (for $35.00) to take a timed 120 question exam and get a report on how well you did in each medical content section

PAEasy

- http://www.paeasy.com

Disclaimer: There are many other online test banks for the PANCE/PANRE, however, these are the only ones that I am personally familiar with, or that were recommended to me by attendees and students.

Useful Textbooks

There are so many textbooks out there; but some are just not useful for reviewing for a broad-based amount of information as on this exam. (Harrison's Principles of Internal Medicine comes to mind).

That said, the NCCPA makes it clear that textbooks are what we should use to study. Recent literature; literature in your specialty areas are *not to be included in your study.*

A review journal such as JAAPA that specifically focuses on articles for certification/recertification is extremely useful:

JAAPA (The Journal of the American Academy of Physician Assistants).

- If you are an AAPA member, this will come to you complete with a picture on the front cover highlighting a topic in the "quick recertification series". I would recommend that you take a quick look every month when it arrives, and even if it is not in your clinical area of interest, I suggest you quickly read it and answer the questions at the end.

I am providing just title and author information for the following texts. Again, these are either resources *I have used in teaching, or those recommended to me by students and attendees.*

Current Medical Diagnosis & Treatment, 2012 or 2013
Maxine Papadakis, Stephen McPhee (Authors)

Ferri's Clinical Advisor 2013: 5 Books in 1, Expert Consult - Online and Print, 1e (Ferri's Medical Solutions) [Hardcover]
Fred F. Ferri MD FACP (Author)

The 5-Minute Clinical Consult 2013 (Griffith's 5 Minute Clinical Consult)
Frank Domino (Author)

I also like to use UpToDate and Emedicine (Medscape) in clinical practice, and while it does use current journal evidence, these are relatively basic sites, easy and quick to read, and provide concise information if you know exactly what topic you want to know more about.

Radiology Review

http://www.med-ed.virginia.edu/courses/rad/

This is the best website I have ever found for teaching others or myself radiology.

It is best to spend your time in this order on:

- Chest Radiographs
  - Start with Chest Radiology
  - then Plain Chest Radiograph (takes a long time to download)

- Orthopedics
    - Skeletal Trauma
    - (and if interested Cervical spine, but not essential)
- Gastrointesintal Radiology first, then
    - Plain film abdominal radiograph (again, takes a while)
- Head CT
- Pediatric imaging
- Cross-sectional radiology (CT)

http://radiologymasterclass.co.uk/tutorials/tutorials.html

This website was suggested to me by a follower on my blog and is also a WONDERFUL review – You will notice the British spelling of things..... very good to spend an hour here to review basic films.

Review of Electrocardiograms

Several good ECG websites exist online, depending on what you need.

If you are weak in ECG, then I would recommend focusing on most common and most life-threatening:

- normal sinus rhythm
- atrial fibrillation
- left bundle branch blocks
- acute myocardial infarction
- ventricular tachycardia
- ventricular fibrillation

One you are adept at recognizing the above quickly; add AV blocks, Hypertrophy, and then the other arrhythmias

ECG Learning Center: http://library.med.utah.edu/kw/ecg/

- This tutorial takes you from the very basics to rhythm strips and twelve-leads.
- Utilize the table of contents to focus your attention on the most common/life-threatening and forget the "zebras" for this exam!

ECG quizzer: http://www.gwc.maricopa.edu/class/bio202/cyberheart/ekgqzr.htm

There is a quizzing function that allows you to move quickly through rhythms that you identify correctly, however, there are also those that will stump you, so be judicious in what you focus your attention on (ECG can be very difficult with myriad nuances; for this exam, focus on the basics)

Contact me if you are interested in "learning" ECG – I have a set of free modules available – about 10 hours of review time though, so NOT for this exam. Just for your future practice!

General Websites

http://physician-assistant-ed.com

This is an exemplary website designed first for prospective PA applicants and now expanding now to assist currently practicing PAs. I am a contributor to this website; but I do not get paid for participation, so I have no conflicts of interest to disclose; except that I participate in developing blogs and respond to queries.

Now that you have passed your test --- **you get 10 years!**

However do you understand the additional requirements that were "tagged on" to our move from 6 year exams to 10 year exams? Most do not. So make sure you review this section (but do it AFTER you pass your test!)

- You will only have to take an exam every 10 years.
- You will have to recertify every 2 years, as always.
- You will need 50 Category 1 credit every two years, as always.
- You will need 50 Category 2 credit every two years, as always.

CATEGORY 1 CREDIT HAS CHANGED:

Every two years (for four two-year cycles) you will have to elect to do 20 Category ! credits in either

- Self-assessment CME, or
- PI-CME (performance improvement)

In every two year cycle, you have to pick ---

You can do PI-CME in years 2014-1016, then self assessment in 2016-2018, then PI CME again in 2018-2020, then exam in 2014 (or any combination of this, with the last 2-yr cycle being your exam)

You will still need to accrue 50 Cat. 1 and 50 Cat 2 in your last 2-yr cycle, but now it could just be attending any old conference, and sitting there (no passing any quizzes)

So READ YOUR NCCPA NEWSLETTERS --- Pay attention to the requirements!

I hope to create some self-assessment projects for credit – so visit my blog or website once in a while for updates.

Index

ABOUT THE AUTHOR

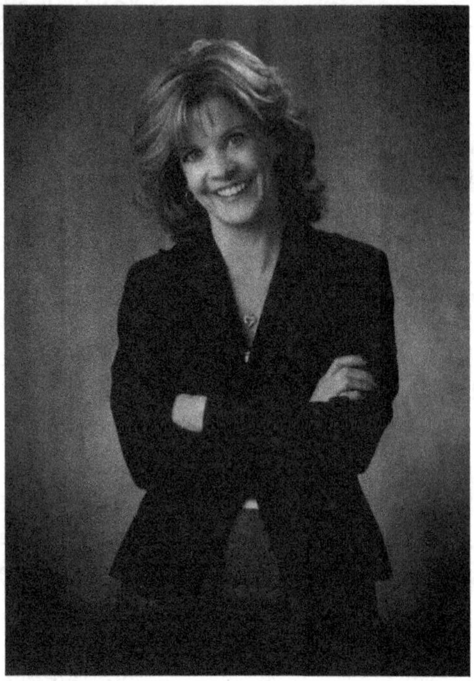

Jackie Kazik has been a Physician Assistant since 1985. After graduating from the University of Wisconsin – Madison, she practiced Pediatrics for two years; then Women's Health for 10 years before becoming full-time faculty at Marquette University in Milwaukee. She left Marquette to return to clinical practice in the emergency department in Waukesha. Soon after, she returned to academia, now part-time, coming full circle back to her alma mater at UW-Madison where she taught Labs & Diagnostics, Women's Health, and Emergency Medicine.

She is now a full-time clinical PA in Emergency Medicine, and continues to teach as adjunct faculty at multiple PA programs around the U.S.

She was the Medical Content Director & Lecturer for CME Resources, Inc., a PANCE/PANRE Review Course, from 2002 to 2013. This has afforded her the opportunity to meet PAs from the entire country and around the world that have helped her increase her knowledge base, provided her with ample "pearls", and helped to improve her teaching expertise.

She has received multiple teaching awards at both Marquette University and UW-Madison. She is most proud of the fact that the students themselves honored her with these awards.